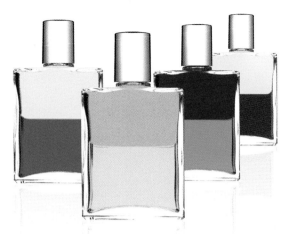

The Aura-Soma Sourcebook

Color Therapy for the Soul

Mike Booth
with Carol McKnight

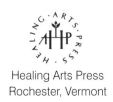

Healing Arts Press
Rochester, Vermont

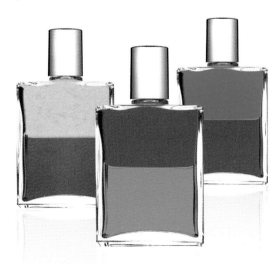

Healing Arts Press
One Park Street
Rochester, Vermont 05767
www.HealingArtsPress.com

Healing Arts Press is a division of Inner Traditions International

Note to the reader: This book is intended as an informational guide. The remedies, approaches, and techniques described herein are meant to supplement, and not to be a substitute for, professional medical care or treatment. They should not be used to treat a serious ailment without prior consultation with a qualified health care professional.

Library of Congress Cataloging-in-Publication Data

Booth, Mike.
    The aura-soma sourcebook : color therapy for the soul / Mike Booth with Carol McKnight.
        p. cm.
    Summary: "A complete guide to the practice of Aura-Soma color therapy"—Provided by publisher.
    Includes bibliographical references.
    ISBN-13: 978-1-59477-077-7 (pbk.)
    ISBN-10: 1-59477-077-8 (pbk.)
    1. Color—Therapeutic use. 2. Aura. I. McKnight, Carol. II. Title.
    RZ414.6.B66 2006
    615.8'312—dc22

                                                                    2006002445

Printed and bound in India by Replika Press Pvt Ltd.

10 9 8 7 6 5

Text design and layout by Peri Champine and Jon Desautels
This book was typeset in Swiss with Berkeley as a display typeface

Right: Light pouring to earth.

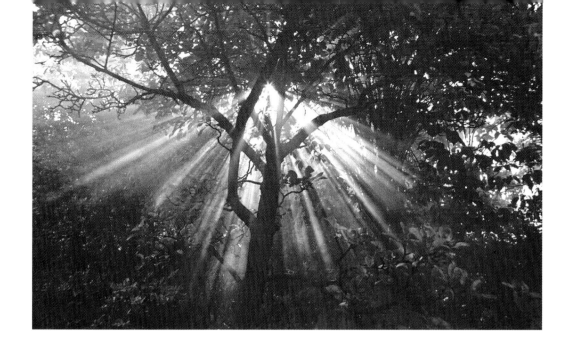

This work is lovingly dedicated to Vicky Wall and Margaret Cockbain; to all of the people who, from the birth of Aura-Soma to its beginning to walk in the world, have been involved in and supportive of its development; to Carol McKnight; and to her three daughters, Ariel, Erin, and especially Kirsten, who have so helped us to bring this book into being.

M.B.

I lovingly dedicate this book to the joy found in the quest to discover who we are and how to live in harmony with one another; to the wondrous possibilities that emerge through creative collaboration; and to Aeonghus, Bridget, and the other animals in our lives, in gratitude for their faithful companionship along the way.

C.M.

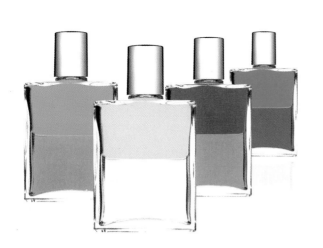
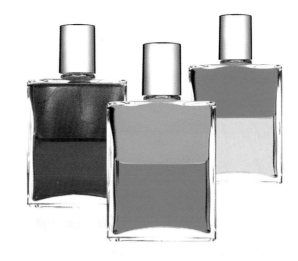

Contents

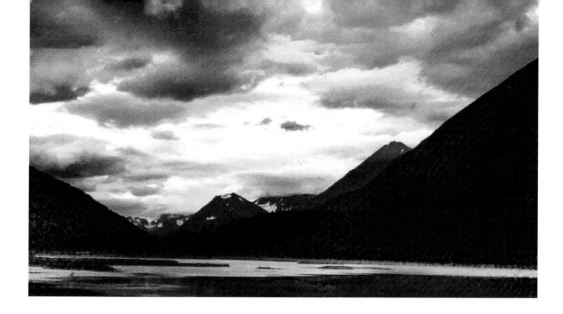

Acknowledgments

Creating this book has been an experience of the Aquarian spirit of co-creative and synergistic effort. Many individuals have given of themselves to help bring it to publication. We would particularly like to express our gratitude to Judi McLaughlin, Nick Vittum, and Christopher Clements for their skill and great generosity in preparing all of the photographs, not to mention their cheerful optimism even as their work extended into the wee hours of the morning. We would also like to thank all of the individuals who offered us their photographs. Judy Taylor and Michele De Santis spent hours researching their archives of beautiful slides; John Buckeridge, Scott Wayne, and Ryan Barolet-Fogarty went out of their way to send images transcontinentally to a stranger met on a plane. Ruth Barenbaum and John Ramsey gave inspiration arising from the wisdom of their own experiences. Elaine Lasker Von Bruns, book-lover and archivist, patiently read and re-read each page for clarity of language. Annabelle Westling Williams and Don McLaughlin offered support and unswerving faith in the project. Ed Besozzi and Irene Paquin helped with the thorough research of documentation; Irene and Ariel Burgess were "Jills of all trades" to support Kirsten Talmage's and our work on the manuscript. Lillith Booth did typing wizardry. We also would like to thank Jon Graham for his openness and encouragement and Jamaica Burns, Jeanie Levitan, and the other people at Healing Arts Press for their patience and skillful midwifery.

Above: Eternal light, outside of Fairbanks, Alaska.

Introduction

Aura-Soma has been aptly called a "non-intrusive, self-selective soul therapy."[1] This succinct phrase perfectly identifies Aura-Soma as a new paradigm in healing, one based on recognizing the inherent wisdom within each of us. Aura-Soma respects and supports that inner knowing, allowing us to create a reflection of ourselves—of who we are and what we need—through our calling to certain color combinations. Because our selections are made from a place of calling and superconscious knowing, they reflect a soul choice, not simply a momentary attraction.

Vicky Wall, the innovator of Aura-Soma, was fond of saying that "the greater guide is within you." The philosopher and mystic Rudolf Steiner believed that in addition to embodying "inner truthfulness and uncompromising sincerity," each person must transcend the personal to "feel and realize as an actual experience that he belongs to . . . higher worlds."[2] Understanding that we can connect to a transcendent aspect of ourselves helps explain how our superconscious self chooses the colors of the Equilibrium bottles in the Aura-Soma system. As you look through the images of the dual-colored bottles in this book, allow yourself to be guided to the four that call to you the most, and trust your inner guidance.

In the Aura-Soma system, the four dual-colored combinations we choose both reveal us to ourselves and replenish us. Who we are is what we express in the world. If we are energetic, we usually do energetic things. If we are given to analysis, we probably think a lot. In this way, we give out to the world, or expend in the world, who we are, and it is this that we need to have supported and replenished. Aura-Soma teaches us that the colors we choose reveal who we are and what we need, and because like resonates with like, they also strengthen us so that we can fulfill our potential. We simultaneously receive and transmit the quality of energy that we embody.

In this sense, the Equilibrium color combinations are an opening to our potential, our birthright, our birth gifts, and our birth obligations. When we come into the conceptual experience, gestation and the journey through the birth canal, our knowledge of our mission and purpose in this life, so clear to us when we were in the bardo—the between life—becomes less conscious. Most of us yearn to be more conscious about our purpose. Our color preferences give us the opportunity to remember. As we discover which color combinations draw us to them the most, our individual color code presents itself, revealing the dharma and the karma of this lifetime and of our soul's journey through aeons of time. It holds the lessons, the opportunities, and the direction and expression of our service in the world.

Consciousness identifies with color and light. The quality of our consciousness within our physicality is expressive of our existence and our characteristics and is synonymous with our color frequencies. Color directly reflects and is reflective within consciousness. In a sense, we identify ourselves in the context of color and light. Upon viewing the Aura-Soma Equilibrium dual-color combinations, we have an opportunity to make visible to ourselves, through color and light, those color identifications.

This sourcebook is meant to be both an introduction to Aura-Soma and a resource for anyone who has been using the system. For those new to Aura-Soma, the picture of all of the bottles at the end of the book provides a vision of the color combinations in the best color quality possible without having the actual living energies of the Equilibrium bottles in front of you. With this chart, it is possible to find the four that call to you the most. We encourage you to look at these combinations and note the order of your preferences to help this sourcebook come more alive for you.

Chapters 1 and 2 give a basic introduction to Aura-Soma, its principles, purposes, and history. To support an understanding of the breadth and depth of Aura-Soma, as it pertains to both our personal lives and our participation in the development of human consciousness, chapter 3 is a study of the colors themselves—their symbolism and their connection with the human body's subtle anatomy. Chapter 4 describes the major Aura-Soma components and how to use them. In chapter 5, we provide specifics about each Equilibrium bottle, including an understanding of their names and, in certain instances, the way those names were derived. These descriptions are at once distillations of the essential meaning and significance of each color combination as we have come to understand it and invitations to trace the bottle's connection to other wisdom teachings. Chapter 6 furthers the discussion of Aura-Soma and its connection to other wisdom traditions, offering readers a point of entry for further research. An example of the abundant meanings a single bottle can reveal is also given, demonstrating that every Equilibrium bottle is like a Chinese puzzle box, revealing surprise after surprise, interacting with our subtle anatomy and physical body to facilitate the expression of our greatest capabilities.

In addition to what you will learn about the Equilibrium system, the colors always speak for themselves. You are encouraged to relate the colors to what you already know and to explore unique ways in which the bottles may be understood. These bottles are first and foremost keys to understanding our beings. As we explore the color combinations in the bottles, these keys to consciousness, we guide ourselves along the path of individuation and, in so doing, help ourselves become more conscious co-creators of planetary evolution.

The Color Rose

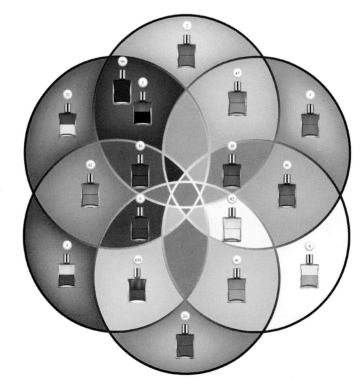

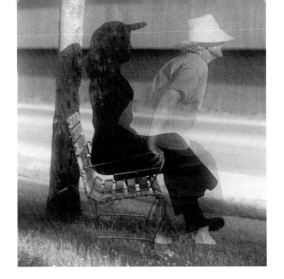

1

Aura-Soma

A Path to Self-Understanding—A Soul Therapy

You are the colors you choose and these reflect the being's need.

VICKY WALL

Perhaps the greatest mystery in life is ourselves. We strongly desire to journey toward ourselves, toward developing a greater understanding of who we are, and toward expressing ourselves in the world in the context of our community. Aura-Soma offers an array of "colored jewels" given to help us achieve our great tasks: the revelation of self and the evolution of consciousness. Color appeals to each of us, whether we are an accomplished adult or a small child. Even those of us who are blind, or color blind, can sense the vibration of the color and be attracted to certain combinations.

The word *aura* means "light" and refers to the facets of colored light within each of us, the potential of our soul—the soul's purpose. *Soma* refers to the being who resides in the body. In Greek, *soma* means "body"; in Aramaic, "being"; in Sanskrit, "living energies," including the electromagnetic field on the periphery of the body. Aura-Soma thus communicates the concept that we are, in essence, beings of light or living energies. As in the perspective of quantum physics—that all matter is light vibrating at different frequencies—human beings are, at the cellular level, bio-photons, taking in and giving out light. This understanding is expressed in the ancient Vedic view and in the Tibetan tradition, both of which describe us as rainbow beings.

As a system, Aura-Soma is a nonintrusive, self-selective color therapy designed to facilitate the connection between our light being and the light of our physical body. This connection, expressed primarily through color, helps us become more aware of the light within ourselves and of the living energies of light that surround us. As Vicky used to describe it, "Insight out, outside in." Through a process of selecting from over one hundred possibilities the four Equilibrium bottles to which we are most drawn, we can learn which frequencies of light most pertain to us. By also learning the language of color, we comprehend what our choices say about our deepest needs and gifts, and we can receive support in understanding our light-body, and that we are beings of light.

Above: Moving toward the light. Woman emerging from statue in Manchester, Vermont.

As we recognize our true colors, we have an opportunity to re-cognize ourselves in the mirror of color. We are given a clue to the color ray upon which we have incarnated.[1] Our choice may reveal our inclinations and the qualities upon which we need to focus. The colors we choose—their meanings and associations—offer a mirror to our soul, granting us acknowledgment of self and encouragement to develop. Each Equilibrium bottle offers both the insights and vigor of color and the associated energies of plants, herbs, gems, and crystals for our soul work.

Greater than each of the four bottles viewed independently is the story line that emerges when we consider the bottles in the sequence of our selection. As we move from the bottom fraction (the bottom color) of our first bottle through to the top fraction (the top color) of the last bottle, the unique color code of our soul's journey through time emerges. Just as life is a constant interplay of change, movement, and stasis, so the weaving of colors through our selections reveals our inherent qualities, how they have moved and developed, and how our talents may be supported and set free of personality and historical or cultural conditioning that may have inhibited their expression. How the colors blend, which ones predominate, and which are hidden or reappear are all part of an unfolding story that we show to ourselves in the mirror of color.

The understandings we receive through Aura-Soma often are both personally relevant and pertain to the collective. That is, while each of us experiences life alone, we participate also in the life of the larger community, and the colors we choose speak to both our unique life experiences and the realities that surround us. Although this book focuses on Aura-Soma as a tool for leading us, individually, toward growth of awareness, there is also something more to it—a direct energy transmission that is a consequence of the energetics of the three kingdoms (the mineral kingdom of crystal and gems; the vegetable kingdom of herbs, plants, and trees; and the hue-man kingdom that pertains to the perception of light and color). This gift of the three kingdoms seems to be specific and unique to the Aura-Soma color system. Our understanding of Aura-Soma is that the energies of the three kingdoms resonate in accord with individuals and their needs, as well as—and this is an underlying principle of Aura-Soma—in harmony for the greater good.

All that we have set down in this handbook is offered as a key to comprehending the meaning of color in support of your journey toward your self. Ultimately, it will be your personal experience of color, the particular associations and insights that you make, that will be most significant. Whatever we seek is what we already have.

Intrinsic Concepts

At the time of this writing more than two decades have passed since Vicky Wall brought forth the first Equilibrium bottles. Since then, many thousands of people throughout the world have found Aura-Soma and begun to explore its promise. Empirically we have learned the basic principles of the system, familiarity with which provides an opening to further explorations.

An array of color choices allows our soul's color preferences to be made conscious in the present. These color preferences are a key to understanding our self—as a soul, as a personality, and as an eternal being. It is said that before the exodus from the Garden of Eden, Adam knew the name of every animal; each had one essential name. In a sense, the word and the object were identical. After the Fall, the one name moved into diversity; arbitrary and conventional names were given, bound to a plethora of languages.[2] Such a diversity of languages can separate person from person. A sense of alienation can result when people call the same thing by different names. Existence becomes fluid, mutable, and transitory. Our personality is like these names, given to change and impermanence, appropriate for certain external situations and particular internal challenges. With our various names, it may be that only a part of us is known or perceived. Yet our color code—which is, in a sense, our intrinsic name—is eternal. Perceiving it can reduce our sense of alienation or estrangement. Our true color code can bring us back to a feeling of oneness with our self, to a feeling of alignment with our soul star, with our dharma, with our soul's purpose. We are drawn to certain colors that reflect our color code through time. Finding them is at once a homecoming and a return to our essential nature, a re-membering.

The quality of consciousness is communicated by color and by our color preferences. The superconscious aspect of ourselves perceives color and light independently of the physical form. This understanding seems to be a part of many of the ancient wisdom traditions. It is exemplified through the Tibetan yogis and lamas, specifically in the Bardo Thodol (Book of the Dead). This treatise by ancient Tibetan masters describes consciousness as independent of physicality, whether as part of transitioning from one state to another while on the earth or at the moment of transcendence at the end of the physical life. It specifically describes the after-death experiences of the soul in which the independent consciousness knows itself in terms of color and light; it is color that helps guide the soul on its journey of evolution.

Through harmonic resonance, colors can support us and nurture us in our life as we express our purpose and potential. Aura-Soma works on principles similar to those of other vibrational medicines. The colors of the bottles are formulated by combining plant ingredients, gem and mineral energies, and natural colorings. Through sympathetic resonance, which can be compared to homeopathy's doctrine of *similia similibus*, or "like cures like," the energetic vibrations of these ingredients have a stimulating, clarifying, and balancing effect on us. When relating to the colors we are drawn to, we see that those colors create a strengthening resonance within our physical bodies and auric fields, helping us achieve positive well-being and personal growth.

A Gift with a Purpose

Humanity seems to be at a threshold of great change and growth. It may be that Aura-Soma is offered at this time so that all of us have the opportunity to discover our color code, thereby developing greater awareness of our life purpose, gifts, talents, and challenges. As we become more personally aware and purposeful, we also are part of a slow wave of change in the collective consciousness, bringing our awareness and clear intention out into the world.

Interacting with the colors of Aura-Soma can be a personally rejuvenating and supportive process, affecting the energetics of our subtle anatomy and physical being. Supplying the needed color, plant, and crystal energetics to the body helps us move away from dis-ease and into a state of more harmonious ease.

The Aura-Soma approach to human subtle anatomy includes eight chakras or energy centers (subtle anatomy is discussed further in chapter 4, page 23). Each Equilibrium dual-color combination may be seen as a chalice of light containing resonances that, when in relationship to a chakra, affect the consciousness of that chakra and can have a direct effect upon the subtle energy systems of the body. The colors help the chakras open and function well as transceivers, easing the flow of energy within our being and better enabling us to express our soul's intention on Earth. Ultimately, Aura-Soma encourages a greater state of relaxation, a clearer receptivity to spirit, and an increased capacity to function and individuate.

Aura-Soma is about color and light, color and life. As we come into alignment, we stand straight—rainbow hueman beings poised between heaven and earth, our head in heaven and our feet firmly planted on the ground, feeling our connection with our soul star and our earth star. Allowing our center to flow freely, letting go of fear and anxiety, we can express our incarnational star.* The "I am" comes to earth. In a sense, this is the gift of Aura-Soma.

---

*The earth star is a point located just below the surface of the earth, which tracks each human being wherever he or she is upon the earth. The earth star is the reason we incarnated here rather than elsewhere. The earth star divides from the incarnational star at the moment consciousness associates with the first cell. In the incarnational star is the potential that exists in the first cell and the memory within our physiology of that first cell. From there is an access point to the open page of the akashic record that pertains to this incarnation.

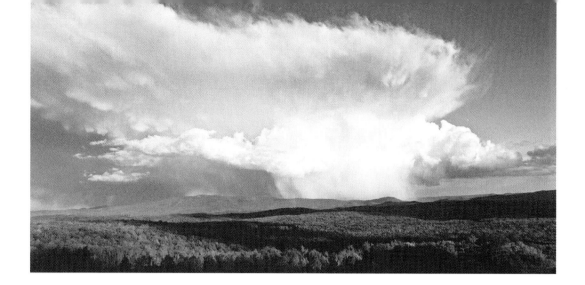

2

The History of Aura-Soma

Vicky Wall, the innovator of Aura-Soma, received the inspiration for the Equilibrium bottles as a consequence of prayer and meditation. In her autobiography, *Aura-Soma: Self-Discovery through Color,* she describes her heritage, and in so doing also identifies the underpinnings of Aura-Soma itself:

> I was born in London, the seventh child of a seventh child. My father and his parents belonged to the Hasidim, a deeply religious sect involved in the mystical aspects of the Bible. My father was a master of the Kabbalah and the Zohar and from his background he inherited a knowledge of the medicinal and healing qualities of living plants and natural methods of healing, which he passed on to me.[1]

From her earliest years, Vicky shared with her father the gift of auric vision, or clairvoyance, a gift that would be enhanced in her later years even as hereditary diabetes blinded her. In her person were combined intuition, an awareness of the subtle anatomy, a kabbalistic heritage, and wisdom from the plant kingdom. This background and unique set of inherent capabilities made it possible for Aura-Soma to be revealed and birthed through her many decades later.

The Birth of Equilibrium

While Vicky yearned for her father to share his kabbalistic knowledge with her, Hasidic rules did not permit him to teach her because she was a girl. To some extent, she comforted herself with the knowledge that they shared the secret of their auric vision, and when she was very young, her father promised that she would one day be able to speak openly of that yearned-for mystery. Sadly, her bond with her father was outwardly severed during her adolescence when she left home because of her stepmother's abuse and took up residence in a Gentile household. Following the rules of Hasidism, she was not able to

Above: Londonderry Mountain, Vermont.
Page 7: (left) North Branch of Middlebury River, (right) magenta bottles.

see her father again. However, her love for him remained strong throughout her life.

As a young woman Vicky worked as an assistant to a pharmacist, who taught her the ancient arts of the apothecary. It was during this time in the pharmacy that she realized the joy of being able to help others. Initially she planned to become a masseuse, but because of the era in which she lived, her advertisements were misconstrued. She trained to be a chiropodist instead and was one of the first women in England to be appointed as a surgical chiropodist. Vicky went on to teach at many of London's teaching hospitals. Eventually her eyesight declined, ending her career. In her mid-sixties, she was registered as blind; she was diabetic; she had had a sequence of myocardial infarcts (heart attacks), which had left her with just 40 percent of her heart muscle; and she and her partner, Margaret, had lost the collected wealth of their professional lives to a friend in a major fraud case. Vicky saw the entirety of these circumstances as a kick from her cushion of complacency—a divine nudge. She turned to meditation and prayer. Early in 1983, she received the inspiration for Aura-Soma. As she described in her biography:

> I found myself suddenly enveloped in the most beautiful cascade of color, which receded and advanced like the ebb and flow of the tide, sighing softly as it went. As it came towards me rhythmically, I longed to remain within it; my whole being was diffused with vibrant new energies and peace. . . . Then came the still small voice . . . "Divide the waters, my child." "Divide the waters?" I repeated and came back to earth with a thud. *What waters?* I thought. . . .
>
> The second night was a repetition with again the injunction: "Divide the waters." Once again, mystified, I came out of meditation quite quickly. On the third night, I began to feel as Samuel in the temple, for I could no longer ignore the voice, even though the commonsense part of me said, *What are we thinking about? I'm not Moses. I'm blind, only forty percent of my heart is working, nearly seventy years old. So who on earth would I be leading into what Promised Land?*

> But I could not dismiss it, and I got up out of bed. For the life of me, I do not remember the next few hours, nor how Equilibrium was actually born. I only know that other hands guided mine.[2]

When, the morning after Equilibrium was born, Margaret asked Vicky what it was for, Vicky replied that she did not know. Aura-Soma Equilibrium was indeed born out of mystery, and the complete understanding of Aura-Soma is still a mystery, an unfolding revelation, discovery, and expansion. What Vicky did say is that she had "no doubt whatsoever" that Aura-Soma was a reemergence of something she had had knowledge of in the far distant past . . .

> Gradually the full meaning and the structure began to make itself known. It was . . . a continuation. All was so familiar and was pouring into consciousness. The old wine had appeared in a new form expressly for the New Aeon. . . . It has been researched for a very long time, back into the very beginning of time, and then searched, re-searched and re-membered. . . . I had been taken to the beginning when God said "Let there be light" and there was light. And light was the life force and the beginning of the life energies, and there I re-searched and thus, remembering, entered the mysterious and magical world of color in the Greater Garden of God.[3]

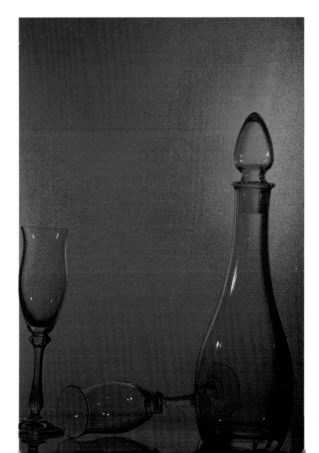

Vicky's love for her father was deep and unconditional. When the waves of color were coming toward her in those first three nights and unseen hands were guiding hers to create the first Aura-Soma Equilibrium bottles, Vicky felt that it was her father's gift. At that time, unbeknownst to her, her father, the master Kabbalist, was already on the other side.[4] Certainly, it was the complete and open love she had for her father that opened the door through which this communication from spirit could come. It was a direct communication and a revelation for our time, a time when it is most needed—a gift of color that is accessible and appropriate at the onset of this New Aeon.

In a passage that could characterize Vicky's personal experience, Rudolf Steiner—the visionary philosopher-mystic, scientist, and father of anthroposophy who lived at the turn of the last century (1861–1925), had access to the akashic chronicles, and communicated with spiritual beings—described the stages whereby "the sublime treasures of the Spirit" can become our own:

> There are children who look up with reverent awe to certain venerated persons. . . . Many occult pupils come from the ranks of such children. What was once childlike veneration for persons becomes, later on, a veneration for truth and knowledge. . . . The Initiate has acquired the strength to lift his/her head to the heights of knowledge only by guiding his/her heart to the depths of veneration and devotion.[5]

Aura-Soma seems to have parallels with other systems acknowledged as divine revelations. For example, there is a related sequencing and patterning between Aura-Soma and the Gnostic tarot and the paths and sephirot upon the kabbalistic Tree of Life. Perhaps Aura-Soma, as a part of an unfolding divine plan, helps bring communication from beings within the cosmic hierarchy to the earth at this time of need.

The Growth of Aura-Soma

That Aura-Soma is an unfolding system is one of its most appealing qualities. As each new bottle is born, the whole of the system expands exponentially, as do the insight and knowledge of the people who work with it. As some levels of information and insight are refined and integrated, other gifts inherent in the system are given or become more evident. Vicky herself said that she was given seven years of "borrowed time" after her last near-death experience to ensure that Aura-Soma would be firmly established. Helped by using Bottle 10, Green/Green,[6] she was able to nurture the gift of Aura-Soma she had received and encourage it

to take its first steps. These two processes of receiving and transmitting are central to the Aura-Soma system. They are consistent with the traditions of kabbalistic teaching in that *kabbalah* means "to receive" and the teaching of the most sacred aspects of Kabbalah is done by direct transmission from teacher to student. Vicky was not consciously aware of this, as she had received no formal training in this discipline. Nonetheless, her enduring bond of love for her father opened the doors to spirit, giving her a direct experience of the living Kabbalah as she received and gave birth to Aura-Soma.

Similarly, Rudolf Steiner trained the natural clairvoyance he had as a child to make it more conscious and to develop his ability to gain knowledge of the spiritual worlds through which the comparable precision and exactness of information concerning the scientific world could be discovered.[7] He conceptualized this "spiritual science" as a method by which other people could attain inspiration and intuition, and he described some of the stages of practice whereby an individual might achieve the ability, similar to his own or to Vicky Wall's, of inner hearing:

> Something begins to live within him which transcends the personal. His gaze is directed to worlds higher than those with which everyday life connects him. And thus he begins to feel and realize as an actual experience that he belongs to these higher worlds. . . . He listens to the voices which speak to him in the moments of inner tranquility. . . . Out of the silence something begins to speak to him . . . it resounds through his soul. . . . An inner light spreads out over his whole external world.[8]

Aura-Soma comes alive through our interaction with the Equilibrium bottles, the Pomanders, Quintessences, ArchAngeloi, and Color Essences. While learning about the meaning of the individual colors can be a tantalizing prospect, significant also is the actual experience that comes from interacting with the core elements of the system. Not only is information transmitted to us from the vegetable and mineral kingdoms, the world of color and light, and the Aura-Soma body of wisdom, but understanding is transmitted from the collective to the personal aspect of ourselves. Our inner knowing is strengthened. We are awakened and inspired as the process of individuation ensues, we become more aligned with our potential, and we too begin to unfold, bringing forth more of our self, and more of our destiny, our talents, and our gifts.

Mike Booth first met Vicky Wall at an earth-spirit exhibition in the Malvern Hills of Worcestershire, England, in the fall of 1984. Mike had previously been involved in a Zen practice and was an artist and potter whose paintings had begun taking the form of mandalas. During his early years, he had been exposed to theosophical teachings through his parents and was therefore familiar with the concepts of the Masters, hierarchy, and spiritual beings (see the discussion of Quintessences, beginning on page 38, for an explanation of these concepts). He had by chance encountered the Kabbalah, in the context of Druidic studies, while in teacher training outside London.

One of Mike's important questions to the mediums and intuitives he met during his childhood was about the significance of the area around the human navel. Mike recognized Vicky Wall, in part, because while many visionaries speak about the colors that surround us, Vicky and Mike shared a perception of the true aura that lies within this section of the body—the golden area that contains the incarnational star, a point of light at the center of the being that contains the memory of the first cell (see "The Subtle Anatomy" on page 23). Partly due to the confirmation of their shared perception, Mike answered the calling to work with Vicky for the next seven years. She had predicted that it would be Mike who would help Aura-Soma walk in the world. He was her constant companion, supporting, learning from, and collaborating with her in bringing the Aura-Soma system to us. With Vicky's passing, Mike accepted the responsibility for continuing to care for and develop Aura-Soma as it is brought through from spirit.

Aura-Soma is an ever-developing system, which might be seen as a mirror of and a parallel to the development of humankind. After Bottle 43 (B43) Mike was handed the responsibility for bringing new color combinations into being. Gradually Vicky withdrew her attention from the birthing process so Mike would grow in confidence in the unfolding of the system before she passed, a transition that was marked by the birth of B78. Bottles continue to reveal themselves to Mike, and at the time of this writing, there are 106 combinations within the Aura-Soma dual-color range.

It would seem that as the needs of humanity shift and change, as the collective of humanity's consciousness evolves, new bottles appear to support and encourage from within that process. For the past several thousand years, one view might be that there has been an overemphasis on issues relating to the first three chakras: the root, the sacral, and the solar plexus. The root chakra relates to issues of survival, the sacral to dependency and codependency, and the solar plexus to issues of fear and power. Much has been written about how humanity is at a point of bridging from three-dimensional consciousness to four-dimensional consciousness, to a collective opening of the heart chakra. Four-dimensional consciousness is being able to put yourself in someone else's shoes—really being able to see from their perspective, understanding why they might think, act, or be a particular way. The heart chakra is connected with a sense of spaciousness, awareness, and unification within the self, going beyond jealousy and envy and entering into the possibility of seeking truth. The Aura-Soma system helps us move beyond the first chakras toward that of the heart.

Perhaps Aura-Soma has been given by spirit to help us evolve in the preparatory period prior to 2012 and through the time after that transition. Aura-Soma may help us with rapid adjustment as consciousness becomes more available, and support us in the integration of energies through that evolutionary leap. As individuals we may become more conscious moment to moment and concurrently become more aware of the beings that surround and work with us.

There is a growing body of empirical data about Aura-Soma, compiled over time, from the experiences of many consultants and teachers around the world. This body of information includes the efficacy of and responses to the Equilibrium bottles—emotionally, psychologically, intuitively, spiritually, and physically. There is also growing empirical understanding about the potentially therapeutic effects of the plants, gems, crystals, and other ingredients that are used to make the liquids within the bottles. During the course of the development of Aura-Soma, individuals felt it appropriate to utilize the Equilibrium bottles, Pomanders, Quintessences, and Color Essences with not only people but also pets, animals, and plants. As Aura-Soma is taught, used, and investigated in the world, there are increasing opportunities to research what is happening. Many individuals have combined Aura-Soma with other disciplines and practices, such as nursing, Reiki, acupuncture, massage, and psychology, thereby enhancing the effectiveness of each. In 1997 the Aura-Soma Art and Science International Academy of Color Technologies was created to promote the study and research of color therapy around the world. To date, it has graduated more than twenty-five thousand students, and Aura-Soma is taught in over fifty countries. Throughout all of these changes, one constant has been the understanding that information is given to be shared. The synthesis of many people's experiences, anecdotes, and research contributes to an evolving understanding of Aura-Soma, and Aura-Soma in turn unfolds in richness as we explore it.

A recent major development in the Aura-Soma system is the beamer light pen, a tool used to introduce the Equilibrium color combinations into the human energy field and to the acupuncture and Jin Shin (Aurajin) points and meridians of the body. By means of the beamer pen, the wavelengths of the energies found in each color combination are amplified through a crystal and focused as a light beam. Light is known to behave both like a wave and like a particle. It may also move in yet different harmonics. The paradoxical nature of light may account for why it can be so simply and beautifully present and also can carry such a complexity of information. The Equilibrium bottles, applied as light through the beamer pen, can have a strong stimulating effect.

Current Understandings

Aura-Soma has been in the world since 1983. Our current understanding is based on what we have witnessed over the past decades, as Aura-Soma has developed. We encourage you, too, to see the system as evolving, and we hope that it will be a springboard for your greater understanding of your path and purpose.

It was shortly after the revelation of Aura-Soma that Dr. Carolyn Shreeve, of Saint Mary's Hospital in London, defined Aura-Soma as a soul therapy in her comparative text on alternative and complementary therapies.[9] So apt was her description that Aura-Soma has become widely known as a soul therapy, indicating that it works at the deepest levels within the self and points to that within us that is not limited by our physical bodies.

Fundamentally, we know that color selections offer the possibility of providing present moment definitions of ourselves as well as describing underlying qualities that may be transcendent. Therefore, Aura-Soma helps us become more conscious of the roles we play, of our personalities, of that with which we identify and of that which goes beyond personality into the essence of ourselves.

One implication of the work of Aura-Soma is that the seeds of karma inherited from the past tend to manifest in the present as particular tendencies. Reincarnation or recurrence gives us the chance to meet the same set of circumstances until we learn to respond to them differently and experience a different outcome. Since our karmic seeds are expressed in the color of our energy fields and respond to external color, we can use our color choices to both perceive problematic tendencies and facilitate our transformation. Karma relates to the patterns of tension or stress which are habitual and with which we identify. These patterns are often passed down to us from our parents, either genetically or from our upbringing. The way in which we uproot karmic seeds is directly related to the way we may be able to overcome their consequences and bring a quality of expression, of dharma, into all that we do. Karmic seeds can be expressed and viewed in terms of color and light. If we have been able to overcome these karmic seeds or patterns, then color will manifest as an expression of the dharmic qualities we bring to our work and daily lives. Both the problem and the solution are reflected in the color.

Aura-Soma enables us to stimulate a remembrance of our essence and helps us undo some of the consequences of conditioning within our personality. In this way, we can give ourselves back to ourselves through the specific vibrations of color and light from the three kingdoms.

The science of signatures is based on a fundamental law of correspondences. Signatures bridge the three kingdoms through the specifics of color and light. The minerals and crystals, the herbs and plants, and the colors all relate in a resonance that crosses many levels of the human experience. Let us consider an amethyst from the crystal kingdom, lavender from the plants, and the violet ray from the world of color and light. Each has the capacity to remind us of relaxation, of calming, and of a greater ease: the amethyst as a self-clearing absorbing stone; the lavender as an herb that 'eases tension, relieves stress, and induces relaxation; and the color violet as the most calming wavelength of visible light.

The core of Aura-Soma, the key that leads to other components, is in the Equilibrium bottles. Vicky referred to them as her colored jewels containing the resonances of the three kingdoms. When they are applied in a band around the body in accord with a chakra, they have an effect on the body's subtle energy system through sympathetic resonance in relation to consciousness. To understand their effect in another way, we can consider the meridians of classic Chinese acupuncture as being the roads or pathways that connect points of light together. The streetlamps upon these roads are treatment points. The application of an Equilibrium combination over one of these treatment points may illuminate not only the streetlamps themselves but also the roads that connect the energy flows between various organs and glands.

Humanity seems to be at a threshold of immense change, offering a real potential for growth. Aura-Soma has been offered so that each of us has an opportunity to discover our color code through time. Aura-Soma as a system has the possibility to help us develop greater awareness of our life purpose, gifts, talents, and challenges.

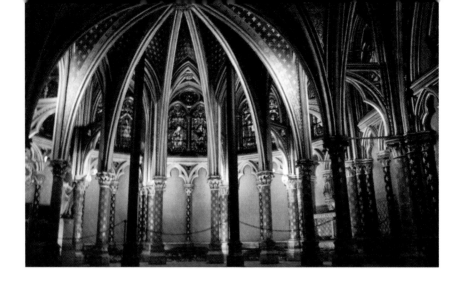

Entering the Mystery of Color

The greater guide is within yourself.

VICKY WALL

The Aura-Soma system works with the spectrum of visible color as well as the information encoded in the sequences of color combinations. The complexity of this information opens door after door. Color is a universal language through which nature speaks. It expresses part of the underlying order and rhythm of the universe. It is a means by which we can draw connections. Understanding the information related to our color preferences can help us in the process of individuation and self-realization.

Let There Be Light

Color emerges from light. In Genesis, it is written that God said, "Let there be Light," and then God saw the light and it was good. Light is special, a truly divine gift. The light of the sun warms us and supports life. We understand from physics that light is made up of many colors, some perceptible to our naked eyes, others sensed by different species, and some we can "see" only with the help of our inventions. Historically, light and color have been used for healing, for example, in the healing temples of ancient Egypt and China, and by the Essenes. The stained-glass windows of the great Gothic cathedrals are a visual testimony to the effect of colored light. When sunlight shines through these windows, the interior of a cathedral is bathed in scintillating light. The interplay of colors creates an atmosphere, while the images, stories, and symbols depicted in the glass impart information. In an era when literacy was not widespread, people could learn from the pictures as they were bathed in the illumined colors. As Steiner said, "Color is the soul element of nature and of the whole cosmos, and we have a share in this soul element when we experience color."[1]

The interplay of light and color seems to connote significance greater than phenomenological. Aristotle, in his *Harmony of Color,* suggested that color is the interaction of light and darkness.[2]

According to Steiner:

> Angels bore light into the darkness, or darkness into the light. They became the mediators and messengers between light and darkness. And what had previously only shone in the light and brought its shadow, the airy darkness, after it, now burst into color, changing from one color to another, as the light appeared in the darkness and the darkness in the light. . . . [The angels] conjured forth colors out of light and darkness . . . [and are] behind the cosmic significance of the bursting forth of colors.[3]

"The colors are acts of light."[4] Thus Goethe, through his personal dedication to the observation of nature, reached an understanding of color. To him, "light and its absence are necessary to the production of color. Next to the light, a color appears which we call yellow; another appears next to the darkness, which we name blue."[5]

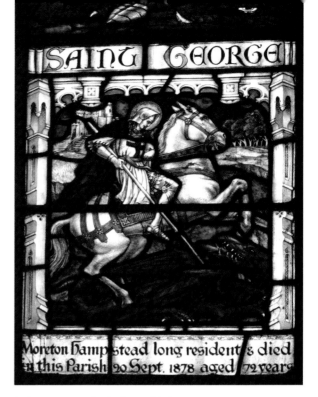

St. George encountering the dragon of darkness.

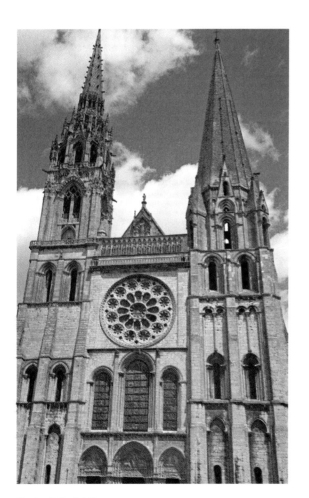

Chartres Cathedral, France.

Certain wisdom teachings would suggest that consciousness has the ability to perceive color independent of the physical body. The Bardo Thodol (Tibetan Book of the Dead) talks of color and light experienced in the after-death state. The Tibetan mentor helps the departing soul navigate through the color choices that present themselves to consciousness, with each color, hue, and tint being representative of certain soul qualities and tendencies. The color choices inform and have an influence on future incarnations, and on eventually being set free from the wheel of death and rebirth. *The Dark Night of the Soul,* by Saint John of the Cross, and the Mayan codices express the same phenomenon: that consciousness that has left the physical body can express preferences in terms of color and light, based on actions performed and experienced in a particular lifetime. This is a parallel by which to understand that our current preferences reflect our eternal color code and transcend the personality. It has been said that our eyes are the windows to our soul. So too are our color choices.

The Language of Color

Light emerges from darkness. Darkness emerges from light. From these phenomena the generation of all color gradations will occur.

RUDOLF STEINER, *COLOR* (119)

12

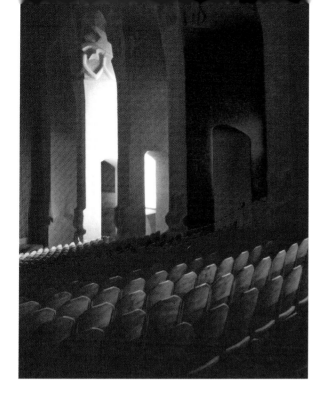

Blue and green light in the Goetheanum, Dornach, Switzerland.

*I wandered lonely as a cloud
That floats on high o'er vales and hills,
When all at once I saw a crowd,
A host, of golden daffodils . . .*

WILLIAM WORDSWORTH

We are all familiar with the language of color. When a child presents to us a bunch of dandelions, or when Wordsworth extols the beauty of a riverbank covered with "ten-thousand" daffodils "tossing their heads in sprightly dance," we have a sense of the optimism and cheerfulness of spring. In the Beatles' movie *The Yellow Submarine,* when the Blue Meanies assault the land of happiness and music, we understand the mood conveyed. We can be amused by the complexity of color meaning, as in the song from the 1950s that proclaims, "It was an itsy bitsy teeny weeny yellow polka dot bikini." In Sweden, where there is so little sunlight in the winter months, many houses are painted yellow, and they glow throughout the year with radiant welcome.

"Colors speak all languages," says Joseph Addison.[6] Red, for example, is the color of passion and blood, of wine and of rubies. Eighteenth-century Scotsman Robert Burns writes, "O my Luv's like a red, red rose," and we sense his undying devotion. In American Stephen Crane's 1895 book about the Civil War, *The Red Badge of Courage*, the hero has the courage (a word derived from the French *coeur*, meaning heart) to passionately commit his heart in the face of danger, to fight for his ideals and to sacrifice his life for them.

Yet red is also the color worn by Santa Claus, an embodiment of abundance and goodwill. In India and China, brides traditionally wear red as a symbol of fertility and happiness. In a red-light district, red has a sexual meaning.

Beauty is in the eye of the beholder. Truth is as it resonates within. We are drawn to certain Equilibrium bottles. The colors we ascribe to them are in the visible spectrum. However, beyond what we are able to perceive with the naked eye, there exist infrared and ultraviolet colors. Color can be described by both wavelength and particle movement, yet its actual nature still holds mystery. Part of the mystery is that, irrespective of our scientific knowledge we respond to color. We may be drawn to some colors more than to others. Butterflies prefer some flowers and frequent others less often. The chameleon matches one plant at one time and blends with another plant at another hour.

At the same time that we learn about color and about our personal color code, we can experience the archetypal significance of colors, the universal meaning as well as culturally influenced nuances. To the ancient Egyptians, a deep blue lapis streaked with gold might designate prestige and respect. The "Blue Stocking Society" of eighteenth-century London, on the other hand, was a derisive term for a predominantly female club of people who were thought to be

Wedding dress adorned with red.

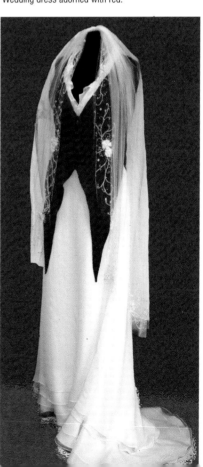

13

pedantic intellectuals, who read scholarly works and wore blue worsted stockings. Whether it is 3500 BC or now, we all live on Earth, under a blue sky, with sunlight pouring through our atmosphere and stimulating the life process of nature to produce green vegetation. As described in "The Subtle Anatomy" (page 23), to come into conceptual experience, we all must meet the yellow star in the blue field. As we begin to unfold our color code and understand how the color choices speak to us, we will find many associations. For example, green reminded Vicky Wall of nature, and she spoke of Green/Green, B10, as "Go Hug a Tree." Another

The impression of warmth may be experienced in a very lively manner if we look at a landscape through a yellow glass, particularly on a grey winter's day. The eye is gladdened, the heart expanded and cheered, a glow seems at once to breathe towards us . . . [but] by a slight and scarcely perceptible change, the beautiful impression of fire and gold is transformed . . . the color of honor and joy reversed to that of ignominy and aversion. To this impression the yellow hats of bankrupts. . . .[7]

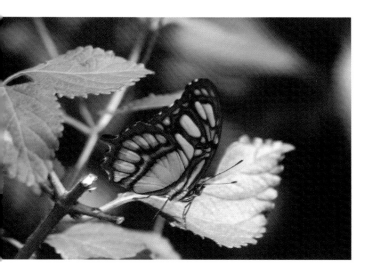

Green nymphalid.

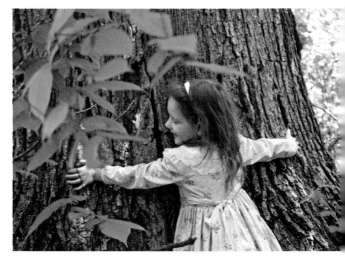

Hugging a tree at the old apple orchard in Shelburne, Vermont.

might hear the tune "Greensleeves," the sixteenth-century love lament to Lady Greensleeves, or be "green with envy," or long to preserve the environment and protect the lush tropical rain forests.

Inherent in understanding the meaning of color is acceptance of the diversity of meaning. We are living with a consciousness that at this time perceives duality and polarity, light and dark, yet can comprehend far greater subtleties along many spectra. An individual of choleric temperament, flushed with anger, could also bring a red rose to his or her true love. It may be helpful, in exploring the language of color, to understand that both polarity and ranges of meanings associated with the colors are ways to remember that inherent in every difficulty is a gift or potential for expressing our talents and for growing in consciousness.

An example of this challenge, the transformative potential of light and dark, of joy and sorrow, is described by Goethe:

There are so many evocative color associations. Consider those of landscapes (the turquoise waters of the Caribbean, the coral desert sands of the American Southwest), those of symbols (the white marble of the Taj Mahal, testimony of a shah's love for his wife), and those of concepts ("Pure as the driven snow"). The Equilibrium bottle color combinations represent the personal and the universal. An individual who chooses Clear/Blue, B12, Peace in the New Aeon, may have been shy and had a tendency to stutter when young. This person may also be a soul dedicated to global peace and truthful communication, values symbolized by the blue and white flag of the United Nations.

Each Equilibrium bottle has two color fractions. Goethe suggests that color combinations such as these have "a certain significance and tend to excite a definite impression."[8] As we select our bottles and apply the liquid to our bodies, we receive a reflection of a facet of the jewel that we are. At the same time we have a sense of our place in the great sea of universal consciousness. Our own heart is reflected in the heart and potential of the earth, and the earth is reflected in us. We are each a reflection and an aspect of the whole. As we discover our bit of the prismatic whole, we help to further the evolution of humanity on the planet.

The Color Rose

Here we will describe all the colors of the Aura-Soma range. It may be helpful to look at the color rose on page 2 as you read through this section. The exploration of the Equilibrium bottles in chapter 5 is based in part on color theory; for example, the list of related bottles has to do with primary, secondary, and tertiary colors and color components.

In Aura-Soma, blue and yellow are considered to be the two primary colors. Even red is created from these two, as when the sun sets in the blue sky or rises in the morning, casting a red glow upon the horizon. In pigment addition, however, red is considered the third primary. Together these three primaries make the secondary and tertiary colors. The colors of red through violet compose our visible spectrum; magenta occurs between red and violet.

Each color can be represented as either a hue (a darker, more saturated, version of the color) or a tint (a paler version of the color). A hue is the grounding of a color. A tint, created by adding light (the "clear" color) to the hue, is the intensification of that color. Interpretively, the inherent meaning of a tint is the same as that of its base color, its hue, though its value is amplified or intensified. The intensity of a color's meaning, from an Aura-Soma point of view, increases when light enters the color and turns it into a pastel. The increase in light is indicative of an increase of consciousness, which has two possible causal factors: First, consciousness grows with suffering and the understanding of suffering. Second, consciousness develops proportionally to an increase of awareness, mindfulness, and presence.

Red

Red is a grounding energy. From the earthing within our physical body to the rainbow of our light-body, the journey to the rainbow of ourselves can begin. Red is about awakening that which lies at the root of our physicality, wherein also exist our survival issues. Have we been given all this complex equipment within our physicality and within the subtle energies of ourselves just to survive, just to deal with the material side of life, or have we been given it for a higher purpose—to develop the light-body, to bring the awakening of the male/female energies within ourselves to

a union that will be a harmony throughout our whole being? Within red lies the answer to this question.

Red represents detachment, a consciousness that has the potential to witness all that occurs upon the stage of ourselves. In red are the energies associated with the emotions of anger, frustration, and resentment. These emotions can be transmuted when we drop the labels we have been conditioned to assign to them and recognize the nature of the energy behind them. Such an understanding can lead to a deepening of detachment, of nonattachment, which is part of the potential of the red.

Red contains the potential for the rising of kundalini, and the courage to allow this to happen. Through working with the emotions of anger or aggressive reactivity, the journey of awakening leads to a broader awareness, to our light-body. The fullness of our being is in the root within the red energy center. As consciousness is

"Commencing the ascent," engraved glass window in Goetheanum, Dornach, Switzerland.

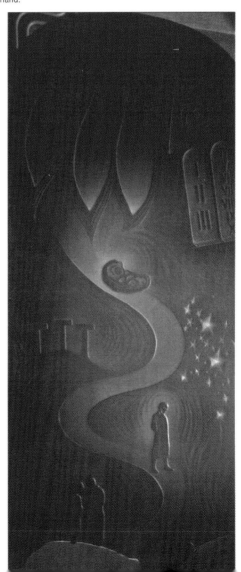

brought to the red, the red turns pink: first rose pink (B23, B104), then pink (B81), and then pale pink (B52). These are progressive stages of intensity.

Passion for life is a fundamental part of the expression of the red energy, but red can also indicate the tendency to say "Stop" or "No more," the energy of pushing away and of aversion. Passion (red) before consciousness (light) is brought to it (before it turns pink) can be the energy of rejection and aversion. As it becomes pink it has the energy of acceptance, of saying yes, of being more at peace. Some aspects of sexuality have inherent the energy of rejection. Perhaps Sigmund Freud had a point when he attributed the root of neurosis to sexual problems. One of the primary causes of suffering comes out of our aversion, and particularly as it is expressed as repressive sexual energy.

Red also connotes the blood of life, of new life, of the life force. A woman's twenty-eight-day ovulation cycle is a clearing of energy, the energy of purification harmonized with natural cycles at the root of ourselves. For many ethnic people, the time of a woman's menses is a time for stillness and meditation, an opportunity to find stillness within during the process of cleansing, a sacred ritual connecting the self to the earth. Red belongs to the earth and is an intrinsic part of our physicality, intimately linked to life itself through the blood, the carrier of oxygen in our bloodstream. Red is a primary color of adornment—rouge upon the cheeks, scarlet lipstick, ruby nail polish—all to enhance the appearance of a vibrancy of life. Light entering red turns red to pink. Pink may indicate both a feminine energy, an internal one of compassion, and a masculine energy of outgoing awakening, a step toward developing wisdom.

Coral

On the color rose, coral exists between the primary red and the secondary orange, and it carries some of the messages of both. Coral has a strong place within Aura-Soma as a tertiary vibration. The concept of coral has to do with inside out and outside in. Living coral is skeletal on the outside and fleshy on the inside; human beings are the other way around.

Coral refers to the new consciousness, the New Man emerging from within humanity, those whose priority to awaken and become *Homo sapiens* is most urgent. These people invite awakening into a life that is independent and interdependent. Coral gives us the understanding of what is referred to in Aura-Soma as the New Christ energy, the inbreathing and outbreathing in the moment of the awakening energy of the Christ. The term *Christ* here does not specifically refer to Jesus Christ of Christianity; instead, it has to do with our potential to awaken to the incoming and

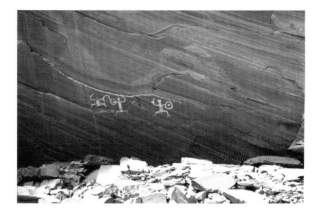

Petroglyph in southwestern United States.

outgoing divinity in our own consciousness, to awaken to deep levels of insight, to develop qualities of love, wisdom, and the wisdom to love ourselves.

In coral is the experience of unrequited love, love that cannot be placed when it is felt, love that is not able to be accepted in the form in which it is given, as when there has been deception and great vulnerability. Unrequited love offers a strong potential to develop self-acceptance and spontaneity.

Pale coral is an intensity of the coral experience, showing the light of consciousness brought into the hue. If coral appears as a pale tint, it can indicate an increased understanding of coral issues or an intensity of suffering from unrequited love, perchance from the inability to express love the way it is felt or when love is undeclared and hidden.

Coral opens the way for networking and cooperation. In Aura-Soma, turquoise is associated with connection, mass-media communication, and networking using new technologies, based on the silicon chip, that are available to connect people globally. Curiously, coral, the complementary opposite of turquoise, is also associated with connectivity, reminiscent of coral growing in the sea as an interdependent community of plants and animals. With pale coral, added to networking are the coral qualities of cooperation and compassionate and philanthropic interaction.

Orange

Orange is the color of enthusiasm, deep joy and bliss, profound insight, and instinctual wisdom. It is the color of expressive sexuality. In the Aura-Soma conceptualization, orange is discussed predominantly in the context of shock or trauma. Orange, a secondary color composed of equal proportions of the primaries red and yellow, is linked to the second energy center of the physical body, at the sacrum, immediately above the red energy center of the root.

Orange is concerned with issues of dependency and codependency. We may create dependent relationships by trying to fill gaps in ourselves from the outside, rather than using the power and force of our insight to recognize the cause of our sense of lack and inadequacy. Our state of dependency is also a fact, not a choice: We are dependent, as humans, on the trees, the grass, and the entire organic film upon the earth that replenishes the oxygen we need for survival. Without oxygen, we would live relatively few minutes. In other words, within the issue of dependency is something involved with survival (red). Knowledge (yellow) of this brings us orange.

Orange is linked to the etheric body, the first body beyond the bio-electric or bio-energetic field, which is still intimately connected to the physical. The etheric body retains a distinct memory of shocks and traumas from the past.

Orange has an effect on healing the timeline that extends both forward and backward. When we are in harmony with ourselves, we will more likely be in the right place at the right time doing the right thing, according to our soul's path and the greater good. When shocks have displaced the true aura, which normally exists in the golden area of our body, we may be out of harmony with ourselves. In this case the true aura moves toward the left side of the body, toward the etheric gap, and we lose the sense of synchronicity. Orange has the capacity to help us let go of past traumas to bring us back into right relationship with the timeline, restoring the opportunity of being well oriented in the right time and place, with the capability of being persistent and dedicated to that to which we commit.

Orange particularly inspires our instinctive gut reactions. These reactions spring from the fundamental truth of knowing and wisdom that lies in the orange. We may experience a zest for life that gives us a sense of being available and optimistic, perceiving circumstances of life with a positive outlook that may become blissful and rapturous.

Gold

Between orange and yellow is gold. Gold is key in the Aura-Soma philosophy and understanding of color. Vicky Wall often described gold as containing the true aura, that which indicates the true essence of self, containing color information about both the personality ray and the soul ray. The true aura, roughly the size of a walnut, is composed of the surrounding personality ray, which formed from the energies that brought the first cell into being, the blending of the genetic lineages of the mother and the father, with the ray's nuances of color expressing the fusion of those streams. The soul ray, contained within the walnut-

like shape in the golden area, indicates what the soul has brought from the deep past as the essence of its being, which will go from life to life until that aspect of the soul's evolution is complete. Gold is our nugget of wisdom.

Different from knowledge, wisdom is the gold of our being, which may need refinement out of denser matter and yet is truly our own. Wisdom may be rarified by a process of inner alchemy and our journey toward ourselves. The refinement of gold is perhaps depicted in the nimbus that appears in the Renaissance paintings of saints and masters, in the Buddhist icons of the bodhisattvas, and in the Tibetan images of lamas and deities. This gold is the realization and fulfillment of the refinement of the raw materials within the temple of the body, which occurs upon the inner planes of being, through inner alchemy.

Within that golden area is also the incarnational star, containing the physiological memory of the first cell from which all of the multicellulared organism came into being. Connecting with this star revitalizes all of our systems, in

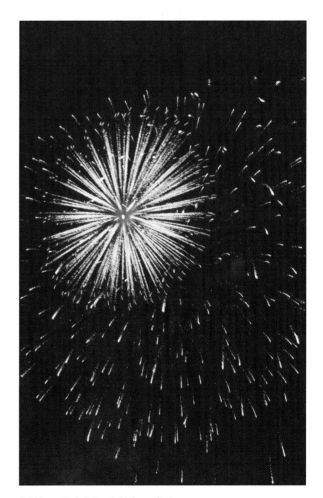

Gold fireworks in Palma de Mallorca, Spain.

much the same way that stem cells are used to remind other cells of their capacity for regeneration. As we penetrate ourselves with the essence of our awareness, regeneration may take place as a reminder of the potential of that first cell.

Gold is the depth of happiness, of confidence as wisdom dawns within us. The fascinating thing about this quality of wisdom is that it cannot be possessed or owned. It is something from which we may learn, whether we are speaking or we are listening to wisdom from another. The nature of gold is, like yellow, to radiate.

Gold is about overcoming anxiety and fears so that we can step into a new moment. Perhaps at the beginning of the golden age, an age of more consciousness and more light, golden moments will occur as a consequence of being in touch with the golden area within ourselves. Gold is also possibly the color most related to the idea of letting go: to let go in the gold stimulates the inner alchemy, the transmutation toward a greater wisdom that may radiate from the core of the being, with profound joy. If that wisdom is realized and lived on a moment-to-moment basis, it may lead to the splendor of the golden nimbus surrounding the head.

Yellow

Yellow is the color of sunlight before it meets the pale blue sphere that surrounds the earth. Without this source of light, life on this planet could not be sustained. Yellow is the source of happiness and laughter within ourselves, the joy of life itself, the joy in the light force within life.

Yellow is also the color of intellect, clarity of thought, and the processes that unfold within the mental realm. In the same way that orange is related to the etheric (emotional) body, yellow is related to the astral (mental) body. Yellow stimulates us to regenerate our mental capacity and our ability to learn.

Yellow has to do with nervous fears. Nervous fear may cause us to experience a knot of contraction created by self-consciousness. That knot tightens with embarrassment, and we experience a sense of separation from self. It is, perhaps, most acutely felt when we are teenagers, when our sensation in our solar plexus, the yellow area of our self, is of an acute sense of self-consciousness. As we let that go and feel more at ease, the repercussions, ideally, would manifest as self-awareness, an emanation of light from the sun within our self.

The Greeks believed that when those who sat gathered in a room closed their eyes, the room would get darker; they believed that light shone from the eyes of those gathered. The light that is born in self-consciousness and develops to self-awareness in the yellow area of ourselves shines through the eyes, the windows of the soul.

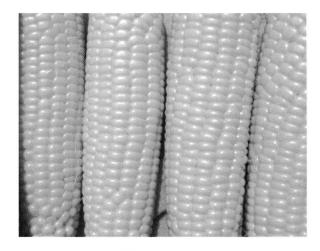

Golden sun-ripened corn in Ripton, Vermont.

Yellow expresses the gathering of the harvest, when the seeds that have been planted and grown begin to be gathered. We reap what we have sown. Yellow indicates issues to do with fear, with control that is exerted through fear, and with power that has become unenviable. In yellow we find the self-consciousness that surrounds the "little" will, or the self-will, the willfulness within the self. Perhaps much of recent history could be seen as a consequence of the misuse of the inner sun, the question of how to express our individual will. Power might best be in accord both with what lies within our golden area and with what is above, with the green and olive aspects of our being.

Olive Green

Olive is between the primary yellow and the secondary green, and as a tertiary color, it contains elements of both. Contemplation of the qualities of an olive tree helps us understand olive. The olive tree can live for many centuries, enduring difficult climates, and it is able to offer the olive branch of peace and its fruit. Olive oil nourishes the heart, keeps our skin lubricated, and, when burning, shines light. The fruit of the olive tree is bitter when first picked. It needs to go through a process of soaking and marinating, with just the right amount of salt, to turn its bitterness into something sweet and edible.

Olive reminds us that as we let go of the bitterness of the past, we may find a sweetness of spirit. We can recall the covenant, between God and man, of the rainbow, the rainbow of our being in which all the colors come together, suggesting that the waters of the subconscious and unconscious mind will not be allowed to fully cover the possibility of consciousness arising. This hope and optimism is contained in olive.

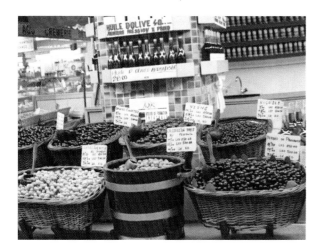

Olive mart in Avignon, France.

Olive expresses the feminine aspect of ourselves, the remembrance of Goddess, the female leadership of the heart. In our heart we might find trust in our intuition, which in turn is guided by our awareness (green) and light and clarity (yellow), which come together in olive green.

O-live is almost like a plea for the life force. The color olive has been used as camouflage by the military in times of conflict and war. We are asked to give up hiding, to overcome conflicts within ourselves, to abandon sectarianism and paranationalism, so that the feminine receptivity may achieve a new level of cooperation.

Our intuition is honored with joy when we recognize its equality with our analytical nature. Olive reminds us of the joy of finding our own space and making space for ourselves. To be aware of our own space while being able to give space to others, as in the context of a therapeutic situation, is to give them the space to grow. When we move a single rose from a bunch of roses, we can appreciate the fullness of its beauty in a new way; we give it space to be.

Green

The two primaries yellow and blue combine to make green. Green is representative of panoramic awareness, spaciousness, direction, and decision making.

In the Aura-Soma understanding of human subtle anatomy, within green is the emerald of the heart. Our heart is an intimate link with the earth. If we rearrange the letters of the word *heart*, we can spell the word *earth*. This is elegantly pertinent. Green issues have to do with the earth: the way we care for it; the issues of pollution; concerns of what we take from, rather than give to, the earth. It is not a coincidence that "green" or environmental issues have

become so political currently, as humanity moves closer to the collective opening of the heart.

As yet the green movement may be a still, small voice within the whole of humanity, but inevitably this movement will grow. The earth can not sustain us if we continue to take from her in an unsustainable way. We need to balance our consumption with efforts toward regeneration. Similarly, our hearts, so intimately linked with the earth, will not sustain us unless we live more in harmony with nature.

Heart disease is of significant concern in Western culture. Regardless of diet and other environmental factors, the heart will not function as it is meant to unless we have harmony and joy in life. Harmony emerges from an intimate relationship with the whole of existence, rather than from the fears and stresses of modern life. With this harmony and balance we manifest greater synchronicity in our life.

Green also symbolizes the green fields and open spaces, the trees and the stillness that trees seem to create as they record the seasons by rings in their trunk and as they solidify light in their beings.

Green expresses jealousy, envy, and those stressful emotions that indicate wanting to be in someone else's space. The positive aspect of this is panoramic awareness, the ability to perceive clearly from the point of view of another, to understand another's position as if it were our own.

Turquoise

Turquoise is the creative communication of the heart, where green, a secondary, is expressed through blue, a primary. In Aura-Soma we associate turquoise with the unfolding process of individuation, as we move through our individual challenges and patterns toward the collective life of humanity. This concept, explored extensively by Carl Jung, refers to the experience of becoming more centered and grounded. As that occurs, we begin to receive symbols, thoughts, and perceptions that exist in the collective mind and unconsciousness of humanity. This information is transcultural and transepochal; it belongs to no one person and is available to all, from any culture, race, or era.

Turquoise relates to the Ananda Khanda, the small center on the right side of the chest. Translated from Sanskrit into English, Ananda Khanda means "the abode of bliss." It is also commonly referred to as "the little center" and "the heart within the heart." Pertaining to the turquoise band around our body, turquoise also connects to the movement of the Ananda Khanda toward the middle of our body, toward our heart. The awakening of the abode of bliss is a process of individuation.

Turquoise is the creativity within ourselves, the possibility of becoming a co-creator with the Creator. As we get in touch with our creative force, linking our feelings with our heart's communication, we may express our heartfelt feelings in song, dance, painting, or poetry.

Turquoise is associated with mass-media communication, networking through the Internet, and the new technologies based on the silicon chip that have revolutionized the world as we know it. Using this chip has allowed us to awaken the global brain, stimulate the neural synapses of global communication, and think of the planet as a smaller, more integrated community.

As the neural circuitry is activated at the outset of the awakening of the global brain, many of the darker bits of the subconscious/unconscious mind are flushed through the neural net. Turquoise also contains these subconscious/unconscious tendencies, which we tend to deny within ourselves and yet we need to bring to awareness and to a new level of responsibility. Turquoise symbolizes a blend of our individual ability to respond and humanitarian independence.

Creativity is the essence of the turquoise experience. Vicky Wall said that since 1966, turquoise and magenta have become visibly stronger in the rainbow, metaphorically and in the sky, symbolizing the New Aeon dawning at the end of an age of darkness. Turquoise promises the possibility of transdimensional communication, of a new appreciation of the gifts of the mineral world of crystals, and of the group cooperation, sharing, and play exemplified by cetaceans.

Blue

Blue, the primary primary, is peace, a peace that is not polarized with conflict or war, a peace that passeth all understanding. The energy of blue is one of affirmation, of saying "yes," of being at peace with what is. Blue represents a communication that comes through us, not from us. As with the wisdom of the gold, the communication of blue cannot be possessed. It comes through us that we may listen in order to gain guidance and serenity.

Blue expresses faith and trust: we have the possibility to trust that what is ours will come to us, without our having to reach forth and grab it, without having to pursue it; with faith, we can know that if it is ours, it will come or return to us.

Blue can depict authority, a natural authority that we each have but can so easily lose when we take it for granted or lack humility. The authority of blue has both positive and negative connotations. The difficulty in blue can be a narrowing of vision resulting in an adherence to our own opinions, with an unwillingness to participate in the ideas and opinions of others. There can come a certain degree of dogmatism, of self-righteousness. If we can

release these things, we have the possibility, particularly as blue becomes paler and more intense, to move in the direction of the higher will.

With pale blue, if we allow it, we may become receptive and transmittive, like a hollow bamboo. The higher will may come to us and through us, inspiring us. Perhaps this inspiration will be aligned toward a higher plan, toward fulfilling our destiny in relation to why we are here and what we are for, becoming like a bee, who knows exactly where to put its bit of wax.

Cooperatively bees build a honeycomb with perfect 60-degree angles, each and every time. Nobody tells them where to put their bit of wax; they follow no architectural plan. The *blue*print showing them where to put their wax is within them. Likewise, if we can get out of our own way, possibly the higher will work through us: we may put our bit of wax in the right place, as part of a cooperative network building the hive of cohesive life on the earth.

Blue also expresses the mother principle, in both our own nurturing capacity and the nurturing of the divine mother who can care for all equally.

From the discussion above, we can see the significance of blue and yellow being the first two primaries. The sun and the sky, as they appear to us on earth, tell the story of the relationship of these two colors. Our individual will (blue) and the higher will (yellow) integrate in all the other colors that are blended from these two primaries. Through combining of pigment and light, green and red are formed from blue and yellow, followed by the subtleties of the rest of the palette.

Royal Blue

Royal blue, a tertiary made by blending the primary blue and the secondary violet, exists in the part of our body that contains most of the sense doors: the eyes, ears, nose, and mouth. Royal blue can bring clarity to each of the senses. The red (in the violet) mixed with blue brings the possibility of detachment from sensory experience, a guardian at the sense doors allowing the potential for clarity.

Royal blue communication is fed in from above, like a ticker tape that might be read and consulted. We have a choice of what to do with this communication; it is our responsibility to decide whether this information is to be shared. Royal blue exemplifies a deeper level of authority than does sapphire blue. This could be an increased sense of dogmatism or utopianism or an awe-inspiring mysticism. The natural authority of royal blue, as a consequence of sensitive and intuitive perception, is clairvoyance, clairaudience, clairsentience, and an ability to be efficient and determined.

Royal blue nurtures our ability to relate. When we develop the capacity to witness, to watch the self, in the midst of all that occurs in our mental and emotional bodies, we can learn to dis-identify with ourselves and our reactions and opinions. Then we do not extend our reactivity beyond ourselves. We develop clarity of our sensory experience in a new way. That is, when we are less centered, our awareness is in what is coming at us or with what we are outwardly engaged. We can watch what is happening with detachment. We are able to witness our self, not in a negative, aloof way lacking in humility, but with full involvement and sensitivity.

Violet

Violet, a secondary, is made by blending the two primaries blue and red. It signfies service, transformation, wholeness, and healing.

The Aura-Soma concept of service is to be doing what we are meant to do, to fulfill our purpose and destiny and to bring our part of the blueprint to earth. Encompassed is the attitude and intention we carry as we manifest our service. Caring and kindness are associated with such service.

In violet is the idea of the shrinking violet, recognized as the little flowering plant that grows in nooks and crannies. This association represents the desire to be invisible and the tendency to hide our light. Not wanting to be seen may be an expression of false ego or inappropriate humility.

Violet can depict grief, whether for loss of what was, for what might have been, or for our identities in the past. Yet in violet is the potential for a total change of point of view, for metanoia: a shattering of all that has previously been constructed to allow a transformation and reintegration of our masculine and feminine sides. Violet represents the veil between this world and the world of spirit. It is associated with transition and an understanding of death and at-one-ment.

As we shine light into the violet it becomes the pale violet of transmutation. The light of suffering and the understanding of suffering with the violet ray support this alchemical process.

Magenta

Magenta, from an Aura-Soma point of view, is the color immediately beyond our physicality. Goethe referred to this color, which joins together the primary red and the secondary violet, as the unseen color of the spectrum.

Magenta signifies love in the little things. This is a key concept in Aura-Soma. The more we practice putting our attention, caring, and warmth into the little things, devoting

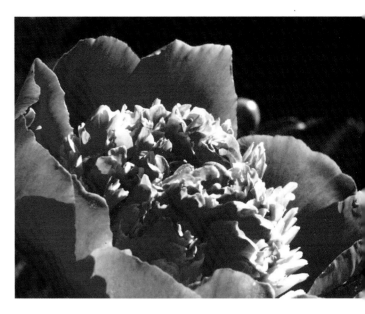

Magenta peony receiving light from above.

appropriate attention toward the details of our everyday life, the greater the possibility of building up an account with spirit, so that attention might be available when we need it in our life. Unless we practice love in the little things, a love that is merged with service, we cannot expect love to be present in the big things. Magenta refers to love from above, to grace. Grace might seem to be a noncausal phenomenon. Yet if we practice putting love into the little things, we may enact a direct relationship with magenta energy coming down from above, with grace from above, that might support our everyday activities. Magenta gives caring to the caregiver.

The Equilibrium bottles generally show a light-full form of magenta, which is something of an approximation of the true color. True magenta seems to be the deep magenta found in the base fractions of the Rescue bottles B0, B1, B78, B89, B90, and B102. The deep magenta, which absorbs all of the colors, can be understood to contain all of the colors. In contrast, the magenta found in B67, B25, or B77, for example, is more a fuchsia pink. This fuchsia represents the magenta as it might appear when it is full of light.

Pink

Pink, a tint, results from light being added to the primary red, and suggests consciousness brought to physicality. Accepting ourselves, suspending self-judgment, allows us to awaken to be who we are. In pink, as we awaken, we find the capacity to accept ourselves as we are, rather than as we might like to be. The skill of detachment fosters change.

When we stop pushing ourselves away, we can allow ourselves to be.

Pink, an intensification of red, could represent intense anger, resentment, and frustration. The light of consciousness present in pink may help us utilize the energy of anger, transforming it to a strong love of our process of awakening, or to a great courage to ground and manifest our feelings of unconditional love.

When we are attracted to pink, we may have the capability to give love and at the same time find it difficult to love and care for ourselves. We may always find a reason to deny our vulnerability, to not care for ourselves. Instead we may choose to offer compassion and tenderness to others. If we could care for ourselves, moving ourselves up the line to receive attention, our love may more unconditionally overflow into the world, and to others.

Clear/White

Clear represents the full spectrum of consciousness, wherein all colors are contained. It can express simple purity and great intensity.

Clear signifies suffering and the understanding of suffering. The light of that understanding is related to the enlightenment of the Buddha, after which he defined his experience of and understanding of suffering in the four noble truths: there is suffering; there is a cause of suffering; there is a way out of suffering; there is a goal at the end of suffering.

There are three causes of suffering, which can be expressed simply: we suffer when we get what we do not want; we suffer when we want what we cannot have; we suffer when we cannot distinguish between these two.

Vicky referred to clear as the well of unshed tears, and this too relates conceptually to suffering: when we feel as if the colors have been washed out of our life. As humans, we are seven-tenths water. Perhaps the well refers to those emotional forms of suffering with which we identify. Suffering does not necessarily equate to sufferers; suffering could exist without sufferers, when there is no personal identification with the experience.

Clear also relates to transparency. Consciousness and transparency seem to be synonymous. Lucidity lies

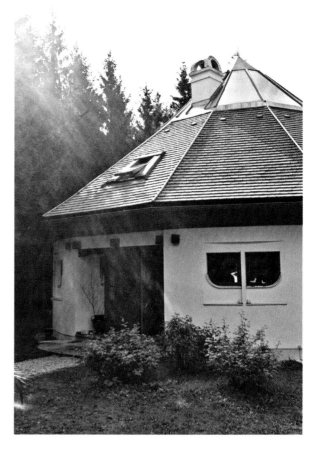

Rainbow light coming to a teaching center in Austria that was designed using sacred geometry.

behind all sensory experience, behind perception. When we look at a mirror, transparency and reflectivity are paradoxically both part of our experience. As in transparency, clear allows all colors to pass through it. If you put red behind the clear you see the red and so clear can be said to contain red. At the same time, clear represents the light and has the quality of reflection.

Although the Pomander and Color Essence that correspond to this color are clear, Vicky named them "white" and we continue to refer to them this way today. When we add light to a color we go from a hue to a tint. When we think about pigments we would add white to a color to achieve the same result. In this way light, or clear, and white are the same thing. So interpretively we view clear as white. Like clear, white too can be said to contain all of the colors.

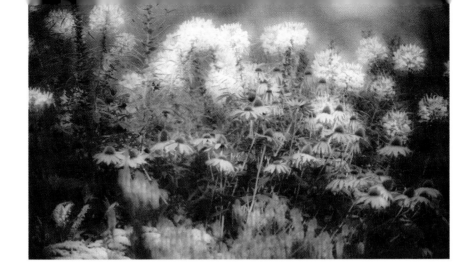

4

The Aura-Soma System

Aura-Soma appeals to many because of the inherent simplicity of the calling by vibrant colors. Yet as we begin to understand the complexity of it, those of us who are compelled to look deeper can find the exploration very satisfying.

The Subtle Anatomy

In Aura-Soma the traditional seven chakras, or energy centers, of the physical body are designated as they are in the Vedic tradition. Aura-Soma also recognizes that within each of the seven major energy centers of our physicality are seven levels that in turn correspond to a minor chakra system within each major chakra; each of these forty-nine levels corresponds to a particular color vibration and its corresponding wavelength.

To function well, these energy centers must operate as transceivers, both giving out and taking in energy as part of their function. In this sense we are describing energy as information, and this information, as far as Aura-Soma is concerned, is taken in and given out as color and light.

The Aura-Soma subtle anatomy includes the incarnational star in the golden area, the earth star in the red area, and the soul star within the magenta realm; the emerald of the heart and the *icosidodecahedron,* a thirty-two-faced polyhedron, composed of twenty triangles and twelve dodecahedrons; the eight major energy centers or chakras (the seven within our body plus one at the soul star, just above the body); and the turquoise center, the Ananda Khanda. Eight colors correspond to the main energy centers: red, orange, yellow, green, blue, royal blue, violet, and magenta.

The root chakra (red) relates to issues of survival, the sacral (orange) to issues of dependency, the solar plexus (yellow) to fear and power, and the heart chakra (green) to a sense of spaciousness and panoramic awareness. The throat chakra (blue) relates to communication and peace, the third eye (royal blue) to clarity and relating, the crown (violet) to service and transformation, and the soul star (magenta) to divine love and attention to detail.

Above: Out of the darkness the colors emerged, first red then green.

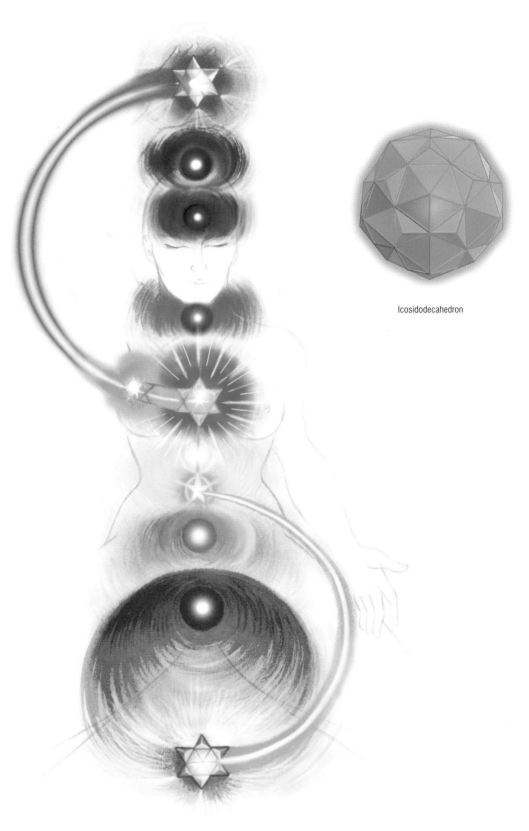

Magenta combinations relate to the 8th chakra, Soul Star

Violet combinations relate to the crown

Blue combinations relate to throat and communication area

Turquoise combinations relate to the throat and heart area

Green combinations relate to chest and heart area

Yellow and Gold combinations relate to the Solar Plexus area

Orange combinations relate to navel area and periphery of body

Red combinations relate to the Base Chakra

Pink combinations for love and creativity

Where possible apply combinations around body to include spine

N.B.
Pink and Magenta combinations have a close energetic assocation

The Chakra (or energy centers) run from the 1st at the base of the spine (Red/Pink) through to the 8th above the crown (Magenta)

Any color applicable to feet

Icosidodecahedron

Gold, the color that exists between the second and third chakras, between the orange and the yellow, is very significant in terms of the subtle anatomy. The golden area of the body contains the true aura. The true aura could be understood as a point of embarkation to the development of wisdom within ourselves. This memory is in the incarnational star, which is an infinite brilliant point of light, like a diamond, at the center of our being, within the true aura. If you were to put a compass on the incarnational star and extend the radius from the bottom of the rib cage and to the top of the pubic bone, all of the area within the circle drawn is called the hara. (The hara includes the golden area, the incarnational star, the true aura, and the hologram of the first cell.)

Three phenomena, existing in relationship to one another like the points of a tripod or triangle, exist within the first cell: the entirety of the genetic lineage of the mother; the entirety of the genetic lineage of the father; and the consciousness that we were before we entered into incarnation. Governed by our karma and our dharma, this consciousness, was attracted into the situation of this incarnational experience with the provided combined genetic lineages.

As we get in touch with our incarnational star we will begin to sense the presence of our inner master. If we are centered within our incarnational star, our teacher is on the inside. If we are not centered, life will present us with experiences to teach us from the outside.

The incarnational star appears as a consequence of going through the conception mandala, the precursory experience to entering into the first cell. This process is the same for all humans. Consciousness independent of physical form first passes through a single point of light appearing on a blue background, which becomes a brilliant yellow pentagram in the middle of a blue sphere. At that point the memory of the bardo and of all the beings we have been and all the beings we are yet to be is partially erased. It is as if a blue curtain or veil were drawn across all of the information contained within consciousness prior to the experience of conception.

The point of light that appears in the blue is the consciousness of the self. It remains a point of access to the lessons we have learned in the past and the ones that we have set for ourselves, and that are set for us, in this particular lifetime. When we connect with this consciousness of the self, this point of light or incarnational star, we have the potential for downloading information and energy that lies above us concerning all the beings we have been and are yet to be.

The brilliant yellow point of light of the incarnational star brings us to the human experience and to the experience of our soul ray for this lifetime. Our soul ray or soul color can be identified by the base fraction of the bottle we feel to be our first selection, as far as our superconsciousness perceives the soul color to be at that point in time. External and internal factors, filters, and conditioning can influence who we are and our ability to perceive that soul ray.

As the yellow incarnational star appears on the blue background at the time of our conception, simultaneously our consciousness experiences the mingling of colors, the merging of the mother and the father in space. The color produced by the mingling of colors becomes the personality ray.

From having no form, from being a being of light, we materialize to come into form, first with the soul ray and then with the personality ray, through which the soul ray will work to develop itself in this incarnation. The primary colors blue, yellow, and red come together as a manifestation of our light being in accordance with our whole history and the future of our soul ray. The soul ray becomes more individual with the appearance of the personality ray, which defines what it is that we are going to work through in order to be able to express what our soul has to express in this life—in other words, our karmic and our dharmic work.

As we reconnect with our incarnational star, our physiological remembrance of the point of conception, the star grows. We become more conscious of and accepting of our physicality and of the inheritance we have received from our genetic lineage. We begin to bring more consciousness (light) to our body, to the red aspect of ourselves, the grounding and earthing within us. Bringing light to the red turns red to pink. Pink then begins to arise from the red.

The earth star is located in the red area. It has to do with our destiny on this planet for this incarnation and contains pre-programmed information about where we will incarnate and in what places we will visit and live. Earth as a being has her own destiny and evolution, but she is linked to us and our evolution. Our recognition of our relationship with the earth and our shared growth and reciprocal maintenance is fundamental for being grounded and for our work with ourselves. With that, we will be likely to be in the right place at the right time, doing what we are meant to do at that moment, in synchronistic harmony with our destiny.

Red exists below the waist, in the legs and feet all the way to the base chakra. Within the red area lies the source of creativity, both the urge to replicate ourselves and the desire to understand ourselves creatively. As the pink rises, it moves through the coral area to the orange and toward the gold, activating the hologram in the true aura. The warming energy of the pink continues to ascend, arching across the solar plexus through the olive toward the emerald of the heart.

The soul star is located approximately one hand's breadth above the top of the head. The soul star contains the full potential of who we are. It is in touch with our self as a being that has existed through incarnations earthly, stellar, and in other forms over many thousands of incarnations. The soul star contains the complete knowledge of who we have been and are yet to be, our individual pages of the akashic chronicles. The particular page at which the book is open has recorded the agreements we made with our guides, teachers, and masters before we came into this incarnation, when we said, "Yes, I will do that," to certain experiences and responsibilities in this lifetime.

When the pink energy touches the golden area, the memory of the first cell within our physiology, simultaneously and synchronistically the magenta energy of the eighth chakra, the information in the soul star, gives a reciprocal response, starting to move toward the turquoise center, the Ananda Khanda. The inherent energy in the heart and in the turquoise center awakens as the pink energy from the earth star and the magenta energy from the soul move toward each other.

The turquoise center can be understood to represent or to be the process of individuation, as described by Carl Jung. This process of awakening develops our connection with the collective consciousness and helps us to be co-creators with all that is.

As the magenta overflows through the turquoise toward the emerald of the heart, the little center on the right side of the chest begins to move toward the middle. There is an inherent stream of energy in our hearts, in the emerald, that is our connection with the earth and with our self as a being of service in the world. Perhaps, for the planet, the plans for the heart and for the earth are the same. In the emerald of the heart the three streams of energy come together leading to the opening of the green, the opening of the heart.

The emerald, from an Aura-Soma perspective, is an inheritance from Lucifer, the Lord of Light who sat next to God. God as a primary phenomenon is the Mother/Father, the creator, and the architect of all that is. When God and Lucifer became separated, Lucifer made the tremendous sacrifice of accepting exile from heaven and losing his role as the Lord of Light. Lucifer did not want to serve the two-legged creatures upon the earth. We carry aspects of both God and Lucifer within ourselves. This is reflected in our opposing impulses of wanting to ground our light, being fully present on earth and then at other times our desire to move into spirit and not be connected to earth. Perhaps at times we have difficulty relating to our earth star and resist

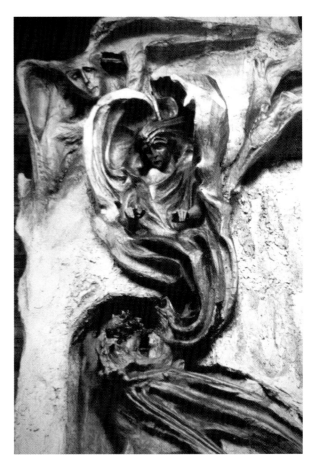

The struggle between Lucifer and Ahriman. This wooden sculpture by Rudolf Steiner and Edith Maryon represents humanity's attempt to balance emotion and reason.

incarnating fully into who it is that we could be and what we are here to do. An opportunity we have as beings on the earth is to find a way to bring the Lord of Light within us into resonance with our hearts. Then the Lord of Light may be able to sit harmoniously next to the godhead within us. The magenta energy can continue its journey to connect with the golden area within us, and the pink energy can come into the emerald of the heart, having moved through the yellow of the solar plexus and the olive of the diaphragm and abdominal cavity. We may walk the path of individuation and our heart may expand.

Color Resonance in the Chakras

When pure white light is refracted through a prism, seven distinct frequencies appear out of that refraction as the seven visible colors of the rainbow. Each of the seven chakras in the body has a direct correspondence to one of those colors. Our attraction to a particular bottle indicates that we have the possibility of fine-tuning the corresponding chakras through their sympathetic resonance with the color, gem, and crystal energies contained in the bottle. In a sense, the Aura-Soma system may assess diagnostically the condition of the chakras.

The relationship between color and the subtle anatomy is profound. As our awareness of color, perception of color, and work with color point in the direction of ease, the implication for all patterns of dis-ease are immense. Whatever patterns of disease lie within our genetic code—our inheritance—have the potential to be eased through work with color and light. At this dawn of the New Aeon, perhaps Aura-Soma has been offered to humanity to provide the tools to aid each us in perceiving our color code and fulfilling our potential to individuate. This could include an examination of the DNA codices into which we have incarnated and therefore is at once an examination of our genetic history as well as how it is that our color code depicts our self as a being of light from what might be called a soul perspective.

The interaction with color in the context of Aura-Soma, through the direct application of the Equilibrium bottles, as well as through the Pomanders, Quintessences, ArchAngeloi, and Color Essences, has a profound effect on the energetics of the subtle anatomy, which in turn has profound repercussions within our physicality. The colors for each of these products are formulated in different ways. The colors, as they are made available in these various forms, have a resonance with the electromagnetic field, the etheric field, and the astral field of the aura, which surround the physical body and with the physical body itself. For greater clarity, we will discuss in detail each of the core components within the Aura-Soma system: the Equilibrium bottles, Pomanders, Quintessences, Air Conditioners, ArchAngeloi, and Color Essences.

The Equilibrium Bottles

The Equilibrium bottles contain colors that are perceptible to human sight as well as the energies of crystals and plants. Part of the inspiration Vicky Wall received during the first nights of the birth of Aura-Soma was the instruction to bring together the oily and the watery parts of plants. In aromatherapy, therapists largely use the oily parts of plants, known as the essential oils. Herbalists, on the other hand, use the watery extracts of plants. In an Equilibrium bottle, the upper half, or fraction, contains oil extracts, and the lower fraction water extracts, so that both parts of a plant are present in the bottle. When the bottle is shaken, the two parts form a temporary emulsion that has a sympa-

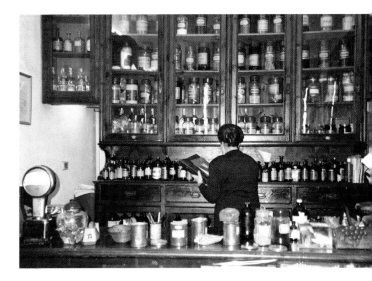
Traditional supply store for color dyes and pigments in Florence, Italy

thetic bio-compatibility with our physical body and is readily absorbed through the skin.

The upper fraction of the Equilibrium bottle represents the conscious mind and the lower represents the unconscious. This correlation was noted by Carl Jung who found that when looking at a mandala with his patients, the upper fraction most often referred to symbolism, imagery, color, and form that was the most conscious for that person, while the lower referred to the unconscious, subconscious, or collective conscious of the individual.

A Trinity of Resonant Waveforms

The trinity of resonant waveforms is comprised of the waveforms of the mineral kingdom, the waveforms of the herbs and the plants, and the waveforms of color and light as they relate to the human and animal kingdoms. The colors are formulated by combining plant ingredients, gem and mineral energies, and natural colorings. Aura-Soma is dedicated to bringing together in the finished preparations the finest energies available from the vegetable and mineral kingdoms. The formulation of the bottles' contents alters over the years as constant listening to the inspirational source enables us to improve the quality of the ingredients and the standard of cultivation. All plant materials are carefully chosen and harvested. Production is overseen in the United Kingdom, and source material is both produced locally and brought in from around the world.

Using farming techniques compatible with the Aura-Soma system, Aura-Soma Products Ltd. (ASPL) grows what it can on its farm in Lincolnshire, England, expanding cultivation as it becomes possible to do so. The botanic ingredients grown by Aura-Soma Products are Demeter registered, meaning that they comply with a biodynamic standard. (Demeter is the Greek goddess of the harvest.) Developed by Rudolf Steiner, biodynamic farming approaches cultivation in accord with his philosophy, and plants raised biodynamically carry an enhanced life force that is in harmony with the spiritual forces of nature. At ASPL's farm, plants are grown in cooperation with both the landscape angels and the devas involved with each plant species' development.

When necessitated by climatic considerations or because production demand outstrips the farm's supply, ASPL seeks other biodynamic sources. If biodynamic plants are not available, organically grown material is sought. If that too is unavailable, we use the best source that we can find, such as essential oils derived from wild plants in renewable environments.

When Vicky was a child, her father often took her for walks and introduced her to the science of signatures, a field of study based on the theory that a plant's usefulness can be determined through the evaluation of clues given by the plant itself (for instance, where it grows, how it looks, and its color), in a manner similar to the work of the ancient Greek physician Galen and the medieval alchemist Paracelsus. The signature of plants is one of the bases for homeopathy, developed in the early nineteenth century by the pioneering German doctor Samuel Hahnemann. Today, the plant extracts used in Aura-Soma preparations are chosen for their therapeutic significance as suggested by each plant's signature.

Homeopathy also applies the law of similars, which suggests that "like cures like." In Aura-Soma the ingredients in the bottles we choose can help us move from dis-ease to greater ease. Through sympathetic resonance, the energetic vibrations of the product ingredients have a stimulating, clarifying, and balancing effect on us. Those colors that call to us create a strengthening resonance within our physicality and auric field, helping to establish positive well-being and personal growth. Furthermore, through harmonic resonance, colors can support us and nurture us in our life as we express our purpose and potential. The plant kingdom and the mineral kingdom relate, respectively, to the flesh and the skeletal structure of our bodies. Water makes up a large percentage of the human body, and the water medium can carry a memory of energy. Water is also synonymous with an aspect of consciousness. While we are in the physical plane, water is the carrier, or the instrument, of consciousness within us. This consciousness of water has been a part of the understanding of many ancient philosophies, as exemplified in Chang Tsu's saying, "I take water

as my element, and it is through the understanding of water that I come to the understanding of truth." Water makes up one-half of the Equilibrium bottle contents and two-thirds of the Pomanders, Quintessences, ArchAngeloi, and Color Essences. It is a key component for carrying intention and consciousness within the Aura-Soma system.

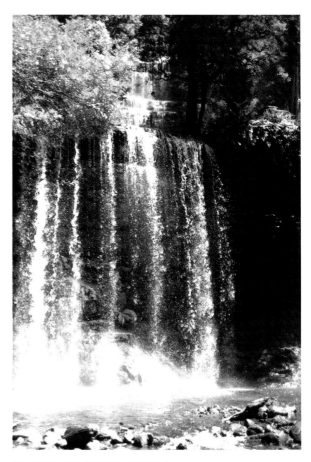

Russell Falls at Mt. Field National Park in Tasmania.

To understand the concept of signatures, let us consider *Hypericum perforatum*, known to many as St. John's wort, as a specific for abrasions to the skin. St. John's wort has a delicate yellow flower. Picking this flower is an unforgettable experience, as the plant exudes a bit of red juice when cut. The plant's signature could thus suggest an association with bleeding. The language of color suggests that a combination of yellow and red can be helpful if we have experienced fear (yellow) and emotional trauma or have the potential or need to use our energy (red) wisely. Not coincidentally, St. John's wort is often also used as a remedy for depression. Similar connotations can be inferred for Bottle 5, Yellow/Red (for more on B5, see page 68).

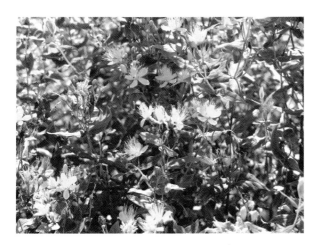

Hypericum.

The moment you see the green jewel you transport your eye back into far distant ages and the green appears to you because divine spiritual beings created this substance out of the spiritual world, out of the green color belonging to the spirit. The moment you see green, red, blue or yellow in precious stones you look back into the infinitely far distant past. . . . And as the jewel takes us back in time we look at the first beginnings of Earth creation before the Lemurian epoch of our Earth evolution, and because we see it being created out of the spirit we see it colored. . . . [T]he divine spiritual beings who created stones long ages ago come alive in the colors and stimulate a living memory in us of their past creations.[3]

Further understanding of the qualities inherent in a plant's color comes from observing how it grows. Johann Wolfgang von Goethe, the early nineteenth-century German scientist, author, and artist, said that "as yellow is always accompanied with light, so it may be said that blue still brings a principle of darkness with it."[1] Based on this, Steiner theorized about the source of pigment:

We have to know, for example, how the yellow works in the sunflower or the dandelion. We have to know how the blue works in the chicory. The processes which make chicory or indigo blue are found in the root, whereas the processes which make the sunflower or dandelion yellow are found in the blossom. I must bring chemistry alive and copy the blossom process in the plant, then I shall get a light color. I must copy the root process in the plant if I want to get a dark color.[2]

St. John's wort and its two pigments offer an example of how plants may reveal their nature and qualities, inspiring meditations, inquiries, and applications, and helps explain why ASPL is so committed to using ingredients cultivated in harmony with the spiritual forces of the plant kingdom and under the auspices of the devas and the landscape angels. The mindfulness brought to each step of farming will affect the vitality of the harvest.

Aura-Soma also works in harmony with energy from the mineral kingdom. Crystals and gems can function as receivers and transmitters. Differing from that of a plant, the consciousness of a crystal is slow and long—a crystal may take more than three hundred thousand years to grow. Much in the life experience of a crystal has been preserved in it and can be "seen." According to Steiner:

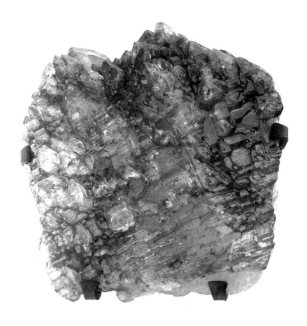

The laboratory guardian: Elestial crystal.

Vicky was inspired to infuse the Equilibrium bottles with the energies of certain gems and crystals through an energetic process. While you might expect the bottles to contain ground-up gems and crystals, we refer instead to the presence of a tincture of the mineral kingdom. Vicky was shown a means to transfer information and energy from crystals and gems to another medium with what has been referred to as a kabbalistic invocation. Originally she did not have any devices or technology to assist in that process. Gradually, as Aura-Soma began to grow during her lifetime, ways were found to stabilize that process with technology that does the job more effectively. Now subtle technology is used to more effectively transfer the resonant waveforms, information, and energy of the crystals and gems into the receptive medium of the water or the oil in the Equilibrium bottles.

A recent development has been the alchemical technique called the spygurik process. This ancient process has its origins in alchemy and the foundations of modern pharmacy. It would be true to say that Parcelsus had knowledge of the spygurik process, and it is from these ancient roots that the present spygurik process has emerged. A Swiss pharmaceutical company cooperates with ASPL in producing spygurik essences from the crystals and minerals that the company supplies. The spygurik essences then are added to the lower fractions of the bottles.

Another example of the continual development in Aura-Soma is the oloid machine, a device used for blending ingredients. Developed by Paul Schatz, the machine is named after the oloid, the shape that occurs when a cube is turned inside out.[4] The oloid is a very important structure in nature. The golden ratio—as it occurs, for example, in a nautilus shell as it spirals outward—can produce a structure similar to that of the oloid.[5] The oloid machines were produced by a Swiss company specifically for ASPL and are unique. The Equilibrium bottles, the Pomanders, the Quintessences, the ArchAngeloi, and the Color Essences are all prepared in oloid machines of varied sizes.

When Vicky made the first bottles, she introduced the ingredients to each other by a very gentle rocking motion of a demijohn (a glass jug holding approximately a gallon of liquid). This process was affectionately called "rocking the baby." The oloid machine mixes the ingredients in a similar movement, merging the molecular surfaces of the components in a harmonious way. The movement of the oloid as it slides the ingredients past each other creates what might be seen as a lemniscate (figure-eight-shaped curve) in three dimensions, perhaps intimating a connection with the infinite. This sliding motion is very different from percussive mixing. The oloid machine provides a very gentle way to achieve a harmonious union of the materials, rather than a homogenizing of the product with sharp blades.

Cooperation between a Swiss company and ASPL also led to the development of an energizing device, called the golden pyramid, that operates pneumatically to create an energetic field around the demijohns. It works in concert with the shambhala, an energizing device that places the multiple potentialities of resonances from minerals, crystals, and plants into the receptive mediums of oil and water. The golden pyramid device contains seven pyramids made of twenty-four-carat gold, each of which contains certain gems. It creates resonances in harmony with the information that comes through the shambhala and stabilizes them through time.

The colors of the bottles, derived from plants and imbued with the resonant waveforms of gems and crystals, have a living quality that is harmonious with our own life force. As our life force is strengthened, so might be our ease in connecting with spirit, for as Steiner suggests, "If we become aware of the fact that things are colored

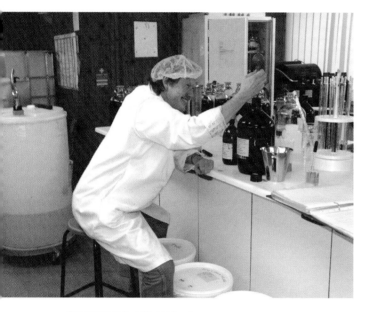

Eric Pelham in Aura-Soma laboratory.

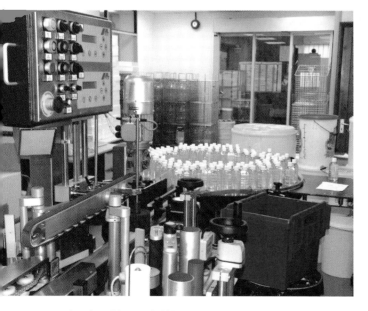

Aura-Soma laboratory in 2005.

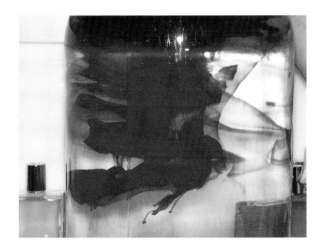

Oils mixing.

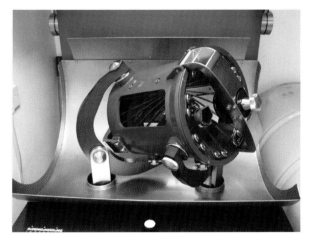

Oloid machine.

because gods are speaking through them, it will engender the kind of enthusiasm which comes from experiencing the spirit."[6]

The Greater Guide Is Within: How to Select the Bottles

Ideally, to select your four bottles you would look at the entire range of Equilibrium bottles. For those who do not have access to the bottles, the picture of all the bottles on pages 296–97 is a good substitute for not having the actual living energies of the bottles right in front of you.

To choose your first bottle, bring your attention to a place about two finger widths above your belly button and two finger widths inside. From that place, from the golden area of the true aura, allow yourself to feel which bottle calls to you the most. Another way to approach this is to imagine that you are stranded on a desert island and this color combination is the one, out of all the bottles, that you would most want to be living with for all time.

Once you have made your first selection, put that bottle out of sight and out of mind. Repeat the process of bringing your attention to the point in the golden area of your being and again discover which bottle, of those remaining in the Equilibrium range, calls to you the most. Do this until you have four bottles, each selected independently.

The first bottle selected is considered the "soul bottle" and represents how we, from a superconscious perspective, view ourselves and our purpose for this incarnation, at this point in time. It is a reflection of our mission and purpose and our life's lessons, showing the beginnings of the lessons that we are growing with in this lifetime. The upper fraction of this first bottle represents the color of the path upon which our soul will walk in this life—it includes the energies and the experiences that the soul will express through our personality ray. The upper fraction expresses our secondary talent, which supports our soul's expression through our personality. It also indicates the context into which we have been born, including our genetic lineage. The lower fraction of the first bottle selected reflects our soul's essence, our soul ray, and our subconscious mind. It may indicate our primary talent, which directly supports the soul.

The second bottle selected represents our greatest gifts and talents as well as the challenges that we have designed for this life. The challenges help us rarefy and actualize the potential of the first bottle. As the challenges are understood and integrated into our consciousness, the gifts that emerge from these challenges are revealed. These gifts are ones that we have selected for this lifetime to be of support as we express our mission and our purpose. The second bottle identifies experiences that were important to our life lessons. It represents a midpoint between our beginning and the present. It can indicate that which needs to be worked with or overcome, that which may block our developing and expressing our talents and gifts. The upper fraction of the second bottle reflects those gifts of which we are more conscious. The lower fraction reflects gifts that we are less aware of—those waiting to be revealed and expressed. The third bottle is an indication of the "here and now," where we have come to with regard to our intention for incarnation and our lessons and talents. It shows how our talents have been expressed thus far, as we have worked with our challenges. The upper fraction will reflect that of which we are conscious, while the lower fraction shows the issues and energies which are more in our subconscious.

The fourth bottle shows that which is right in front of us, in our near future, that we can turn to next, that which we are drawing to us and creating for our next step of development and expression. While this bottle reflects the energies that are coming toward us from the future, it also can be an expression of that which we could have now, but tend to put off until "tomorrow." It can be an indicator of what is possible and available to us now, the positive energies and impulses that we could have if we allowed ourselves to let go a little of certain patterns and open ourselves to change. This bottle can indicate our superconscious perception of the complete picture formed by the preceding three bottles—the most likely positive resolution as well as the confirming realizations and energies moving toward us. As with the other bottles, the upper fraction indicates what is more openly expressed and apparent, and the lower fraction shows that of which we are less aware.

There are many ways to interpret the selection of the four bottles. The descriptions of the individual Equilibrium bottles in chapter 5 will give you a further sense of the breadth of interpretive information available. To gain an even deeper understanding of the various ways of interpreting bottle selections—including emotional, psychological, mental, spiritual, archetypal, energetic, astrological, and numerological interpretations—it is helpful to attend an Aura-Soma training workshop or consultation.

Based on our bottle selections we may be guided to other helpful tools within the Aura-Soma system—Pomanders, Quintessences, Air Conditioners, ArchAngeloi, and Color Essences. When selecting any of the Aura-Soma tools, remember that the greater guide is within you. Some people make new selections once a week, others only once a year, or once a lifetime. Many find that it makes sense to finish using the products chosen initially and then to reselect or return to an Aura-Soma practitioner for another consultation.

For the Greater Good: How to Use the Bottles

There are many ways to experience the Equilibrium color combinations. You could imagine swimming in the bottle, letting your imagination immerse you in the colors. You could visualize the colors, breathing them in and exhaling them to surround yourself with a transparent cloud of your favorites. The bottles might sit by your bedside, where the sunlight and moonlight could illumine the colors, allowing them to dance and glisten in your room.

Aura-Soma engages us at our sense doors. While it is intriguing to look at the color combinations and see which ones call to us, it is more effective to actually use the Equilibrium bottles, Pomanders, Quintessences, ArchAngeloi, and Color Essences. Ultimately, for an interaction guided by experience, it is best to contact an Aura-Soma teacher or practitioner. An Aura-Soma seminar or consultation offers the opportunity to receive that which is there to be transmitted from spirit at that moment. Such an opportunity can also occur when we use a bottle, actually applying the contents to the physical body. We receive that which is appropriate for our growth. There is the aroma from the lovely essential oils, the feel of the liquid luxuriant on our body, the visual pleasure, a sound audible to some, and stimulation of our intuition. Furthermore, the intricacy of the system can allow our mind to be busy, while our actual felt and sensed experience of the colors, liquids, and aromas can bring rapid growth, balance, and support in our journey toward ourselves. Steiner would explain this living experience and participation in this way:

> We must bring to life what is in the color, not by practicing color symbolism, which is the worst possible thing, but by actually discovering what is in color, in the same way as the power of laughter is in someone who laughs. . . . The essential thing is to know how to open our souls to what speaks to us out of color.[7]

For example, a green and violet bottle would have to do with the violet outlet of the green energy center and the green outlet of the violet energy center, two levels of the heart and the crown chakra. Let's say that two friends choose these colors, one selecting Green/Violet (B17) and the other Violet/Green (B38). In discussing the difference, the first realizes that she approaches situations with great openness (green in the upper fraction) yet inwardly feels quite reserved. The other tends to evaluate situations and stay aloof (violet in the upper fraction) yet feels quite willing to let others be who they are. The colors describe qualities and points of tension. The colors in the bottles help bring clarity to the associated chakras. Colors carry the frequency on which a clear "picture" may be obtained. They help balance our system, restoring the wavelengths within through resonance with their own pure wavelengths.

The bottles and other parts of the system have been created with the intention that they will be activated for our greater good when we use them. In the case of the Equilibrium bottles, this process starts when we shake our selected bottle with our left hand. The bottle should be held with the thumb supporting it underneath, the middle finger placed over the top of the open bottle, and the ring finger and forefinger on either side of the bottle. The pinkie finger does not touch the bottle. Shaking the bottle, in effect, begins a re-balancing of chakras through a harmonic analysis of the 144,000 nadis, or energy points of the body. This is the level at which the sympathetic resonances work. Once we have activated the bottle for the most helpful of the multiple potencies of plants, gem, and crystal energies within it, we then apply the temporary emulsion of the oil and water. First we shake a few drops onto the palms and rub our hands together. Then we apply this liquid in a complete band around the part of our body that corresponds in color to the ingredient colors in the bottle (as indicated by the illustration on page 24), or as described in the individual bottle description pages in chapter 5. (The section "The Color Rose," page 15, gives further refinement with information about the secondary and tertiary colors.) When the Equilibrium combination is applied to the physical body, the skin absorbs the energies of the ingredients, and the color is radiated into the auric field. In this way, the precise color combination we choose works to restore clarity to a related chakra or to otherwise nurture growth. This self-selective aspect of Aura-Soma is fundamental to understanding how the system works.

There is a repercussion in all the levels of our being that supports our individual development. As you breathe in, imagine yourself breathing in the color you have chosen. As we inspire the colors with our breath and embody them with their application, we bring ourselves into a greater state of equilibrium and alignment with our karma and our dharma. Furthermore, interpreting the meanings of the colors can help us grow in self-awareness.

The Pomanders

Before Aura-Soma was born, while Vicky was practicing as a surgical chiropodist, she collected herbs on her various travels, reminiscent both of her walks with her father and of her time in the pharmacy. She preserved these herbs in glass containers and kept records of what was in each, without plans for their usage or purpose. After the birth of Aura-Soma, Vicky reviewed her collection of herbs. She realized that essentially she had collected herbs that related to the seven levels of the seven major energy centers, or chakras, of the human being. These forty-nine herbs (seven groups of seven) became the basis of all of the Aura-Soma Pomanders.

While Equilibrium bottles work with the physical body, balancing and aligning our physical energies, Pomanders work within and affect the auric field, specifically energizing the bio-energetic and electromagnetic fields surrounding the physical body. They are intended to introduce the positive energies and messages of their specific color and to be protective.

A Pomander exists for most of the colors found in the Equilibrium range. Each Pomander is conceived from all forty-nine herbs in an ethanol base. Seven of these herbs relate directly to the color of the Pomander, while the other forty-two relate to all that is not that color and they are present in a less material form, as more minuscule, subtle potencies. The original white Pomander, the first to be developed, is an exception; as white contains and reflects all colors, the white Pomander has an equal balance of the forty-nine herbs. In the red Pomander, for instance, the herbs present would be the ones predominantly related to the red energy. Some of these relationships are quite complex. The medicinal herb St. John's wort (Hypericum perforatum), with its yellow petals and the red dye from the stamen of the plant (please see page 28), fits perfectly with the yellow aspect of the red, the third level of the first energy center. However, this plant would also be appropriate for the red aspect of the yellow, the first level of the third energy center.

A plant is rather like a human being: its roots are in the earth, and surrounding it is an auric field similar to the bio-energetic and electromagnetic field of humans. If a leaf is cut, Kirlian photography of the leaf will show it in its original, uncut form at an energetic level. This phenomenon supports the rationale for using herbs and plants as restoratives to the human bio-energetic and electromagnetic fields. Beyond the bio-energetic and electromagnetic fields is the etheric body, the first of the intangible fields beyond our physicality. Certain of the Pomanders, particularly the orange and the coral, have a specificity of effect that extends beyond the bio-energetic field to the etheric. Other Pomanders, higher in the spectrum toward violet, also affect some of the more subtle bodies, though still predominantly working through the bio-energetic and electromagnetic fields.

The Pomanders are reenergizing, affirmative, and protective. Their action aligns with the intention that as we protect ourselves, we protect others. Confirming and reenergizing our electromagnetic field is a step toward building strength in the field of light that surrounds our physicality. This intention is carried forward in other parts of the Aura-Soma system.

The Individual Pomanders

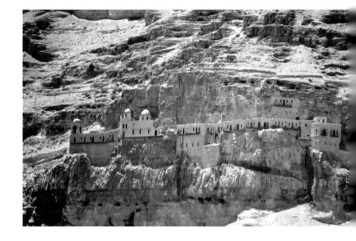

Deep Red Pomander

The deep red Pomander harmonizes the base chakra and is helpful for grounding after meditation or any therapy session. It provides the strongest protection against energy sapping, being both energizing and restorative of physical energies when you are fatigued or depleted. Deep red is particularly useful in situations when it is difficult to come into the body, say after a psychotic episode, or essentially whenever there has been a disconnect, such as after electrocution. It can de-stress the electromagnetic field and help reduce all kinds of fears linked to survival issues, including money and health. It can activate the right half of the brain and brings in deep feminine intuition. Warming and energizing, deep red can have an aphrodisiac effect. It can be used in house clearing by neutralizing psychic activity. It acts as a protective during rituals and sacred dances and protects participants against negative energies arising in sacred sites and power places that have been misused in the past.

The deep red Pomander protects people who work with gems, balancing electromagnetic polarities in the body. Deep red also protects against geopathic stress, negative ley lines, and psoric water and helps restore polarities that have been upset by any of these.

Red Pomander

All of the qualities of the deep red Pomander are also found in the red. Red is better suited for everyday situations, whereas deeps red is better suited for extreme situations. Red particularly supports awakening. It stimulates the hormonal system, bringing back energy in a gentle way. It also can help us overcome disappointment and shyness.

Coral Pomander

The coral Pomander has an awakening energy. When we have had difficulties in relationships, especially when we have not felt acknowledged and valued, coral can help us value ourselves more. Similarly, when we have experienced unrequited love, especially of the self, coral helps us to love parts of us that seem most difficult to love and to feel how we then respond. It helps us learn to love and care in a new way. The coral Pomander stimulates a spirit of cooperation and noncompetitiveness. We may accept our responsibilities with a sense of joy rather than hardship. When we accept our fears, we may move closer to synchronicity and a healing of the timeline. Coral and orange both have this effect. Curiously, the coral Pomander is useful for relieving altitude sickness.

Orange Pomander

Between the electromagnetic field and the astral body is the etheric body. Through the etheric body, to which both the physical body and the orange Pomander relate, past and future experiences may be touched. Using the orange Pomander allows the informational content of past experience to be available without necessarily bringing the emotionally cathartic aspects of the experience into the present. This opens the door to insight. By seeking backward in time and resolving situations in the past, we can come to increased synchronicity in the present. We may be more in the present, if we release conditioned patterns from the past.

In situations of shock, the aura may move toward the etheric gap, located at the bottom of the left rib. The gap is an escape route of sorts for the aura after extreme trauma. The

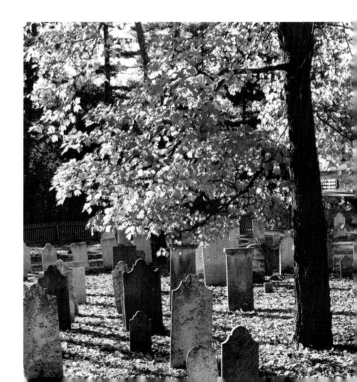

Right: Graveyard at the former Webb estate, Shelburne Farms, Vermont.

orange Pomander helps restore the aura to its proper location in the golden area of the body, sealing the etheric gap.

The orange Pomander also regulates temperature. If the aura feels warm or cool, work on the etheric body with orange. It is a specific that can help with bed-wetting and for those prone to nightmares. As orange is significant for dependency, in some circumstances parents may find it helpful to share the Pomander with their child.

The orange Pomander brings a more relaxed point of view to people who encounter difficulties with technology and electrical appliances. It is useful as a regression protector and memory shock absorber. In regression work, to protect the user who opens the door to knowledge from the past, use first the Saint Germain Quintessence and then the orange Pomander.

Gold Pomander

The gold Pomander helps us reconnect with our instincts and discover our innate wisdom. Gold allays irrational fears and phobias and can assist with peer-group difficulties, connecting each to self-confidence. Gold facilitates in breaking habitual and emotional patterns, be they mental, emotional, or physical, and addressing the fears that lie behind these patterns. With the wisdom from gold, we may realize what leads to the pattern and how to release our addictions. Gold may help with extreme anxiety in written and oral exams, making it easier to remember learned information. The gold Pomander supports the assimilation of food and energy. It assists in letting go of deep irrational fears and in easing tension in the solar plexus. Gold connects us to our incarnational star.

Yellow Pomander

The yellow Pomander brings in the sunshine and acts as an antidote to the blues, nervousness, and anxiety. It can unlock a remarkable sense of joy. It can allay feelings of negativity, cynicism, repulsion, or depression and can uplift us when we are suffering from a lack of sunlight and feel like hibernating. Through its connection with sunshine, the yellow Pomander may help in cases of jet lag, sickness, and travel sickness.

Yellow helps us develop self-knowledge. It both helps us learn and stimulates our intuitive knowledge. The yellow Pomander is a specific for releasing patterns of addiction and detoxifying. Yellow is important for assimilating the energies of food and water. We are nourished not only by food but also by the entire energy field of the environment, which we receive as prana primarily through our solar plexus. The yellow Pomander feeds the wavelengths of herbs and gems to restore, regenerate, and balance that area of our body.

Olive Green Pomander

Both the emerald green and the olive green Pomanders invite a feeling response. They are useful for emotional issues and go to the heart of things.

The olive green Pomander helps us overcome anxieties, fears, and disappointments that have to do with our feelings. It encourages feminine, heart-centered leadership and cooperation instead of competition, yet it enhances our ability to stand up for our truth. The olive green Pomander can bring clarity to our path when we are at a crossroads or in the process of decision making.

Olive is an antipollutant and disinfectant. In our subtle bodies, it is useful for clearing jealousy, envy, and other difficult emotions and for resolving issues of space, including both agoraphobia and claustrophobia.

The olive Pomander can open the way for us to find a new space, to let go, especially if we are feeling strong emotions and reactivity. In a business or therapeutic situation, the olive Pomander facilitates transition from one circumstance to another, while helping us to be centered and integrated in the new moment. Olive aids in the grace of transitions, bringing an awareness of the sacredness of each new moment. In Christian terms, this could be defined as a sense of the presence of the Holy Spirit. When we bring our breath to the olive center of our diaphragm and abdominal cavity, we may experience being in the moment in a new way.

Olive expresses feminine intuition, a knowing that arises out of caring for something. A fear of giving space may arise when we feel overwhelmed by shadows or by what is hidden. The olive green Pomander helps us stay balanced and assists us in enabling the space to come into balance so we are not tempted to manipulate or control that which is arising. One quality of feminine wisdom is compassion. In cases of nervous fear, olive encourages compassion, bringing wisdom into the heart and releasing fear, helping us find our own way.

Emerald Green Pomander

The emerald green Pomander is wonderful for the heart chakra, opening and calming the heart, helping to expand our breathing, and supportive of any breathwork. It nudges us in the correct direction to connect with the truth of our own heart. In a confrontational situation or when we have difficulty with other people, emerald green brings a clarity to our communication of our feelings.

The emerald Pomander provides the space for us to find our own way and to free ourselves of outdated ideas. It helps us when we are at a crossroads of our life and enhances our clarity in finding new directions.

Emerald green soothes feelings of agoraphobia and

Page 34, top: Greek Orthodox monastery built in the late 5th century, above Jericho, Israel. Legend says that the monastery was built around a cave chapel where Jesus sat during the temptation.

claustrophobia. It may provide a sense of peace, and a sense that our space is protected and respected. Therapists and consultants may more easily preserve boundaries between clients and themselves using the emerald green Pomander.

Emerald green is an antidote for those who feel spaced out. As with inoculations, when a little of a virus is given to stimulate our antibodies, a little green can be an effective antidote to a spaced-out, ungrounded moment.

Both the olive green and emerald green Pomanders link time and space. Thus, they support our memory. When we are beginning to seek and search, the emerald green Pomander can lead us to a new beginning and awareness. It can allay our fears, bringing a quality of peace into our space. It helps us keep our balance when we have encounters and shifts into the fourth dimension.

Emerald is an antipollutant and disinfectant for both the environment and our subtle bodies. It also links us with nature and trees. This Pomander helps us connect with the grid structure of the earth, the energy lines of the earth, and find the resonances between our own heart and the earth.

Turquoise Pomander

The turquoise Pomander is the Aquarian Pomander, facilitating communication of New Aeon wisdom. This Pomander releases creativity, encourages communication from the heart, and eases the flow of inspirational, mass-media communication from one person to many, as in radio, movies, plays, and public speaking. It can alleviate stage fright and technophobia. It enhances communication with crystals and devas and facilitates our rapport with computers and silicon-based technology. Turquoise is supportive of all creative pursuits, such as writing, painting, and dancing.

Turquoise refers both to the process of individuation and to the unfolding of individual development that comes with the meditative process. It helps our development to be a creative one, encouraging us to be with ourselves and to disengage from unhealthy patterns and reactivity and instead become more familiar with how we are from moment to moment—to stop our pattern of replaying and reenacting dramas and conditioning that are not of our own individual nature.

Turquoise can help when we do not know how we feel, allowing us to express what lies in our heart. At the same time turquoise protects us from an excessive experience of vulnerability as we express love and caring. It can assist in counseling. Turquoise encourages independence and the ability to take responsibility for our feelings and actions and yet, at the same time, to creatively be in touch with the collective archetypal world in our mental body.

Sapphire Blue Pomander

The sapphire blue and royal blue Pomanders support the highest communication of love, fostering inspiration, devotion, and trust of our inner guidance. They help us find spirit in the worldly and deepen our experience of inner peace so that we can be clearer, expending less energy in our own preoccupations. Energy is freed for us to do what we need to do.

Blue represents the mother of us all as well as the father principle. The blue Pomanders guide us to alignment with the Divine plan, providing protection for the communication that comes through us, rather than from us.

Transition is made through the blue energy. Blue is the journey backward and forward from death to life to death. For those suffering from terminal illness, it can bring calm, peace, and tranquility. Both the sapphire blue and royal blue Pomanders will bring peace to the transition and will bring energy to support the return to life. They can be helpful for those working with death and dying or rebirthing and midwifery. The sapphire Pomander is particularly appropriate during transitions.

The sapphire blue Pomander nourishes our meditation, protecting and bringing peace. It can be helpful for particularly sensitive people or for those who have difficulty with authority or are in authoritative roles. It helps us remember our natural inner authority, so as to not be intimidated by situations in which authority exists externally.

The sapphire blue Pomander eases the accommodation of role reversals in families, for example, if the father has the responsibility of nurturing the children and the mother is the breadwinner. For a hyperactive child, the sapphire Pomander offers soothing. Sapphire also relates to the throat, providing support for those who speak publicly or teach groups.

Royal Blue Pomander

The royal blue Pomander, relating to the brow and the third eye, fosters the development of the higher mind functions such as clairvoyance and telepathy. It provides protection when we are receiving inspiration. The more informed the communication, the more we need protection: as increased light is generated, the dark will become more interested. Royal blue helps utopian idealists who like to build castles in the air stay grounded. When we are deeply depressed, royal blue, by taking us out of our interior isolation, opens us to our imagination. By amplifying our perception of all of our senses, the royal blue Pomander can enhance our pleasure in art and music and our enjoyment of life.

When we are having difficulties in relationships, royal blue helps us relate. For those already working with sound,

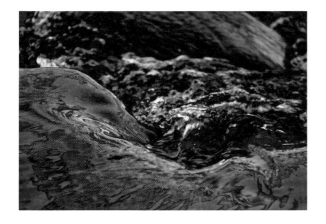

chanting, mantras, and toning, royal blue can increase sensitivity.

Note: Both the sapphire and royal blue Pomanders have a strong peppermint content. Please, if you are using a homeopathic treatment, take care when using the blue Pomanders. The peppermint in the Pomanders can neutralize a homeopathic remedy.

Violet Pomander

The violet Pomander opens our perception and awareness of the higher realms, helping us connect with our mission and purpose. We can become more conscious of why we are here and what we are for; we can witness the way we do what we do, and the way we are to do what we are for, while we are incarnate. The violet Pomander delicately helps us know how we may serve and sacrifice in the context of peace. It gives accessibility to the akashic chronicles.

Violet calms situations, balancing the flow between the two hemispheres of our brain. It supports dynamic relating, and it is beautiful to use before meditation. It also supports transformation and making things whole.

Deep Magenta Pomander

The deep magenta Pomander can be helpful when we have given all our energy to others and now need to receive caring for ourselves. It gently provides the energy we need, bringing love from above into the auric field. This Pomander leads us to self-knowledge, to discovering our task and life purpose. Combining the energies of the primary red and the secondary violet, the tertiary magenta Pomander is energizing and soothing at the same time. It assists us in staying focused, investing in the right account within ourselves. As we put care into the little things in life, big events are more likely to take care of themselves. The deep magenta Pomander can be useful when a nuclear

family breaks up. It gives us energy to clear up and bring order to the details in our life that tend to be put aside for more important, or seemingly more important, things. With this Pomander we may more gracefully do everyday tasks with love.

During times when it is difficult to attend to details, deep magenta is supportive, offering us the caring that helps us attend to everything we are doing. The deep magenta Pomander harmonizes our intellect and our instinct, opening us to an increased quality of consciousness and understanding. It builds our energy and is supportive and very protective after depression. With this Pomander, we can more easily tune into nature and focus in deep meditative states.

This Pomander stabilizes bodywork on particular reflex or energy points, such as in acupuncture and reflexology. It seals energies at the completion of a session. Applying several drops to the points that have been worked can help the energies to continue to flow longer.

Pink Pomander

The pink Pomander surrounds us in a loving atmosphere, helping us to bring out our best, to love ourselves the way we are and not the way we would prefer to be. It nurtures our emotional well-being by bringing warmth. Pink represents the basic ground upon which we all function. Caring makes everything possible. Pink is a specific for harmonizing group energies and for neutralizing aggression. The Pomander is appropriate to use at the beginning of any group work or meeting to foster more harmonious interaction and mutual respect.

Pink protects us when we have opened to love and true love, helping us to believe that we are loveable, and

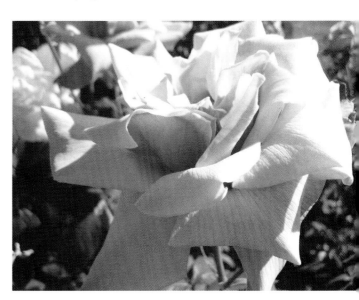

Above: Autumn sky reflected in swift river along Kangamangus Highway in New Hampshire.
Right: Pink rose with light catching it on the banks of the River Derwent in Tasmania.

helping us to sustain a flow of love to others without moving into irritability and reactivity.

Pink is harmonious with, supports, and amplifies the energies of rose quartz, a significant crystal energy in the Equilibrium bottles.

Original White Pomander

The first Pomander that Vicky made is called the original white Pomander. It appears in a white bottle because white contains all the colors of the rainbow, and it has all forty-nine herbs in equal proportions. It has a medicinal smell, predominating from the oils of cajeput and bay.

The principal crystal energies in the white Pomander are clear quartz crystal, selenite, and apophyllite. As it is harmonious with quartz, this Pomander is good for cleansing, clearing, and reprogramming quartz.

The white Pomander's function is to clear, balance, and protect the whole electromagnetic field and all the chakras. It is useful for everyday application. It can be detoxifying, restorative, and refreshing when we find ourselves in a polluted environment, whether emotionally, mentally, or physically, or when unhelpful odors leave us feeling unclean. It provides an energetic cleansing that makes it possible to bring in the light and sustain other energies that would otherwise be adversely affected by the contaminated environment.

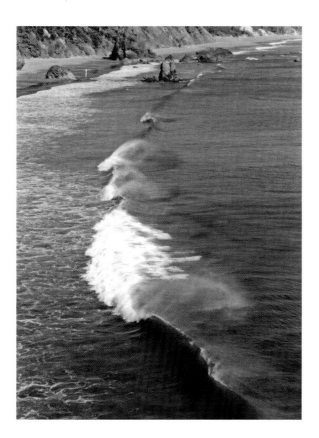

How to Select and Apply a Pomander

Most frequently, the color in the base fraction of the first bottle selected suggests the color of the Pomander that will be most useful. There are times when other Pomanders may seem to be needed or appropriate and that is fine. Often our response to the aroma of the Pomander will also be indicative of which one we are needing.

To apply a Pomander place three drops in the palm of your left hand and rub both your palms together. Reach your hands above your head, imagining that you are offering the Pomander to the world, out of the left hand, around the world, and back into your right hand. Gently offer the energies of the Pomander through your energy field, beginning at your crown and moving through every chakra and energy station. Rest for a while at your heart, offering caring to all that concerns you, and then move through the solar plexus to the root. Offer the energies to the earth, imagining the energies of the Pomander connecting with your earth star and penetrating deeply into the layers of the earth. Then, with your palms together, bring your hands up to your face and allow yourself to take three deep breaths of the aroma into your own body.

The Quintessences

Like Pomanders, Quintessences are preparations including herbs in an ethanol base. They work specifically with the astral fields beyond the etheric body. The etheric body could be seen to relate to the emotional body and the astral fields to the upper and lower mental bodies; energies move through the emotions to the mental realms, or through the etheric to the astral. The astral fields contain the possibility of invocation of the Ray Masters. The Quintessences facilitate the flow of energy from the inner planes and invoke the most positive energies of the color ray to which they are connected. Reciprocally, from deep within us, there is invoked into manifestation our own related qualities. We may more easily recognize and accept our own inner beauty. Let us examine this concept from an Aura-Soma point of view.

Each Quintessence (with the exception of Holy Grail and Solar Logos) is paired with one of the Equilibrium bottles in the Master Set (B50 through B64); both the bottle and the Quintessence bear the name of a Master. When the Equilibrium bottles of the Master Set were born, Vicky said that each had a personification. With further inquiry, she brought forth, in many instances, names similar to those used by the early Theosophists Madame Blavatsky, Annie Besant, and J. G. Senet. Vicky was surprised to learn that the names she attributed to these pale color combinations were names

Wave cresting with rainbow at Nookie Point on the Oregon coast.

Theosophists had earlier attributed to the Masters. Masters are highly evolved beings who at one time or another, sometimes multiple times, have been incarnated. Partially from gratitude for what they received from their earthly experience, Masters have committed to help humanity.

One of the understandings within Judaism that was close to Vicky's heart was the possibility that we can have a direct relationship with God, the Father, the Creator of all that is. This direct relationship precludes intermediaries between humans and God. At the same time, she was comfortable with the concept of Masters. She explained that each human being has a direct line, a direct connection, a golden cord to the source of all that is. That cord can never be broken. Any prayers, meditations, and questions from a guileless heart would be received and noted within the consciousness of all that is. From there we may receive a response. Just as the power from a power station needs to be transformed before it reaches the socket in front of a toaster, so this response to us may need to be transformed. The Masters are an expression of the transformers between us and the source, to help ensure that we do not end up as burnt toast.

A request from us goes to the source. Out of compassion, there is a step down in the energy before we receive the answer. The hierarchy of the Masters, at an energetic level, is that step down.

Vicky perceived that all the Masters of the hierarchy are cooperative at this point in time in a way that they have never before been. By using any of the Quintessences, we can be in touch with the whole of the hierarchy. In a sense we cannot use the wrong Quintessence, because each Quintessence is a point of shared accessibility. We can conceptualize this as a central telephone exchange: a call comes for the specific Master whose number has been dialed. The Master knows whether the phone needs to be answered or not; also, if that Master is unavailable or not the appropriate Master for that call, then instantly the appropriate Master is available to answer, should an answer be required.

Each of the Master bottles also has the potential to help us get in touch with our inner master. The concept of the master within is discussed on page 55. It is concerned with going to great depth within our self, through the mental emotional layers. This process is informed by the inner teacher, which we can contact through the incarnational star within the golden area of the self. As a consequence of the unfolding of the turquoise process of individuation, as these processes become deeper and the turquoise becomes lighter, we reach the teacher's teacher, what could be called the master within.

At this point of contact is a change of being: the master within is in touch with our inner wisdom. Metanoia, a transformative violet process in which we let go of conditioned patterns of identification, our belief systems, and our ideals and completely reevaluate, has happened. Enhanced synchronicity occurs. The appropriateness of all that is appears unquestionable.

The Individual Quintessences

In this section, each Quintessence is described. The Quintessence's corresponding Equilibrium bottle in the Master Set is also noted along with its color, the color it "aligns" with, and a keynote.

In addition to their association with the Master bottles, the Quintessences are also associated with the pastel bottles such as B44, B66, and B74. If all of the fractions within our selection of four Equilibrium bottles are hues, provided we have not chosen a bottle in the Master Set, then the Quintessence that aligns with the color of the base fraction of the first bottle will be most helpful. However, if there is a Master bottle, or a pale or tint fraction in one of the bottle choices, then another Quintessence takes precedence. The Quintessence associated with a Master bottle closest to the here and now position, the third position, is most appropriate. This can be an indication that the soul is particularly aligned with the focus of a particular Master at this time, or that this Master is especially available and supportive now. If there is not a Master bottle in the third position, then the Quintessence that aligns with a Master in the fourth position is the next most appropriate, followed by the second and then the first positions. When there is a pale color in both the upper and lower fractions, the Quintessence that goes with the lower fraction should be considered first as it helps that which is subconscious become conscious. The aroma of the Quintessence and our response to that can also be indicative of the most appropriate Quintessence.

El Morya
Pairs with: B50
Color: Pale blue
Aligns with: Blue
Keynote: Thy will be done through me.
El Morya offers the finest layer of protection, allowing us to release the imposition of the "little" will (our personal will) so that we may actualize our destiny in alignment with the higher will. This Quintessence increases communication through the astral and etheric bodies, invoking peace: I will that Thy will be done through me from heaven to earth. It helps us to come to that point of allowing divine will to be done.

In calming the subtle bodies and bringing peace, El Morya makes information accessible to our consciousness in the astral body. As we become more peaceful, energy is released.

El Morya inspires creative communication and stimulates our creative abilities. It can be helpful if we have always had problems with the Mother/Father archetypes, or if we have difficulty developing these models within ourselves. It may help us find greater clarity in situations with our parents. El Morya offers the nurturing of the Mother and the wisdom of the Father. It stimulates a feeling of being at one with all things. Thus it is an antidote to feelings of loneliness: we recognize that we are all one, rather than each alone. El Morya offers grace, ease, and a strengthening of our connection with divine will, which enables us to align our self with our purpose.

Kuthumi

Pairs with: B51
Color: Pale yellow
Aligns with: Yellow
Keynote: Love and wisdom. A nurturing of angelic-human-devic communication.

The word *kuthumi* sounds like "Come to me," and it is considered to be an invocation of the positive energies of the future. This Quintessence points toward enlightened self-knowledge. It relates to the Maitreya Buddha, who looks after the future. Kuthumi is a member of the White Brotherhood, a group of beings who have become enlightened while on the earth plane and have committed to helping all human beings evolve in consciousness.

Kuthumi helps humans find their role between the angelic and the devic kingdoms, so that we may understand the divine plan through our intuition from the angelic realms and then ground it on earth. Saint Francis exemplified this process and is one of the principal associations with the Kuthumi energy.

Kuthumi supports us, as humans, to be a communication link between the angelic kingdom and the devic kingdom of minerals and plants, of the elements of fire, water, air, and earth. Devas belong to the earth. At this time the devas are in chaos as a result of a lack of caring and attention from humans. Kuthumi helps us attune to plants and connect with devas, angels, fairies, and other beings especially when we are engaged in gardening, meditation, and healing work. This offers us the opportunity to be in the right position in relation to the hierarchy and order of creation.

Kuthumi represents the intensification of our little will to the point that negative self-consciousness is released and positive self-awareness blossoms. It amplifies and supports our ability to see through processes and to understand backgrounds and connections. Kuthumi helps us communicate with our familiars, or personal symbols.

Often familiars are animals, such as the witch's black cat, an eagle, or a unicorn. We may become more receptive to the energy of these animals.

Kuthumi brings luck into our life by drawing in positive qualities. It relates to Pythagoras, helping us understand science and numbers. It invokes those energies into the auric sphere, giving us a different understanding of forms and energies. It also brings wisdom and unconditional love.

Lady Nada

Pairs with: B52
Color: Pale pink
Aligns with: Royal blue and pink
Keynote: Unconditional love.

Lady Nada relates to the sixth energy center, the third eye, and is depicted as two petals. *Nada* in Sanskrit means the sacred sound, the inner sound, or the sacred note *om*. Nad Yoga is the yoga of attunement to the voice of the silence. Lady Nada helps us to hear and to be heard, thereby improving our capacity to relate. For those working with sound, Lady Nada links music and our voice, fostering our integration of light and helping us to better comprehend the intermingling of light and sound in the auric sphere.

Lady Nada supports healing with love by helping us to let go of negativity at a deep level. As we allow the negative aspects of our personality to be digested by the spark of divinity within us, we may experience a kinder response from the universe. Our thoughts about ourselves create our reality. Lady Nada is the most mitigating and soothing of the Quintessences, reducing aggression within and around us. When we profoundly accept ourselves—when, with the caring of the pale pink, we dissolve whatever we feel resistance to, both internally and externally—then there is no resistance to react to us.

Lady Nada brings the pure love of the Divine Mother, the highest vibration of unconditional love. We may have a personal encounter with our truth. Truth becomes the living truth. Divine wisdom comes from acceptance of this experience of truth.

Lady Nada helps change negative energies to positive ones in all respects. It cleanses the auric atmosphere and environment of negative vibrational states, bringing in a nurturing love and transmuting negative energy to positive. It clears aggression from our auric sphere, subsequently protecting us and thereby changing the behavior of the aggressor. It also can restore a flow in communication that has been blocked or impeded.

Lady Nada connects to the moon and its function of removing negative energy from Earth. The Quintessence can be of help if we find that the rhythm of the moon negatively affects us. It will enhance meditations undertaken during the full moon.

Hilarion

Pairs with: B53

Color: Pale green

Aligns with: Pale green and emerald green

Keynote: A space for the new. The Way, the Truth, and the Life.

The Way means that, with increased self-knowledge, our direction, our own way becomes clearer. The Truth of the green is an expression of our own truth. The Life reminds us that as we become more conscious, more light-filled, it is important that we manifest our own facet of the light in our life.

Hilarion helps us create inner space, whereby we are able to know our self better. It allows us to find the peace and space we need to make decisions. Hilarion also clears space, affording us an opportunity to step into the present anew, as we release outdated identifications. This Quintessence encourages the higher feeling aspect of our heart. If we let go of all that we have felt in the past, we can develop a new understanding. In a time of stress, Hilarion offers stillness in which we may find a clarity of direction.

As we come to understand the world with both our thinking and our feelings, Hilarion opens the door to our own wisdom and truth. Then a true integration of the self becomes possible.

Hilarion may clear and protect us against environmental pollutants as well as inner and outer deception. Hilarion's focus on truth allows us to refresh aspects of our being that we are not usually able to reach with other Quintessences. Hilarion gives us the opportunity to truly understand our light-body. It is significant among the Quintessences because, being connected to the Master bottle B53, it is also related to B8, Anubis, Yellow/Blue, both by number (5 + 3 = 8) and by color (yellow + blue = green). This connects it to the development of the light-body, or the lightness of our being, through the system of Aura-Soma. Anubis as guardian of the threshold would, along with the forty-two assessor gods of Egypt, weigh the heart of the deceased against a feather. If we live the truth of our heart, if we do what we love to do, we will be filled with lightness. Our hearts will be light. The feathers of the wings of our light-body will remain intact.

Serapis Bey

Pairs with: B54

Color: Clear

Aligns with: Clear

Keynote: Purification and new beginnings.

Serapis Bey offers karmic absolution, an opportunity to perceive our karma in a new light, not as a burden, but as a way to healing. Serapis Bey is the light itself. As discussed on page 22, the color clear (light) represents suffering and the understanding of suffering. When we deeply dis-identify with our self, we gain more understanding of the light. For example, after his enlightenment more than two thousand years ago, the Buddha's first statements were about the causes and understanding of suffering. When we shine light on a subject, we may see that it is not what we thought. Serapis Bey releases us from past karmic seeds by absolution of our subtle bodies, shining light on past experiences so that we may be more illuminated in the present. This Quintessence gives a depth of understanding into conflict, pain, and all suffering.

Serapis Bey is particularly useful for therapists, who can use it to cleanse the space between sessions and to protect, harmonize, and seal the client's aura so that he or she may more easily integrate the experience. It is good for detoxifying and balancing on all levels. It is best to use pink with Serapis Bey. The compassion, caring, and self-acceptance offered by pink, as in the pink Pomander or the Lady Nada Quintessence, facilitate comfort with the light of Serapis Bey.

This Quintessence is especially useful when we are working with quartz crystals, which are the keys to the mineral kingdom. With Serapis Bey, we can enter the inner dimensions of crystals and energetically cleanse them. Serapis Bey can also be helpful when we are beginning something new.

The Christ

Pairs with: B55

Color: Red

Aligns with: Red

Keynote: Reenergizing, protection, and caring.

The deep red of the Christ offers sacrificial love with a new degree of caring and loving. Light shining through red turns it into pink, the pink of unconditional love. Lady Nada, with the highest vibration of unconditional love, is the consort of the Christ.

We may each have a personal experience of the Christ by allowing this consciousness to touch us. The Christ consciousness is not specifically connected to the historical figure who lived two thousand years ago. Here we refer to a possibility Rudolf Steiner thought would be significant as we move from the twentieth to the twenty-first century: that many individuals would have a personal experience of the Christ energy in their auric sphere. It could be described as the Christ consciousness in the Buddha body. Any person, whether Christian, Buddhist, Hindu, tribal, agnostic, atheist, and so on, could achieve this development.

The Christ Quintessence brings an understanding

of our own purpose in life and clarifies our relationship to the earth. It helps us take responsibility for grounding our light, for ourselves, on earth. We may make personal inner connections with the Source. The Christ is the awakened I Am: truth expressed through one, the word made flesh, the Logos. The Christ Quintessence encourages our awakening as kundalini energy arises from the root chakra, the red energy center, and moves toward our crown. This Quintessence helps us know what we are for and what we want to communicate. It is of support for talking and writing, for manifestation through words.

The Christ Quintessence supports the emancipation of women and helps balance the male and female energies within each of us. It is useful in polarity therapy. It offers remembrances of Christmas energies and aromas, of the cedars of Lebanon, and of ancient embalming fluids.

Saint Germain

Pairs with: B56
Color: Pale violet
Aligns with: Violet
Keynote: Healing, meditation, and transformation.
Saint Germain offers the lilac flame of transmutation (see chapter 5, note 44-a). It is a catalyst to the transformation of negative energies into positive ones. It helps us transform our self into a catalyst and transformer, able to be a healing force in any situation. This Quintessence vibrates with the declarations of the French Revolution: liberty, equality, and fraternity (and in this case sisterhood as well). It invokes high energies to bring well-being to all our major energy centers and balance to the male/female aspects within our self.

Saint Germain has a calming effect on the etheric, astral, and electromagnetic fields. It helps us to detach, to dis-identify, to step outside of our self. We may allow energies to come through us, without becoming too involved with them. We may respond rather than react. When we are calm and impartial, the best can come through us. At the same time Saint Germain brings forth all the actors—all our qualities—onto the stage of our life. It allows the energies coming from the future to permeate the present. With the possibility of dis-identification, we may experience the positive and more difficult consequences of invisibility. Humility is a positive aspect; however, being reluctant to stand in our own personal power and authority is a negative aspect. Saint Germain helps us address these issues and bring a transmutative capability into each moment.

Through the energy of transmutation, Saint Germain helps us purify issues related to the root chakra, such as those to do with survival, security, health, and finances. Through its encouragement of detachment, Saint Germain is useful for therapists doing hands-on work, encouraging them to allow healing energy to come through them to their client. The Quintessence also can clear lingering emotional problems.

Saint Germain encourages healthy breathing. When we fully let go of our breath and breathe out, then new life, as a new breath, can come in fully. As we more completely let go, we are more free to be reborn in the moment. As the amethyst helps return things to their natural state, this Quintessence helps us to return to our natural state. This Quintessence is of help in rebirthing and regression work. It helps us change our energy, such that our anxiety or sense of overstimulation can be transformed into spiritual energy. It also offers the keys to higher knowledge, an opportunity to touch mind upon mind.

Pallas Athena and Aeolus

Pairs with: B57
Color: Pale magenta
Aligns with: Magenta
Keynote: Creative expression of love and beauty.
Pallas Athena and Aeolus offers the love of, and awakening to, beauty, a higher truth. This Quintessence makes heaven and earth available to all. It is helpful for dream work, supporting us in dreaming more consciously, dreaming things the way we would like them to be. Pallas Athena and Aeolus helps us remember the content of our dreams, so that we can draw inspiration from them and decode them by gaining insight into our own dream symbolism. Both in our dream life and in our wakefulness, Pallas Athena and Aeolus helps reveal that which is usually hidden that we would do well to release, helping us to dream dreams, to see visions, and to create, whether through pen, paint, music, or dance.

A Quintessence on the magenta ray, Pallas Athena and Aeolus reminds us to use our energy caringly and to practice using appropriate energy for the small things. If we do not like how our life is, if we would like to overcome old patterns, we can choose to change the way we use our energy. Then the energy—the attitude and caring—that we give to the little things in life will be there for us when we need it for more substantial moments.

Pallas Athena and Aeolus helps us connect with shamanistic traditions, particularly those carrying ancient wisdom and concerning our relationship to the earth. Pallas Athena and Aeolus relate to North American Indian traditions, to the Aboriginal song of the earth, and to the gods and goddesses of ancient Greece and Rome. Pallas Athena was chosen as the patron of Athens for her gift of the olive tree. Aeolus, ruler of the winds, offered a safe journey and helpful winds to Odysseus on his travels.

Pallas Athena and Aeolus also helps us find our right livelihood, so that we can be in harmony with our world. This

Quintessence helps us in our journey toward our self, toward our own awakening. By following our true path we will come to our right livelihood, a pertinent responsibility on the path of individuation. Part of awakening, of individuating, has to do with the material side of life, understanding our material, earthly concerns. Pallas Athena and Aeolus helps us both to find what it is that we are to do, what indeed is our right livelihood, and also encourages a prosperity consciousness, or an understanding that we have what we need.

Orion and Angelica

Pairs with: B58
Color: Pink
Aligns with: Pink
Keynote: Fresh beginnings and endings.

Orion and Angelica are two great angels who open and close each day: Orion, with the sacred blue of space, brings in the night and draws the sun across the sky (see note 58-a). Angelica, with the sacred pink of cosmic love, brings the dawn. Angelica gathers impurities in us and on the earth and deeply clears negativity.

The Quintessence Orion and Angelica helps us tune in to synchronicity, so that we can be in the right place at the right time. It also has a journeying energy, useful for all travelers as we move through time and space, and especially for air travelers. It can help us avoid jet lag by aligning all our subtle bodies, so that they all arrive at our destination with our physical body at the same time that the plane lands. (For this purpose, apply Orion and Angelica to the wrists before the plane takes off, at the crossing of each time zone, and after landing.) This Quintessence also brings light into our astral body.

Orion and Angelica helps with the beginning and ending of projects. When we are having difficulty taking responsibility for the light that we carry, we may find that we dislike the smell of this Quintessence. It can be useful when we are doing earth healing work and to alleviate geopathic stress.

Lady Portia

Pairs with: B59
Color: Gold
Aligns with: Gold, yellow
Keynote: "Judge not lest ye be judged"; clear seeing brings right action.

Having the discernment and discrimination to see our self, others, and specific situations in a just and balanced manner is a great gift. Clear seeing enables us to grow in consciousness, to know the right course of action, and to formulate accurate thoughts. Clear seeing may also bring a tendency to be self-judgmental and self-critical or an urge to criticize or judge others. When we are hard on ourselves, we invite criticism from others. We can learn to develop compassion. Being merciful with ourselves is a measure of compassion. Even the most subtle ways in which we may judge ourselves may interfere with our development. Mercy and love with true clarity are exemplified through this Quintessence. Lady Portia can help us develop a balance of discernment (and its appropriate expression) and compassion.

This Quintessence's associated Master bottle, B59, is a more intense version of B22, Yellow/Pink, the Rebirther's bottle. With this connection, the Quintessence offers the energies to support letting go and relinquishing control. It helps with rebirthing therapy and with overcoming our birth trauma. It helps us release fears. If we are not centered within our self, Lady Portia can help us restore a sense of balance. If we find that we are working constantly without a break, Lady Portia can help us be more merciful with our self. It encourages self-recognition. Lady Portia eliminates negative vibrations, quickly clearing the environment and bringing in light. This Quintessence also helps us express our thoughts clearly, informed by discriminative wisdom. Through gold, Lady Portia links with the central sun of our being, the solar plexus.

Lao Tsu and Kwan Yin

Pairs with: B60
Color: Pale orange
Aligns with: Orange
Keynote: Compassion; release from the past.

Lao Tsu, a master alchemist, offers the ability to transmute and transform energies. Kwan Yin is the goddess of compassion and mercy. This Quintessence facilitates regression work, helping us bring forth information from past lives. With the compassion of Kwan Yin, we can understand, accept, and appreciate our past experiences. We then may feel a deep peace. This Quintessence also releases our memories of ancient Chinese wisdom.

With the Lao Tsu and Kwan Yin Quintessence we may understand what lies behind a disease. It brings to the forefront of our consciousness the most cooperative, merciful, and communicative aspects of our self. We may undo a problem and find the gift that exists within it. Often when we change our attitudes and our thinking, we will change tendencies and circumstances in our life. This Quintessence helps us release patterns of tension in our body, emotions, and mind. This improves the functioning of our energy centers. In turn we may experience a sense of compassion and of being nurtured.

Lao Tsu and Kwan Yin brings the healing flow of mercy and compassion from the Mother/Father God. If shocks were associated with any of our experiences in earlier incarnations, Lao Tsu can help us clear those shocks and experience an alchemical transmutation of the energy of the past situations. This Quintessence may be especially helpful in relieving shocks associated with sexuality. Also, when we have not been recognized for the value of our best effort, whether as a young person in school or as an adult in a similar situation, Lao Tsu and Kwan Yin can compassionately mitigate and transmute our shock and disappointment to something positive and life enhancing.

Sanat Kumara and Lady Venus Kumara

Pairs with: B61
Color: Pale coral
Aligns with: Coral
Keynote: To see into the depths of things; to bring an awareness of the divine into the everyday.
The Kumaras offer the Mother and Father principles at the highest level. They are currently responsible for the in-flowing of all the rays to the earth. They express the law "As above, so below." In other words, all that we experience is concurrently in the divine, the angelic kingdom, and the Source, as well as in the plant, mineral, and animal kingdoms.

As administrators of all the rays, the Kumaras can help us connect with any ray. Therefore, when you are unsure about which Quintessence to choose, use this one. This Quintessence helps us discover what lies at the root of a particular circumstance, whether emotional shock or abuse, problematic conditioning, a challenging genetic lineage, or anything else. It helps us find a positive female/ male role model within us. It also helps us redress imbalances with the left and right sides of our body, with the left and right sides of our brains, and with the universal Mother/ Father principles. At this time, the Kumaras are especially active in helping us build bridges between the spirit world and this one. As we are each a spark of divinity, the secrets of the universe are held within us. The Kumaras nurture our ability to be conscious of this spark, so that we may participate in the divine plan with increased awareness.

This Quintessence brings a new octave to the higher level of vibrations. If we dislike the smell of this Quintessence, we may be having difficulty letting go, perhaps of emotional shocks.

Maha Chohan

Pairs with: B62
Color: Pale turquoise
Aligns with: Turquoise
Keynote: To bring an awareness of what, from our feelings, we need to say.
Maha Chohan is the Greater Teacher, the only Master Being who has not incarnated. He is the teacher of the other Masters and was the lord of civilization in Lemuria, an ancient land whose people, among other attributes, focused on creativity through color and sound.

The Maha Chohan Quintessence helps us be in touch with our creativity and feel a sense of cooperation with the Creator and with the creative force within existence. It helps us reach our own inner teacher, so that we may hear what our inner master is communicating to us as we progress in our process of individuation. We may more easily hear the whisperings of our heart and release those feelings that we need to express. Through our inner teacher we find our personal connection to the master energy within the feeling side of our being. This opens the way to an appropriate access to the collective unconsciousness and to a feeling of communication and relationship with the angelic realms.

Maha Chohan enhances our inspiration when we are working with mass media or expressing ourselves through improvisation with music, dance, and theater. It is of help when we are giving an intuitive massage. This Quintessence may support the flow of communication when we have to speak impromptu.

Maha Chohan supports the expression of New Aeon wisdom and facilitates heartfelt connections between ourselves and others. It encourages an awareness of positive qualities for light workers and Rainbow Warriors, increasing the life of the feeling being. Being pale turquoise in color, Maha Chohan gives the aquamarine energies to the Aquarian aeon, the Atlantean resurgence, powerfully working in this long-awaited period of time to manifest the law of a new civilization of light-conscious ascending souls. Genetic-engineering experiments are now being done with animals and plants as they were in the distant past in Lemurian and Atlantean times. A remembrance of this genetic engineering and the potential for misuse of power exists in the memory banks of each of us. The Maha Chohan Quintessence helps us address these concerns about the abuse of power, particularly in relation to genetic engineering. It helps us resurrect pre-scientific knowledge and strengthen the link between spirit and mind.

Djwal Khul

Pairs with: B64
Color: Emerald green
Aligns with: Emerald green
Keynote: Seeking the Truth.
Djwal Khul is the Tibetan Master who helped Alice Bailey in her writings published by the Lucis Trust. Djwal Khul is the most ardent of the seekers, a seeker of truth for truth's sake. His Quintessence supports the search for truth beyond the subjective reflection of the seeker, as in the case of Narcissus, to an objective truth. Djwal Khul is the seeker of Truth and Purpose.

This Quintessence helps us find inner space and the correct balance between inner and outer space, so that we may have the room to find our own direction and the truth that is within our own heart. It offers an emerald protection for our heart. It stimulates green within each of the seven major energy centers, supporting us in creating balance and harmony in our subtle bodies. With Djwal Khul we may stay grounded while opening to our intuition, lest we be overpowered by the information we intuitively receive. If we feel very sad, it gives us the space to develop clarity and self-acceptance.

The seeker, Djwal Khul, helps us understand the rhythms, laws, and patterns of nature. This Quintessence helps us understand astrology and the esoteric. It is useful for those of us who know intuitively that we occupy space beyond the earth.

Holy Grail and Solar Logos

Color: Pale olive green
Aligns with: Olive green, pale olive green
Keynote: To be receptive and listen carefully.
The Holy Grail and Solar Logos Quintessence increases our capacity to be receptive and open and to allow communication to flow through us. Pale olive is a bridge from the solar plexus to the emerald of the heart. In all the aspects of our being, this Quintessence can help us be receptive to the unfolding of our creative feminine intuition. With its support, we may remember that whatever we seek is within us.

There is a relationship between Lady Nada, the Christ, and the Holy Grail and Solar Logos Quintessences. Lady Nada, with pale pink, is about self-acceptance. Lady Nada was considered to be a consort of the Christ. Clear/Red shakes to a color similar to Lady Nada, B52, and shares the same issues of self-acceptance. Acceptance is similar to the concept expressed by the word Kabbalah, "to receive." As we become more receptive, we are likely to find the grail cup within ourselves. The Holy Grail and Solar Logos Quintessence helps us discriminate what is true for ourselves, so that we may gain confidence in the voice of the Logos.

To Apply a Quintessence

Place three drops on your left wrist and gently rub your wrists together. Extend your arms above your head, offering the energies of the Quintessence to the world. At the same time, feel for a sense of contact with spirit. Then gently bring your hands down and cross your wrists over your crown. Continue to open and close your arms, crossing them over each energy center, as if you were folding the energies around you. When you come to your heart center, rest there for a few moments with your hands crossed at your wrists. Then continue on, drawing the energies through your lower energy centers and finally offering the Quintessence to the earth. Then move your hands in backward spirals, moving out from, and upward in front of, your body until you again give the energies away to the world. Finally, bring your palms together at your forehead and deeply inhale three times the aroma of the Quintessence into your body.

The Air Conditioners

Air Conditioners come in spray bottles. They are essentially Pomanders and Quintessences formulated at a strength to make them suitable for a room spray. These sprays condition the air around us, working on the atmosphere; they bring to the space the qualities of the particular Pomander or Quintessence they contain. Each Pomander and Quintessence has a corresponding Air Conditioner. Archangels Michael, Gabriel, Raphael, and Uriel also make their energy available through the Air Conditioners.

The ArchAngeloi

The ArchAngeloi are the most recent component of the Aura-Soma system. As spirits of fire in the spiritual hierarchy, they seem to have appeared at this point to help us step free of conditioned patterns and to stimulate dormant seeds significant for the unfolding of the higher plan on the earth. They, like other angels, are messengers of the divine, functioning as a high order of mediators between humans and the divine. ArchAngeloi particularly support the folk spirit of a country or a group, guiding and overlighting the land and those who are helping to bring forth the essence of that place. The ArchAngeloi work with us particularly during points of transition, giving guidance through the etheric body and helping to awaken us to our part in a greater plan.

They are of the appropriate intensity and vibration for our personal auric field. Spraying the liquid of the ArchAngeloi into your auric field invites the energies of the archangels into your aura.[8]

The Individual ArchAngeloi

Like the Quintessences, the ArchAngeloi are paired with specific Equilibrium bottles, in this case bottles B94 Archangel Michael, B95 Archangel Gabriel, B96 Archangel Raphael, B97 Archangel Uriel, B98 Archangel Sandalphon,

B99 Archangel Tzadkiel, B100 Archangel Metatron, and B101 Archangel Jophiel.

If you choose a bottle in the range of B94–B101, it is a specific indication of an ArchAngeloi that would be appropriate. Other ways to choose the ArchAngeloi include through the color relationships of our bottle selection and through the matrix sequence as discussed in the section on matrices and the tarot (see page 272). Certain archangel bottles appear more than others in the matrices. By examining which of these archangels are present in the matrices corresponding to your bottle selections, you can determine which ArchAngeloi will be most helpful. Our response to the aroma of the ArchAngeloi is another way to make a selection.

ArchAngeloi Essence Michael

The ArchAngeloi Michael essence can help us develop the qualities of trust and faith, so that we may release restrictive patterns of intense fears and anxieties. We may let go of habits of worrying and confusion and experience peacefulness and clarity. We may more easily open our hearts, becoming clearer about why we are here and what we are for. We may step more fully into our harmonious role in the unfolding greater plan.

ArchAngeloi Essence Gabriel

This essence may help us bring our potential, our path of destiny, into reality. As we release patterns of grief and longing, of sadness and anxiety, we may become conscious of a newfound hope and sense of freedom. We may become more conscious of a source of inspiration within our self that warmly and attentively emboldens us to live a life that is true to our nature.

ArchAngeloi Essence Raphael

This essence supports us in developing our intuitive perceptions so that we may experience a deep soothing peace and an awakening to our inner voice. As we detach from the outer sense doors (our five senses by which we perceive external reality) as we release patterns of critical perception and detach from involvement with distractive influences, we become more aware of our inner sensing and of insight fed in from above. Our attention may turn to thoughts of the good of all concerned, of our community, while at the same time we are also more at ease, in greater equilibrium, with the male/female energies within us. We may find that we are less inclined to hold back, analyze, and theorize, and more able to be an instrument of peace, expressing our quality of truth in relation to our community.

ArchAngeloi Essence Uriel

This essence, like Raphael, fosters an experience of deep inner peace and clear intuitive perceptions. We may become aware of our own habits and of patterns in the collective, of anxiety and confusion, which, when released, allow us to express our true, soul-inspired self in the world. This essence may help us to be more open and receptive to our perceptions, which will support us in expansively sharing our wisdom in a heartfelt way.

ArchAngeloi Essence Sandalphon

This essence may help inspire us to develop a profound capacity for compassion, an understanding of interdependence and the potential for cooperation in our hue-man family with the network of energy and life on and of Earth. As we, both in our personal lives and as participants in our greater communities, move away from reactions of conflict and competition, we can experience greater wholeness and an acceptance and appreciation of diversity. The transformation of long-held belief systems arises and esoteric knowledge that exists in our ancient memory banks may become more available.

ArchAngeloi Essence Tzadkiel

This essence helps us find a new understanding, experience, and expression of love. Barriers of reactivity and anger are dissolved with self-acceptance and caring toward others. Recent history has repressed empathetic, heartfelt leadership by the feminine. As we release bitterness and discouragement about this, we may find a new hope, a hope supported by this essence and by the Great White Brotherhood. Dissolving frustration, we may experience a rebirth of the possibilities of expressing peace and love. We may develop a new appreciation for the feminine, both externally within our culture, and internally in relationship to the female/male qualities within our self.

ArchAngeloi Essence Metatron

This essence contains the most intense light and also the depths of the dark—two aspects of the whole. ArchAngeloi Metatron can help us perceive, understand, and strengthen the totality of our qualities, talents, and potential. As we see clearly and are transparent with ourselves, we can come to understand who we are. As we look into our inner shadow, we can reclaim our projections and appreciate that what we had attributed to "the other" is a part of us, a reflection of self.

Through its numerical relationship with B10, this ArchAngeloi helps us to be aware of the wheel of life, the laws of nature, and cause and effect. As we express our light in the world, with the appropriateness and caring that arises

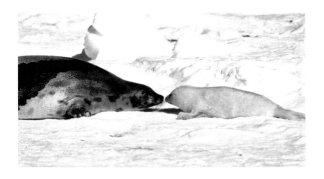

from within, we can know that there is a ripple effect from each of our thoughts and actions. We may find ourselves guided to the right place at the right time for the unfolding of our personal destiny and at the same time we may cooperate with Gaia's development and the stabilization of the planetary grid energy patterns.

ArchAngeloi Essence Jophiel

This essence may help us consciously experience a sense of peace, trust, and calm. As we develop greater faith in that possibility, we may feel a sense of spaciousness and new hope that allows us to release restrictive patterns of cynicism and self-blame. We may open our heart to love in a new way. We may appreciate who we are, joyfully allowing our self, our true aura, to be expressed in the world. We may feel led back to the Garden of Eden as existing, in a sense, in the

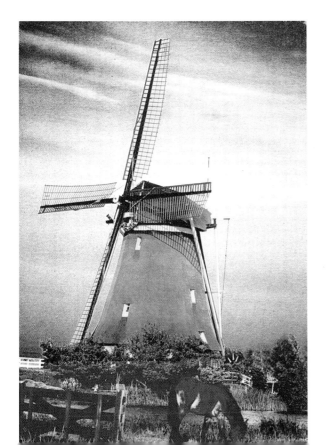

garden of our own heart. A sense of alienation, yearning, and exile seems to be part of the human condition. Perhaps as we feel a greater sense of harmony with our own self, an inner joining and union, our outer experience will reflect this. Coincident with our own individuation process, we may grow in the context of our community, being able to express qualities of openness and love. This may lead to an appreciation of diversity and an understanding and inclusion of each person's and each group's natural authority and value as we share this life on our home of Earth.

The Color Essences

Like the Pomanders, Color Essences relate to and represent the colors in the Aura-Soma range, and not specific bottles. The Color Essences carry the energetic qualities of each color. They form a contact between the mental and emotional subtle energy of the upper and lower astral fields and the electromagnetic field immediately around the physical body, in the area between those affected by Pomanders and Quintessences. They work specifically from the layer related to the Ananda Kanda (see page 19). The Color Essences have a centering quality that facilitates our connection to the earth, that helps us to be practical and to ground our full being in our intended creative endeavors.

Color Essences were developed to support the work of the Equilibrium bottles, helping us to integrate the energies of the plant, mineral, and color kingdoms. We can choose the color we wish to use based on the color of the Equilibrium bottle with which we're working, or we can make our choice based on the chakra to which we feel we would like to attune at the time. In addition to supporting the colors that we are already working with, Color Essences are also a way to experience colors that are not already in our color selection, if we feel a need for a particular color.

The Individual Color Essences

Red Color Essence

The red Color Essence offers energy, awareness, and passion. It strengthens and reinforces the auric field, helping us stay with our own energy rather that being overconcerned and overempathetic with others.

Ingredients include: Cherry, Copper Beech, Ruby, Petrified Wood, Iron

Coral Color Essence

The coral Color Essence is strengthening to the psyche, giving a grateful recognition of the value of community. Openness in times of stress encourages greater protection

Left: Harmony in the garden, Holland, symbolic of a return to the Garden of Eden.

and well-being. Coral offers an opportunity for cooperation, compromise, and interdependence on each others' unique gifts. It can balance all the chakras: with less fear, energy flows more smoothly and we may notice qualities we did not know we had. Coral facilitates group decision making.

Ingredients include: Strawberry, Mulberry, Desert Rose, Coral

Orange Color Essence

The orange Color Essence supports interdependence and interconnectedness in relationship, while helping us to maintain our own inner truth and worth. It offers deep insight leading to bliss.

Ingredients include: Physalis, Mandarin, Orange Selenite, Copper

Gold Color Essence

The gold Color Essence enhances our sense of connectedness, of being part of the greater whole. As we search for and realize our own inner worth, we find fulfillment.

Ingredients include: Primrose, Bamboo, Amber, Gold

Yellow Color Essence

The yellow Color Essence helps clarify our perception of boundaries. It can offer clarification in times of confusion. It offers the stillness of a broader view, rather than the overactivity of dualistic thinking.

Ingredients include: Daisy, Mahonia, Citrine, Pyrite

Olive Green Color Essence

Confidence in the still, small voice within the depth of our self stabilizes as we breathe into the golden area of our being. The light from there rises. The olive Color Essence smooths the passage of that light toward an opening of the heart.

Ingredients include: Red Cedar, Olive, Moldavite, Carbon

Green Color Essence

The green Color Essence supports the manifestation of love in concrete activity. It helps us give ourselves the time, space, and direction we need and likewise respect those needs in others.

Ingredients include: Russian Ivy, Oak, Emerald, Sulphur, Jade

Turquoise Color Essence

The turquoise Color Essence supports the communication of heartfelt experience. Insight, inner growth, and self-knowledge may arise as we express ourselves creatively in all aspects of life.

Ingredients include: Blue Flag, Poplar, Turquoise, Iodine

Blue Color Essence

The blue Color Essence provides peace and a nurturing energy that may also bring clarity. The color blue symbolizes the breath. The blue of the sky, the breathing in and out of the calm air, can give a sense of presence in the here and now.

Ingredients include: Borage, Walnut, Mulberry, Sapphire, Lava

Royal Blue Color Essence

The royal blue Color Essence is cleansing, centering, and calming. It can help us to recognize patterns and gain an overview of events.

Ingredients include: Forget-me-not, Fir, Lapis, Platinum

Violet Color Essence

The violet Color Essence offers well-being and service through greater understanding and new insights, as we begin to honor the mystery of existence in each moment.

Ingredients include: Pansy, Mistletoe, Amethyst, Cobalt

Magenta Color Essence

The magenta Color Essence encourages unconditional love, even in the little things.

Ingredients include: Lavatera, Blackthorn, Opalite, Clay

Pink Color Essence

The pink Color Essence stimulates our ability to receive love and to feel love. It diminishes fear and is helpful in situations of grief resulting from loss or abuse. Pink can help us to be more in touch with our feminine intuition.

Ingredients include: Pink Rose, Honeysuckle, Hawthorn, Rose Quartz, Calcium

White Color Essence

The white Color Essence is strongly cleansing and harmonizing on all levels, facilitating our capacity to see, feel, and sense ourselves anew, with more clarity and insight. It helps us recognize our gifts and what we have to offer, and it supports the bringing of light into any situation. In helping us to more accurately see the reflection of ourselves without judgment, it allows us to be with others more easily.

Ingredients include: Lily of the valley, Magnolia, Quartz, Moonstone, Silver

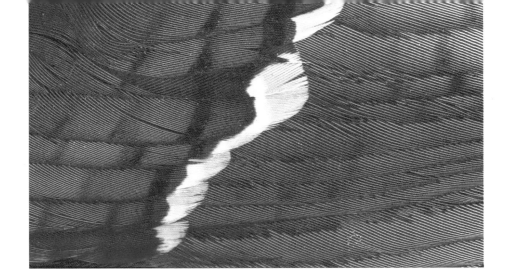

5

The Equilibrium
Color Combinations

*If the eye were not sunny, how could we perceive light? If God's own
strength lived not in us, how could we delight in Divine things?*

GOETHE

Understanding about the color combinations of the Equilibrium bottles is a two-way unfolding: it is a personal journey, and it also taps into universal consciousness and information. As we perceive our own color code, we embody our colors and are able to spread our wings. We can discard conditioned patterns that we have outgrown, recycling them as compost for the next stage of our development. We can awaken to the brilliant jewels that we are as a part of universal consciousness. The heart of the self reflects the heart and potential of the whole. Please enjoy yourself as you look through the following pages, and allow yourself the opportunity for a journey of self-exploration into the world of color.

How to Read the Following Pages

On the following pages each of the Equilibrium bottles is presented along with a good deal of information. This information about each color combination can be read as a beginning or an entry into understanding the individual bottle, and as an invitation for you, the reader, to begin to perceive intuitively what that color combination means on a personal basis. The information here represents a synthesis of experience with the Equilibrium range and includes the salient points that have emerged.

Each bottle has a number, a name, a keynote, and, for most, a tarot relationship. The story behind the name and, when helpful, the history of the bottle is included, along with information about the circumstances in which the color combination might be relevant and the characteristics or circumstances that may lead a person to be called to each particular combination. In addition, we

Above: The natural blending of color in nature shown here on the wing of a blue jay.

note guidelines for the use of the combinations; in general, they should be applied in a complete band about the body, in the locations noted for each bottle.

The Color Language

As you study the qualities of each bottle, we encourage you to read the description as a dialogue between the two fractions in each bottle, a description of the dynamic relationship between the two fractions, and a description of the synthesis of these upper and lower fractions. Even when the same color appears in the top and the bottom, a relationship exists between the conscious and the unconscious, subconscious, or collective mind.

We also suggest that you consider the qualities of the individual colors in the bottle and the qualities of the "shakes-to" color. In the interests of brevity, we have not duplicated the descriptions of each color's qualities in each bottle description. As you become familiar with the language of color, you will see that many of the descriptions are a dialogue reflecting how the two fractions interact and impact each other. This relationship develops as we explore the colors in a four-bottle sequence.

The Name of the Bottle

A teaching of the Western Magical Tradition is the significance of a name. To know the name of someone, the name of a flower, the name of an Equilibrium bottle, is to know that which is named more fully. A name is a part of the person or thing or system that it identifies and hence carries its energy. The process of naming the Equilibrium color combinations has been a part of the growing understanding of what they represent and of the energy they carry. As the names and the stories behind the names have unfolded, so the complexity of the meaning of the bottles has become clearer.

The name Equilibrium itself is of note. Equilibrium connotes a sense of movement rather than stasis, a living dynamic. The middle pillar of grace and will of the kabbalistic Tree of Life is called the "pillar of equilibrium," reconciling and balancing the dynamic tension and opposing energies of the pillar of force and pillar of form.

The names, as with the entire Aura-Soma system, have evolved as more is revealed and as people work with the system. In some cases, Equilibrium bottles have received new names, like middle names or nicknames. Each name presents us with an energy that gives the possibility of decoding another level of understanding for the bottle it identifies. Those readers who are familiar with numerology will recognize the concept that a person's

name and the numbers related to the letters in that name have a particular vibration or interpretation. Each name has meaning of itself, its own story, and also its specific energetics.

The names of the Equilibrium bottles may help us understand the multiplicity of the bottles and may also give us a clue as to their usefulness in the world. Some of the names will link us to the contents of the bottle; some will link us to other disciplines and teachings; some will be anecdotal, having arrived from the experiences of people working with Aura-Soma. In any case, when we know the name, we may know more of the qualities of the bottle it identifies. As you read through this section of the book, it is our hope that you will find that the name of each bottle is a door opening, a different way to come to know the color combination. Yet still we need acknowledge that within the whole offering from spirit that is in Aura-Soma, we are contacting but a small part of the energetics of the bottle. Going beyond the physical is the aura of the bottle, the jewel of light. Contained in that pure charge of auric light is a synergistic totality including all that we have mentioned here and more.

The "Shakes Together as" Color

The "shakes together as" color is the color that results when the upper fraction and lower fraction are mixed into a temporary emulsion. When we choose a bottle to use, the procedure is to shake it by holding it in the left hand in the pharmaceutical grip, i.e. with the thumb supporting the bottle, the middle finger on the top and the ring finger and pointer finger on either side. When the resulting color is close to the same color as another one of the bottles in the collection, we have noted that with a "shakes to" line.

By shaking the bottles we learn more about the energetics of the Equilibrium bottle through the language of color. Conceptually, when the two fractions are shaken together, that which is in the lower fraction, the soul ray, representing the subconscious or less obvious, is brought to the upper fraction, the personality ray, representing consciousness, and is expressed in the outer reality, in the world: our awareness may be directed toward that which was previously less conscious or hidden. At the same time, that which is conscious is offered to the subconscious: light and attention are brought into our innermost experiences. Through this process a greater degree of self-awareness and integration may develop.

The Tarot Card

The traditional tarot deck has seventy-eight cards, of which there are twenty-two major arcana and fifty-six minor arcana. The minor arcana are in turn divided into four suits: wands, swords, cups, and pentacles. The major arcana represent the archetypal steps for every soul going through a process of growth and development on this earth plane. The minor arcana depict the ups and downs, the events and struggles, along that path, related to the worlds of fire (inspiration), air (intellect), water (emotions), and earth (practical life).

Traditionally the suit of wands is linked with the fire world, the element of fire, with its qualities of warming, of sparking inspiration, enlightening, and of quick movement. The suit of swords depicts the air world, the world of the mind and intellect, of discernment and discriminative faculties. The suit of cups is linked with the water world, the emotions, receptive, flowing, cohering. The suit of pentacles represents the earth world, the world of practicality, of grounding and manifestation.

That each Equilibrium bottle would be paired with a tarot card was a concept given to Vicky and Mike. Each tarot card and its meaning sheds some light onto the meaning and significance of the color combination it is related to, and reciprocally, the Equilibrium bottle will give additional insight into the meaning and issues of a specific tarot card.

In Aura-Soma, each of the bottles numbered 0 through 99 is paired with, and has an ascribed relationship with, a tarot card, and an additional name assignation through that pairing. Bottles 0 through 21 are paired with the major arcana from the Fool to the World, while bottles 23 through 78 are paired with the minor arcana. Aura-Soma further augments the traditional tarot in that an additional twenty-two Equilibrium bottles are joined to the twenty-two major arcana. B22 is paired with the Fool, and bottles 79 through 99 are paired with the Magician through to the World. In Aura-Soma we call bottles 0 through 21 the outward journey or the first level of the tarot, and bottle 22 and bottles 79 through 99 are called the return journey or the second level of the tarot. Each of the major arcana represents a journey from one place to another, an encounter with an aspect of our self, or a struggle, or a skill to be developed. The outward journey leads toward understanding something, toward developing our self, growing our soul expression. It is in a sense a journey toward the self. The return journey describes how we may give that understanding back to the world, or how we can express who we are related to that quality in the world. It is a reminder that we understand more completely who we are as we share what we have to offer in the world. Such an evolutionary step, marked by this innovation to the traditional tarot, is of considerable significance.

Yet it is important not to think of the tarot outward and return journey as a linear progression. Every experience in life offers an opportunity to find out about ourselves and to grow. As we integrate those experiences, inevitably we are different, and that is who we are: our self, with our experiences as a part of our being. Often, when we can share from that experience, the real or more profound understanding of that learning takes place. Through expression we can discover what we actually know or who we are. The return journey speaks to this type of understanding. In fact, as indicated on the individual bottle pages, the two bottles that relate to each of the major arcana are to be viewed as a pair. If we are drawn to B0 or B22, the bottles related to the Fool, both bottles would be considered in our understanding of our color code. It is as if they are two sides of a coin, in that as we learn we teach, and as we teach we learn. In other words, the bottle most intimately related to B0 is B22, and vice versa, even though this relationship could be difficult to perceive through analysis of color alone. The concept of the return journey is in accord with the Aquarian aeon idea that, rather than gathering information and experience for our self, integration of learning happens more easily when we can share who we are and what we have found. The significance of the relationship between the Equilibrium bottle and the tarot card with its symbolism is explored both on the individual bottle pages and in the section on the matrix and the tarot.

Related Number

Bottles can also be connected to one another through a number relationship. The language of numbers is another essential part of the Aura-Soma system (see page 280). Although it is not possible to list all of those number relationships, some key ones are important to mention, such as the effects of zero. Adding a zero to a bottle number ($1 + 0 \rightarrow 10$) amplifies the meaning. Part of the meaning of B50, for example, would be an amplification of the lessons of B5: trust and faith in the greater will may develop from dealing successfully with trauma. This type of zero-amplification connection can be contemplated even when there is no apparent color relationship between bottles, although, curiously, B50 is an intensification of the blue color which in turn is the complement to B5's shake-to color. B1 has a relationship with B10 and with B100. Similarly, if the sum of the digits of the number of a bottle is equivalent to the sum of the digits of another bottle, say

B38 and B92, these bottles will also have a relationship. Additionally, the theme of the bottle of that sum, here B11 (3 + 8 = 11 and 9 + 2 = 11) will be part of the story of these two bottles. B101 would also be connected to B11. Here the zero, the Fool, makes a space for a different experience of the themes of B11.

The Keynote

The keynote synopsizes the interpretations of each Equilibrium bottle, giving an entry point for understanding and summation of the most relevant points about that bottle.

Related Bottles

Each bottle is related through color to other bottles. For each Equilibrium bottle we have listed other bottles to which it is connected through hue, tint, or through hidden or contained colors. They are by no means the only related bottles. The related bottles are included to assist the explorer of color in understanding color relationship and how the story of color unfolds in Aura-Soma. As you begin to go more thoroughly into the interweaving of the colors in one bottle, you will find that other bottles are implied or contained, and that the degree of intensity of the situation is suggested by the tint.

The significance of the closest tint and the closest hue categories is comprised of intensification, understanding, practicality, and grounding. A *hue* is a more saturated color; the *tint* is paler, lighter. In general, the hue of a color is considered to be more grounded. A tint is a color to which clear has been added. The clear is considered to intensify, or amplify, the meaning of the hue, or to be more ethereal. For example, B44, Lilac/Pale Blue, the Guardian Angel is the tint of B37, Violet/Blue, the Guardian Angel Comes to Earth. B44 is a lighter, less grounded version of B37. Consider also, for example, B5, Yellow/Red: The yellow and red in this bottle progressively intensify to the tint of red in B22, Yellow/Pink, to the tint of both red and yellow in B59, Pale Yellow/Pale Pink. The meanings of the bottles are progressively more intense also; the light of insight (the lightening color) represents increasing understanding about the qualities of yellow and red.

Several tints or hues could be included for some Equilibrium bottles. A master bottle is often listed as the closest tint of a particular color combination. Again, in the interest of conserving space, only some may be listed; others might be equally appropriate and relevant. As clear contains all the colors, white light refracts to all the colors, B54, Clear/Clear, is not listed unless particularly relevant; in turn, all of the other bottles could be shown with B54.

A related bottle may "contain" or have hidden within it another bottle. By this we are considering the colors that combine to compose the colors in the particular bottle. For example, B16 has two violet fractions. Violet is a secondary color composed of blue and red. Therefore B30, blue/red or B29, red/blue would both be hidden or contained in B16. Consulting the Color Rose on page 2 will help with this study.

We noted earlier (see page 14) that blue and yellow are the first two primaries. Therefore, B2, Blue/Blue, and B42, Yellow/Yellow, contain few bottles, although they themselves may be contained in, or be the components of, many of the Equilibrium bottles. In fact, since there are essentially only two primaries, blue and yellow (red is created from these two, as when the sun sets in the blue sky or rises in the morning), all colors emerge from a combination of these two colors. However, this is a complex concept, and for now, in order for the descriptions to be most comprehensible and insightful, we will not draw attention to the yellow or blue within each color combination. Only the most relevant or distinct related color combinations are shown for each particular bottle.

The "shakes to" color refers to the color that becomes visible when the upper and lower fraction are mixed into a temporary emulsion. If there is a bottle whose color is very close to that temporary color, that Equilibrium bottle is listed as the "shakes to" bottle. The significance of that color is part of perceiving the meaning of the Equilibrium bottle being studied.

Conceptually, when the two fractions are shaken together, that which is in the lower fraction, representing the subconscious or less obvious, is brought to consciousness and expressed in outer reality. Awareness may be directed toward that which was previously less conscious, more hidden. At the same time, that which is conscious is offered to the subconscious. Light and attention are brought into the innermost experiences, into the subconscious. A greater degree of self-awareness and integration may develop. Consider B26, orange/orange with B5. When B5's yellow and red are shaken, it becomes a temporary orange. B5 is contained, and hidden, in B26. As we work through our fears and survival issues we may heal our timeline. The Reverse category lists bottles that are exact or nearly exact upside-down versions of the bottle being studied. This reverse presentation has interpretive implications. The lower fraction may portray the soul's qualities, and the upper the inclinations and tendencies of the personality—how we present ourselves. If the colors are presented in a reverse way then, while we would have inherent in our color code the qualities of both the upper and lower fraction colors, what we might be conscious of and what we might be dealing with could be different. We could have different inner resources or outward concerns that would have to do with the same essence.

The related bottles are to be considered as a snapshot in time, being those that we thought were most relevant as of this writing. With growing understanding, with events in the world, with humanity's development, and as new bottles are born, other bottles may become more relevant. The related bottles are not necessarily definitive or prioritized but, from our understanding, are key to the study of color now.

The Images

The images on the following pages have been chosen for their relevance, beauty, synchronicity, and humor and to offer a global presence and perspective. Some are symbolic, some literal. In some cases they have a color relationship to the bottle with which they are featured. In some instances they were chosen for their significance in relation to the name of the bottle or for an esoteric or punlike relationship. Naturally, they were taken at different times in different regions and are of varying photographic quality. As the Equilibrium bottles are a doorway to a greater understanding of ourselves, please consider the pictures with pleasure, and as a doorway into a greater understanding of the bottles. These images are intended for readers to use as a springboard to stimulate their own creativity and joy in seeing. We hope that you read the text and look at the images with that in mind, and that you find yourself inspired. We also hope that the information, wisdom, and caring shared here stand the test of time. We hope that the following pages help us all to see the world differently and to enter the world of color and light in an enjoyable way.

During a class in the early years of Aura-Soma, a student came into class announcing that she had never seen the yellow of the center yellow lines on the highway as clearly as she did upon leaving class the afternoon before. Undoubtedly we all have that sort of experience when we begin attending to the world of color and light. Colors take on an added significance, as if the whole world were talking to us in a dance of color and image.

The search for images for this book has been an incredibly joyful and fun-filled experience, hampered only by the constrictions of space on the final pages. There were of course an infinite number of possible images to yearn for and choose from. Each of the pictures shown here has been a gift, offered in a spirit of generosity and kindness. We wish to give thanks and pay respect to the vast amount of energy and time donated to us for this photograph-collecting endeavor. At first we searched through our own archives of photographs and selected photos that were relevant. Gradually, willing friends and family began searching through their own photograph albums, looking for the blossoming star-gazer lily or the last trip to Athens. As these things go, friends began to introduce us to their friends and family who might have photographic resources.

Through this process, several amazing people stepped forward to offer pictures and help for this book. Three "chance" meetings on an airplane brought other images to these pages. The experience of collecting and working with the images to offer them here was an expression of co-creativity, synchronicity, and caring that epitomizes and carries the vision of the Aquarian aeon. It was through the grace of this spirit of cooperation that we obtained such a profusion and variety of images.

Sequences and Sets

Not only do the colors within each Equilibrium bottle find their most energetic meaning in relation to each other, but the bottles themselves exist in relationship with other bottles. In some cases we have come to see that a particular sequence of bottles holds special meaning; in others, we know that particular bottles can be grouped into a set for specific purposes or understanding. We describe frequently recognized sequences and sets in the Aura-Soma range below. Others may emerge as the system continues to reveal itself to us all.

The Rescue Set

The Rescue Set includes all of the bottles with deep magenta in the base (B0, B1, B78, B89, B90, B100, B102, and B103) as well as B3, B4, B11, B20, B26, and B87. Deep magenta is expressive of love in its essence, expressed through all things. It is the source. The Rescue Set represents the opportunity to connect with the integral part of the primary purpose of existence. Vicky's conception of the word *rescue* as an opportunity to "re-cue" or re-center ourselves is also a way to further understand the Rescue Set. The bottles in this set are helpful for whatever condition or circumstance we may find ourselves in.

The Chakra Set

The Chakra Set includes those Equilibrium combinations that correspond most directly to each chakra: B1, corresponding to the brow; B2, to the throat; B3, the heart; B4, the solar plexus; B5, the root; B20, the crown; and B26, the sacral.

It may be surprising to some that B5, yellow/red, is the designated chakra bottle for the root chakra (red). B6, red/red, would appear to be the most relevant for the root chakra. Instead, it is part of the Extended Chakra Set. When the chakra bottle does not exactly match in color, it is because at times when the chakra above, represented by yellow in the upper fraction, or orange in the "shakes to" color is opened, the chakra below can open. Therefore, most helpful for the root chakra would be the yellow/red, with the energies of both the sacral and the solar plexus chakra also available.

The Extended Chakra Set

The Extended Chakra Set includes the bottles of the Chakra Set in addition to those colors that were not part of the original Chakra Set but fill in the gaps in the range of the colors: B6, B10, B16, B41, B42, B43, B67, B87, B91, and B96. B96, a recently arrived archangel bottle, is the first time that royal blue has appeared in the base fraction of a bottle. Its appearance adds a component to the Chakra Set. The Extended Chakra Set may help us see the complexity that links the systems of the chakras together.

The Tantric Illumination Set

This set includes B6, B11, B23, B52, B55, B67, B69, B71, B77, B80, B81, B84, B89, B100, and B104. All of these Equilibrium bottles have pink, red, or magenta in their base. These bottles mirror the opportunity for finding a union of the male and female aspects within ourselves at a time when this opportunity is great. The prerequisite for experiencing such inner harmony and union is our ability to accept ourselves as we are, and each of these bottles relates to varied levels of self-acceptance. As a whole the set deals with the concept of how duality can come together toward unification, and the bottles can be of help in understanding that merging and unifying principle. Self-acceptance, harmony, and merging as an inner experience may be mirrored in an outer expression. This set draws attention to the possibility of tantra and the unified field—through this illumination may emerge.

New Aeon Child Set

This set includes B11, B12, B13, B14, B15, and B20. This set is described in some detail in Vicky Wall's book, *Aura-Soma*.

While this set is appropriate for a child, as its name indicates, it is also appropriate for the child within each of us.

B11 opens the door to a deeper understanding that, through the acceptance of our self, we may get in touch with our inner child. As we understand our essence and take responsibility for our thoughts and feelings, we may experience a lightness of our being.

With B12 the child, or inner child, begins to enter into a situation of deeper understanding. In essence, we begin to digest our personality. Through this initiatory process, our development of individuation unfolds. We assimilate aspects of our personality, of our being, and make use of them in the growth of our essence. As we become inwardly more peaceful with ourselves, we are more encouraged in this process and we can gain faith and trust in how it will occur.

B13 supports letting go of the identities within our personality so that something from a deeper level may be born. This letting go of identification with the past is a continuity of what takes places in the initiatory stage of B12.

In B14 we may get in touch with the intention behind coming into this incarnation. In the clear/gold of B14 is the potential of the beginning of a rebirth, where more consciousness is available to understand ourselves and our soul's purpose, to understand why we are here, what we are for, and how it is that we are to do what it is that we are here to do. The gold in the lower fraction helps us connect with the incarnational star in the golden area of the body. B14 reminds us to be with ourselves after the letting go in B13.

B15 shows the beginning of getting in touch with how we have put our energy and purpose into action. This action, which is sometimes called service, is a deeply transformative process in relation to the light of consciousness. B15 also indicates a preparedness to face the shadow, that which lies in the subconscious/unconscious mind, and to shed light on that within ourselves that has been difficult to accept.

B20 manifests a four-way energy connection. The child comes together with the angel that we are at the same time that the man and the woman within us come together. The male and female within are the collective lineages that come through the lineage of the mother and father, the left and right brain, and the left and right side of the body. After the letting go in B13, there is a realization of the process of unfolding in B14. The child is reborn in the context of the star. The four-way energy connection of B20 occurs if we encompass what is contained within B15. As we prepare to look into the shadow of our self, at what we have denied, there is an increased opportunity for the angel that we are to become connected to our self.

The Extended New Aeon Child Set

This set includes all of the bottles of the New Aeon Child Set plus B55, B77, B86, and B100. These extended bottles emerged later in the sequence of the Equilibrium range and include those with tertiary colors in the base fraction and clear in the upper fraction, showing a further refinement of the New Aeon Child Set. The extended set also includes the outward and return journey pairs to the bottles in the set, that is, B89, B90, B91, B92, B93, B98, and B8. These relationships will become more apparent as you read the descriptions for these individual bottles.

The Master Set

In Aura-Soma, the bottles revealed between B50 and B64 are called the Master Set. The concept of Masters is common to many spiritual traditions. It recognizes a culture of beings that may be available to communicate with us while we are in incarnation. The order in which the sequence of Masters has emerged, and the colors each are associated with, gives insight about the colors and also an understanding of the nature of each individual Master.

There is a Quintessence associated with each of the Master bottles, which expresses energies and qualities related to those of the Master bottle. The function of the Quintessences, as described in the section starting on page 38, is to be invocative; to help us invite into our auric sphere the qualities, teachings, and vibrations of a particular Master. The bottles confirm the relationship within the subtle fields of that color ray and awaken a cellular memory of the Master vibration. Through the incarnational star, the point of communication with our inner teacher, we may receive knowledge and energy. The inner teacher is able to be in touch with the master within our self, who in turn is in touch with that which goes beyond our self and is a culture of beings and of wisdom.

Each of the Master bottles has the potential to help us get in touch with our inner master. A traditional image of a horse and a carriage gives us an understanding of the inner master and its position in relation to ourselves. It is described as follows:

The carriage has two doors, four wheels, and a driver who sits on top. Inside is a person being taken from one place to another. The horse is pulling the carriage and has a direct mechanical connection to the carriage. The reins connect the horse to the driver, and the driver uses them to guide the horse.

The horse represents the emotional body. Currently in Western culture, the emotional body is not particularly educated after our early childhood. Even during those years many of the models we have for our emotional education are themselves not well schooled. Consequently much of the horse's education is impoverished. Little of the emotional food for the horse is of a positive nature. The higher emotions, such as compassion, are qualities that many of us do not really experience in our early childhood. Therefore most of us are pulled along in our life by an immature, undereducated horse that lacks appropriate internal discipline.

In this image, the driver represents the intellect. In Western society and actually in much of the world, the driver, the intellect, is overeducated. Great emphasis is placed above the shoulders, where we tend to think the mind exists. Usually our brain is considered to be the source of our thinking and being. Most of the conditioning and education we receive from our early schooling through to higher education tends to be directed toward our brain and the knowledge that is related to the intellect. The driver is overeducated. Often he does not know what to do with much of his information. He has information, but he may not have connected it to the rest of his being; it is disconnected, especially from the carriage, which is symbolic of the physical body.

Although the driver is sitting on the carriage, the relationship between the two tends to be separate. The driver's main responses to the world, to phenomena both internal and external, are limited to those arising from a mental understanding.

The undereducated horse and the overeducated driver are connected to each other by the reins. If the driver does not know where he is going and the horse is undereducated, the driver will have difficulty controlling the horse. The horse does not intuitively understand what the driver really wants. Equally, the driver is not able to clearly express his wishes because he is not fully in touch with his emotions, with the horse. Although the driver and the horse are indeed connected by the reins, that linkage may not be effective: perhaps the reins are too limp or too tight. The thinking and feeling aspects of ourselves are not well integrated.

As mentioned, the horse has a mechanical connection to the carriage. This represents a direct connection

The color rays.

between the horse, or the feeling and emotional body, and the way we are in our physicality. The four wheels could represent the four elements of the physical base (the elements of fire, air, water, and earth) that we experience through our five physical senses. The condition of the carriage is an expression of how we look after our body. Some carriages have painted exteriors, some are a bit shabby, some are in different states of disrepair, and some are tidied and well maintained. There are many disciplines, such as exercise and breathing, that we can undertake that will affect our physicality, giving it the condition we wish it to have. Our conditioning, rather than the integration of the driver, the horse, and the carriage, may influence how much attention we give to the carriage and its general condition.

The possibility exists within this metaphor for the three aspects to cooperate. The driver may begin to be more in touch with the horse and less focused above the shoulders. The horse can become educated and be able to be more responsive to the instructions that are now coming from a different place within the driver. The carriage begins to understand: the physical body awakens, becoming more alert and beginning to function better in each of its seven major energy centers.

All along there has been someone sitting inside the carriage, going for the drive. This is our inner master. The master is always present, whether or not we recognize it. The master sits inside the carriage waiting for us to give him or her a little bit of attention. Until that time, he or she is a still observer of what takes place in our life. He or she is not in a position of judgment; he or she does not do a great deal more than sit quietly, watching whatever takes place. However, a considerable shift occurs when we begin to give attention to the driver or to the horse or direct some of what the carriage is doing toward the inner master. Until then, this being sits silently inside, waiting for love and attention, waiting for caring and for a response. When we begin to feed the master, an initial beneficial response occurs in the different aspects of ourselves: within our physicality, the driver, and the horse. As soon as the master is contacted, a rapport develops among all three.

Our task is to touch that place inside where the inner master is, to find out where he or she is going, where the carriage should be heading. The inner master carries the instructions regarding the direction of the carriage: the unfolding of our destiny and the progression of our timeline. He knows how our potential, which came into incarnation, can really express itself in the world. While the driver, the horse, and the carriage—together the vehicle through which our soul's expression may take place—are all an essential part of what that inner master could become in the world, they do not know on their own where they are going.

Aura-Soma may be able to help us to develop a relationship with the master within. Each inner master can be seen to wear a coat of a particular color. In turn, each of us represents a different facet of a diamond, a different facet of the light that is reflective of our purpose, of our mission, of why we are incarnate and what we are here to do. These varied facets of light are seen as colors or rays, and they are all a reflection of the one pure light. We each have a master sitting deep within ourselves who is of a particular facet or color. Aura-Soma, and specifically the Quintessences and the Equilibrium bottles that represent the Master Beings, point to the horizontal aspect of the vertical transmission that the Masters' vibrations carry. In other words, they expand in space the possibility we each have to hear the still, small voice of the master within. When we have greater quietness in the mind, when we allow the quality of stillness to be in our being, we can better hear that still, small voice. *Mind* in this sense is our entire mind-and-body experience. By listening, we can invoke the qualities of the Masters to express themselves in our life.

The function of the Equilibrium Master Set and the Quintessences is to help us get in touch with the function of that master who sits quietly inside of us. As we look at color, as we look at the light reflected to ourselves, we may recognize the color of his or her clothes: we recognize that which lies at the deeper levels of ourselves. The aromas and energies of the Quintessences and Master bottles may help with this process of recognition.

This is another way to understand the idea that the colors we choose reflect our being's needs. Essentially, our needs are to understand why we are incarnate and what we are here to do. This perception and expression of our karma is a great part of what our life is. The karmic seeds that we planted in the past will have consequences in our current life until we have grown to the point that we can be in touch with the vibration of our inner master. Then we may step from our karmic path, planting the seeds of the past in terms of good or bad, right or wrong, to our path of dharma, that of being able to unfold why it is that we are here.

Dharma is the way, the unfolding of our destiny. As we step onto the dharmic path, the inner master begins to manifest in our life. This is also the manifestation of the witness, that capacity of each of us to watch ourselves from the point of loving compassion and caring, from warmth rather than judgment. Watching ourselves the way a parent might lovingly watch a child is an expression of the energy of the inner master. We begin to establish an appropriate watchful alertness, which enables us to see what we are doing and how we are doing it. We can observe the way in which we approach things, particularly that which is related to the root, sacral, and solar-plexus chakras. These activities may be difficult to witness, as they relate to powerful issues of survival, dependency, fear, and power. We may tend to be fully identified with issues related to the root, sacral, and solar-plexus chakras. As we begin to move toward the fourth chakra, to the heart, we may more easily be in touch with who is inside the carriage. When we bring caring and compassion toward what is on the stage of ourselves, we can move toward what is going on inside the carriage. We are able to witness the events and patterns with ourselves.

In the Master Set a particular order of color unfolds, commencing with a sequence of primary and secondary colors. The first Master bottle is pale blue, the pale blue of sky that appears to surround this planet, providing atmospheric protection for the earth and for ourselves. The next Master represents the second primary, yellow (B51). Then these two primaries combine through light to offer the pink (B52), and then through the addition of hue to offer green (B53). All the colors combine to the white light of B54, followed by the responsibility for grounding that light on earth in B55. And so the sequence continues.

The Archangel Set

As we meet the beginning of the New Aeon, the archangels have appeared through the Equilibrium sequence. This group now includes B94 through B104. The bottles of the Archangel Set are a gift from the future to inspire us now for the evolutionary possibility of the present time. They help us link with our greater purpose and our individual purpose in terms of consciousness. This in turn links us with other archangels and the ArchAngeloi, which have to do with our greater purpose and our individual one. Archangels have the gift to see what is right, rather than what is wrong. They can hold the pattern of the potential with which they are concerned firmly, strongly, and clearly. This is one way to understand their fiery nature—that they can continuously inspire the creation of that which they are overlighting. Archangels do not place a value judgment on humans for their actions. Instead, they constantly offer us the energy to help create that which is harmonious.

Angels and archangels can also be understood as different aspects of our beings, as part of the complexity of the nature of the being that is our self. We may be in touch with a small operative factor within the larger picture of existence. The destiny opportunity for us as humans is to get closer to our inner angel. There is an order to creation, and we exist within that order with certain possibilities. Having incarnated as a human, we have an opportunity to become closer to the angel that we are, to refine the being that exists within us. Through the interface of color, we can come to know the refinement of our being as expressed in color and light.

The angel that we are is in touch with a large being that deals with the greater purpose of our existence. *Archangel* is another term for that greater being. The archangel groups together classifications of angelic beings and therefore human beings. These groups are based on a shared set of purposes or qualities that are aligned with the function of that archangel. Archangels help us understand the refinement of our being, the potential that exists within the gross material of existence in which we are accustomed to living. They help us understand why we are here in this particular form.

The conscious possibilities that exist for us as humans may be an expression of the angel or archangel within which we find our being. This may be more clear when we consider the importance of selecting an Equilibrium bottle by which one calls to us the most. Something within us calls to us. The bottle would be selecting us, rather than being selected by us. The calling to us from within, is relevant to the concept of angels and archangels.

Closures . . . and Openings

It is our hope that what you have read so far has deepened your understanding of what the world of color can mean to you. As you begin to work with the bottle descriptions and explore the bottle sequences, you may receive inspiration on many levels—from the spiritual world, from the devas of color and light, and from the plant and the mineral kingdoms. The support is there for your journey toward yourself. As we step toward our destiny, mission, and purpose with a sense of joy and love, perhaps we can help the evolution of each other and of our earth, the planet that nourishes us and gives us such a perfect training ground for soul development. In the spirit of the New Christ consciousness, the co-creative, cooperative qualities of the coral, our individual growth supports our shared growth and the growth of community. We can awaken to the brilliant jewel that we are as a part of universal consciousness, using the discarded conditioned patterns as the compost for our next stage of development. The heart of self is reflected in the heart and potential of the whole.

We hope that what is offered here will bring you pleasure, curiosity, wisdom, and perhaps amusement. Please enjoy yourself as you look through this section, and allow yourself the opportunity for a journey of self-exploration into the world of color.

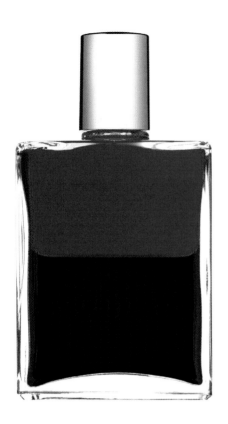

BO Royal Blue/ Deep Magenta

Name: Spiritual Rescue

Shakes Together As: Deep Magenta

Tarot Card: The Fool

Keynote: May help to bring clarity into our feelings about our life. To be able to see our part in the creative process.

In instances of spiritual crisis, this combination, part of the Rescue Set, may be helpful. Vicky Wall often played with words, and she suggested that the word *rescue* be considered in two parts: *re* and *cue*. A cue is an implement used in the game of pool to guide a ball into one of the pockets around the table. Vicky said that to "re-cue" means to "re-center," to bring something to center again. In the case of the first Equilibrium bottle, the re-centering is spiritual.

Zero, the number of this bottle, represents a complete circle from which everything originates: existence itself. This concept—everything and nothing—is implicit within Spiritual Rescue.

A dimension of B0 relates to those who do "rescue work" during the night. These may include people who leave their physical body when asleep, either consciously or unconsciously, to journey to the "other side" to help those in need. B0 is of benefit to these "rescuers," who may wake up tired in the morning because of all their efforts during the night.

In life, we are continually coping with what may be seen as "outside" ourselves. Spiritual Rescue can help us remember to make steps within, which are needed for us to rescue or re-center our spirit. It brings about the possibility

Page 59: Foxtail pine tree in Sierra Nevada. These trees attain great ages of over 1500 years, and after dying will stand for centuries more. This tree died almost 1000 years ago and the wood has become sculpted by the wind. The secret to the longevity of these ancient creatures is probably climate and the resins in the wood.

Below, left: Morocco. "Fools walk in where angels fear to tread."

Below, right: Arenal Volcano, Costa Rica.

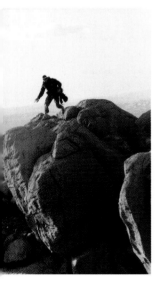

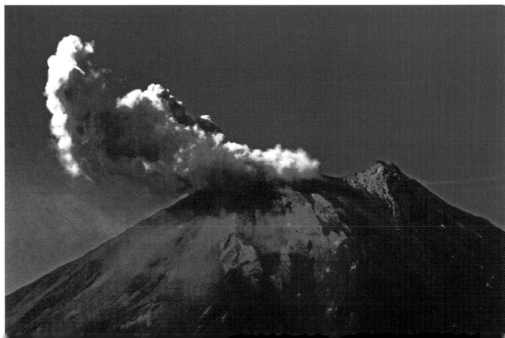

Related Bottles

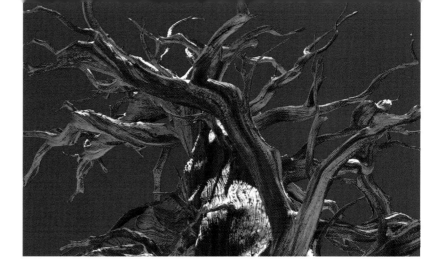

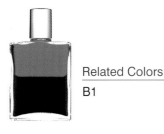

Related Colors
B1

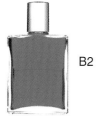

B2

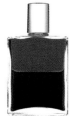

B89

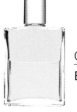

Closest Tints
B57

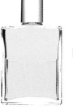

B58

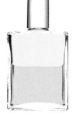

Return Journey
B22

of intuitive insight into the practicalities of our everyday life. It also can bring a sense of deep peace even when our resources have been depleted.

Spiritual Rescue can help us distinguish between spirituality and psychic phenomena. With royal blue's support of higher mind function and clarity, sudden difficulties with the senses may also be resolved. The gifts that we associate with royal blue are of the psyche, and in relation to sensory experience they manifest as clairvoyance, clairaudience, and other sixth-sense experiences. These gifts can be seen as the fruits on the outer branches of the tree of our spiritual being. On occasion we may become more interested in the fruits on the branches than in the tree itself. Spiritual Rescue can help us center on who we are, rather than grasping for the fruits at the tips of the branches. It is important to understand the aspiration to be ordinary, to remember the whole of ourselves or, in this analogy, the wholeness of the tree: its roots, trunk, branches, and leaves, as well as the fruit. To be ordinary is not to enter into spiritual ego, wherein there are more traps than in ordinary life.

The deep magenta appears to be black; it contains all of the colors, representing the complex patterns that lie in the subconscious/unconscious mind. The potential clarity from royal blue helps us perceive with detachment these patterns, which lie in the shadow (deep magenta) within ourselves, and thereby help create change. Detachment is a skill developed within the red energy. In this color combination is found the faith to be able to overcome all obstacles; the energy to succeed from the red in the upper and lower fractions; and the trust to get out of the way to allow warmth and caring to be expressed in the little things of life, a gift of magenta.

Choosing this bottle may suggest illusions, delusions, or apathy that can result from being lost in royal blue; difficulty in finding our direction; or lack of the will to succeed. The red in the lower fraction may indicate that we are holding on to past anger that still gets in our way. We may not want to look into the shadow within, and we may not believe there is one. Spiritual rescue offers deep peace even when our resources are depleted.

Apply this oil along the entire hairline and around the ears. In acute cases B0 can be applied everywhere on the body.

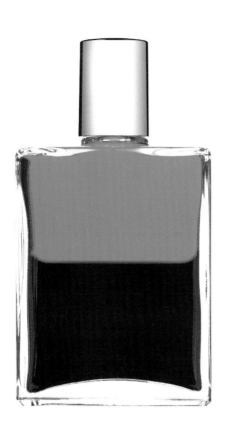

B1 Blue/Deep Magenta

Name: Physical Rescue

Shakes Together As: Deep Magenta

Tarot Card: The Magician

Keynote: A peaceful communication with what lies within ourselves. Helpful communication.

In the early days of Aura-Soma, attention was given to how a bottle might help on the physical level. Both Vicky Wall and Margaret Cockbain, Vicky's constant companion and friend, were hands-on therapists and were accustomed to assessing the efficacy of products according to how they might be appropriate to the physical body. During those early assessments, Blue/Deep Magenta was found to be helpful in many situations, "rescuing" users from a variety of symptoms. Thereby B1 gained the name Physical Rescue and became part of

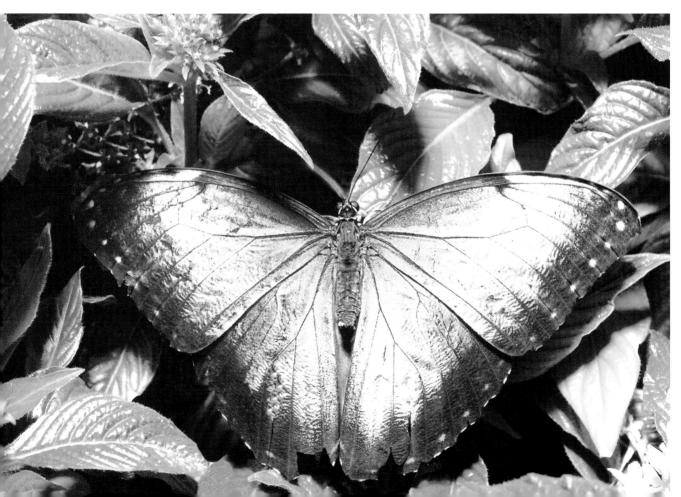

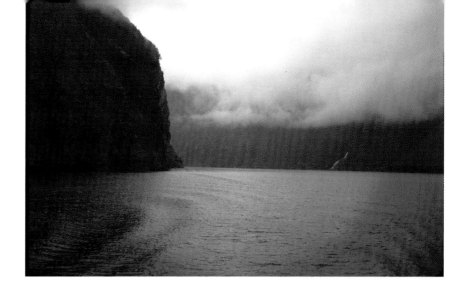

Related Bottles

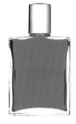

Related Colors
B2

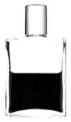

B100

Closest Tints
B103

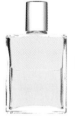

B58

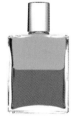

Return Journey
B79

the Rescue Set. It is also part of the Chakra Set and relates to the crown chakra and the third eye.

Physical Rescue helps us more naturally and easily come in contact with our physicality. This means that we are able to let go of or release our tensions, to become real to ourselves. When this happens, we become more peaceful (blue), more able to deal with what our life, our physicality, presents to us.

When we are more at ease, we are more likely to be free of dis-ease. Deep magenta contains all the colors, representing the whole of our physical body. The result of finding peace, ease, or calm in the conscious mind (the blue in the conscious mind) is relaxation of the entire body, a precursor for concentration or meditation. To truly relax physically, to find peace and calm, requires trust or faith, another key concept associated with blue. With trust, peace and ease may be gained in the physical base.

B0 and B1 are similar in color, the difference being a little bit of red in the top fraction of B0. If we consider how these bottles affect us, it is interesting to remember that spirituality depends on the state of our physicality. While we are in human form, consciousness is dependent upon our physicality. Perhaps Physical Rescue may help us remember our physicality in the same way that Spiritual Rescue helps us remember our spirituality.

When we choose this bottle, the blue on top signifies that we have peace and trust. As the color of the throat chakra (see B2), blue suggests that we have the ability to listen and to communicate clearly. The deep magenta of divine love indicates that we endeavor to put our caring and warmth in all that we do; it is easy for others to feel nurtured just being with us.

The blue in the upper and lower fractions could also suggest an acquisitive tendency. This may indicate that we are holding on to the difficulties of the past and are reluctant to let go. We may crave the peace of blue but think it is for others, not for us. This might be a reflection of guilt or unworthiness we feel in the shadow inside ourselves. It could be from not believing in our selves, not seeing our own value.

B1 is usually applied along the entire hairline and around the throat, neck, and ears. However, B1 is one of the few Equilibrium oils that can be applied to any painful area.

Above: Norway fjord.
Left: Stone carving of Quetzalcoatl, the feathered serpent in Teotihuacán, Mexico.
Page 60: Morpho butterfly found frequently in South America. Morpho, an epithet for Aphrodite and Venus, refers to the iridescent beauty of the wings. Both magicians and butterflies are capable of morphogenesis.

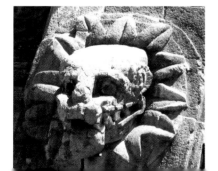

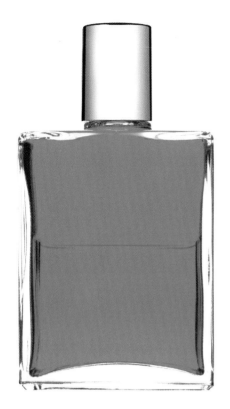

B2 Blue/Blue

Name: **Peace Bottle**

Shakes Together As: **Blue**

Tarot Card: **The High Priestess**

Keynote: **Peaceful communication that comes through us rather than from us. A nurturing energy. A natural authority.**

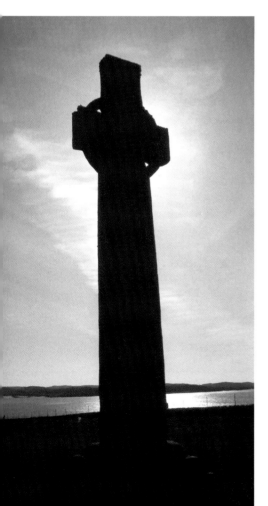

Blue represents the expression of peace. The cloudless blue sky is like a peaceful mind without any thoughts or distractions. Blue is the peace of calmness, of stillness, of a state of mind that is beyond thinking. It has been expressed as "the peace that passeth all understanding," a primary energy that is present deep within each of us, beneath all our sensory experiences and thoughts. The key for us is to get in touch with that peace.

We always have the opportunity to recognize our own reflection, especially if we have the calmness within to see the reflection in the mirror. Peace and blue give us that opportunity. When we become peaceful and calm, we can experience an absence of identity. When all the tensions have been released, there remains a quality of attention that is not dependent upon thinking or feeling, that is just peacefulness, almost as if there were "no one there." The scope of help available to us through Blue/Blue includes letting go of identity. Here we find the possibility of letting go of the tensions and patterns with which we identify, which lead us away from peace.

The Peace bottle may help those in transition. While the word *transition* is often used to refer to the final transition between life and death, it also relates to many small transitions we go through in life: from childhood to adolescence and on to adulthood; from one job to another; from one relationship to another. Each of these changes is a transition between roles within which we have some identity. Change in identity is only a change of consciousness; this is true whether we are in the body or out of it, passing from life to life, or going through different identities while in the same physical base. The necessary accompaniment to any of these transitions is the "peace that passeth all understanding," which brings peace to us in the experience of transition. Peace and trust in the conscious mind can help bring those same qualities into the subconscious/unconscious mind. If we become free of tension, then peace becomes possible.

With the blue qualities of nurturing and trust in both the top and bottom fractions, this bottle suggests we have an ability to nurture others and an immense faith easily communicated to others. By allowing the higher will to come to us or through us, a communication gift of blue, we can know that we are nurtured from above. (Please review the distinctions between the colors turquoise, royal blue, and blue on pages 19–21.)

Related Bottles

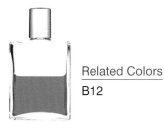

Related Colors
B12

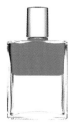

B60

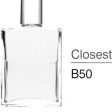

Closest Tint
B50

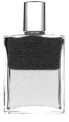

Return Journey
B80

On the other hand, because blue connotes the nurturing of both the female and the male, challenges with the mother or the father may exist. These may be reflected in our discomfort with the female and male models within us, resulting in an absence of peace and a tendency to hold on to our problems. Because blue is associated with the throat chakra, making it a member of the Chakra Set, we may have difficulty communicating or fail to pay attention to communicating.

As we explore the other bottles, it will be apparent that B2 is hidden within many of them, as blue is a primary color.

Apply B2 along the hairline, on the neck and lower jaw, and around the whole throat/neck area. The lower line of the blue band of color is the collarbone. It may seem strange, but B2 may help prevent stretch marks when applied to the area concerned. With teething babies, externally apply the combination around the jaw area. The peace of the blue makes this bottle particularly useful at bedtime.

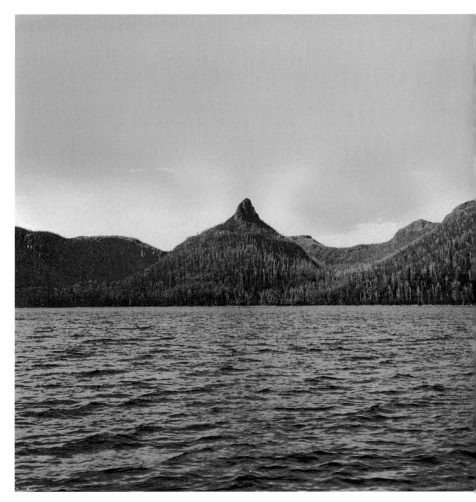

Left: Standing cross on Iona, Scotland, where Saint Columba (Columcille) first brought Christianity after saying goodbye to his beloved Ireland.
Right: Lake St. Clair in Tasmania, named for a relative of the Sinclair family from Scotland.

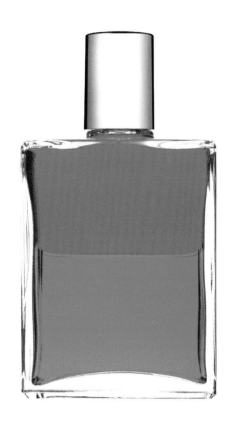

B3 Blue/Green

Name: Heart Bottle/Atlantean Bottle
Tarot Card: The Empress
Shakes Together As: Turquoise
Keynote: Creative communication, especially in relation to the earth, the earth's grid and magnetic structure.

Popularly, the Atlantean myth is of a pre-Egyptian civilization with an advanced technology, based on silica and crystals, that provided a plentiful power source.[3-a] The Atlantean era is considered by many to have been an important age in human development, when great emphasis was given to healing, meditation, and the development of consciousness. Color, light, and crystals played a large part in the development of these processes. Atlantis is also a symbol of harmonious civilization. The civilization destroyed itself by using its technology for unwholesome purposes.[3-b]

When shaken together, B3's blue and green combine to create turquoise, the color associated with Atlantis. It is the turquoise of the sea of the collective consciousness, or the subconscious or unconscious mind. This bottle depicts the green landmass surrounded by the sea from which, mythically, Atlantis came and into which it disappeared.

The turquoise created by the blue and green suggests creativity. Creativity can act as a release, so that what lies within us can be brought forward. B3 is linked to the heart chakra or fourth chakra. The heart is where creativity can find its expression in the world. To give to creativity is to give space within the heart.

In a way creativity is fostered by a sense of peace. Peace in the conscious mind brings the opportunity to reveal the space within the depths of ourselves. If we have made space within the depths of our selves, we have more of an opportunity to consciously realize peace and manifest our creativity. This bottle offers us the possibility to become more peaceful in relation to being upon the earth, within physicality. It is through this possibility that we gain the opportunity to become more individual (a turquoise concept) and more grounded, as the green emerges from the ocean of peace.

This bottle also represents a transition into the fourth dimension, which concerns our relationship with time. This is not the linear sense of time but, rather, the ability to be present within the self, or to be more aware. When we let go of the past and come into the present, we become more heartfelt, more Atlantean. Our hidden fears (the yellow hidden in the green) could be part of the negative legacy of fallen Atlantis. These fears need to be overcome so that humanity may evolve upon this planet during the time we are now facing. If we are able to let go of our fears, then we may be able to be more responsible in relation to the

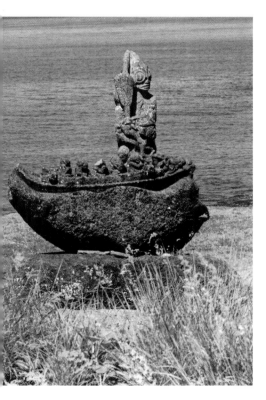

Related Bottles

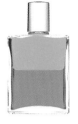

Reverse
B88

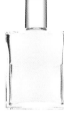

Closest Tint
B101

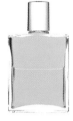

Shakes To
B43

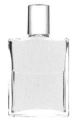

Return Journey
B81

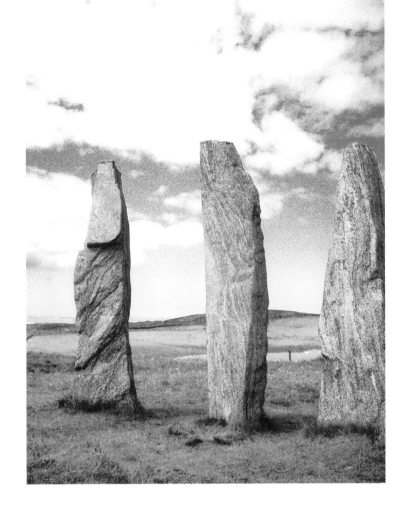

beings of the earth. Furthermore, this bottle may help us establish contact with Atlantean incarnational experiences.

B3 can be effective in animal healing, wherever the ailment. It is of particular use to those of us who deal with animals on a regular basis. Those of us choosing this bottle in the first, third, or fourth position may gain great benefit from physical, practical work.

This bottle may indicate that we can express our feelings (green) and communicate them peacefully (blue), that we are decision makers with a love of nature, or that we are in a position to offer new opportunities to others.

When used to reveal issues, the green in the base suggests that we have discomfort with the emotional side of life, or that we often deny our feelings and have difficulty communicating our feelings. Other challenges concern making space to do what we need and making decisions. We may have difficulties related to a lack of nurturing from our parents (see also B2).

B3 is part of the Chakra Set and the Rescue Set. It should be applied across the entire chest area in a wide band that starts at the collarbone and extends to the lowest rib, including the spinal column on the back.

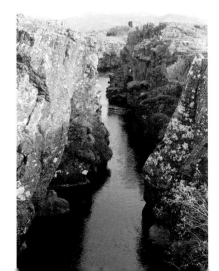

Above: Three standing stones of the Callanish Stone Circle, Isle of Lewis, Scotland.
Left: Two plates of the earth meet in Iceland at the site of the first parliament building.
Page 64: Stone carving by the sea on the island of Niku Hiva in the Marquesa Islands, French Polynesia.

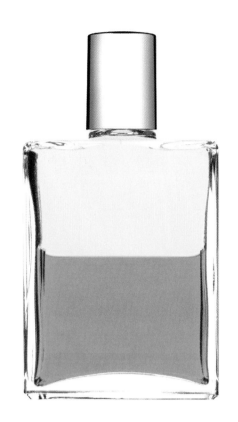

B4 Yellow/Gold

Name: Sunlight Bottle
Tarot Card: The Emperor
Shakes Together As: Golden Yellow
Keynote: Knowledge: that which can be acquired, and wisdom: that which we already have.

B4, known as Sunlight, relates to the solar-plexus chakra, which is the source of light within our being. From the solar plexus, the light can shine, if we let go of anxiety, tension, and fear, if we let go of past and future, and if we allow ourselves to come into the present. Then it is possible to enjoy the celebration of the moment, of the here and now.

Ancient Egypt, from 10,000 to 3500 BC,[4-a] was the next great civilization to evolve upon the planet after the fall of Atlantis. Ancient Egyptian civilization is known to have been concerned with the worship of the sun and solar consciousness. Yellow, which was hidden within the green base of B3 and is now evident in the upper, conscious fraction of B4, is the thread that links Atlantis with Egypt. As may have been the case in Atlantis, history tells us that in Egypt, power may have been used at the hands of the few to create fear as a means of control over many people. This theme shows us the path of yellow, connecting fear and self-awareness, the withholding and the shining of our light. As B3 does for Atlantean incarnations, B4 may help us establish contact with incarnations in ancient Egypt.

The Sunlight bottle is about the possibility of refining the golden wisdom within ourselves, within the golden area of the body, the solar plexus or hara, so that we may realize our wisdom. Chosen in the first, third, or fourth positions it often indicates that we have great strength and knowledge in the conscious mind (yellow) and an immense wisdom (gold) within our depths. We may have

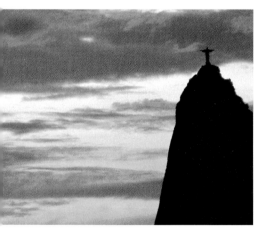

Above: Christ the Redeemer on Corcovado Mountain in Rio de Janeiro, Brazil.
Right: Pyramid of the Sun in Teotihuacán, Mexico.
Page 67: Resting Buddha, Wat Yai Chai Mongkhon in Ayutthaya, Thailand. The temple itself was established in 1357 by King Ramathibodi. It was to be a meditation site for monks returning from pilgrimages to Sri Lanka. Each position of a Buddha has a different meaning reflecting a different moment in Buddha's life. This reclining Buddha with his head lying in the palm of his right hand and his head to the north, symbolizes the passing of the Buddha into nirvana.

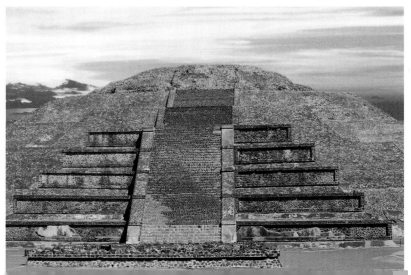

66

Related Bottles

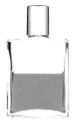

Related Colors
B14

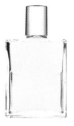

B42

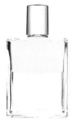

B70

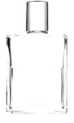

Closest Tint
B51

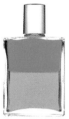

Return Journey
B82

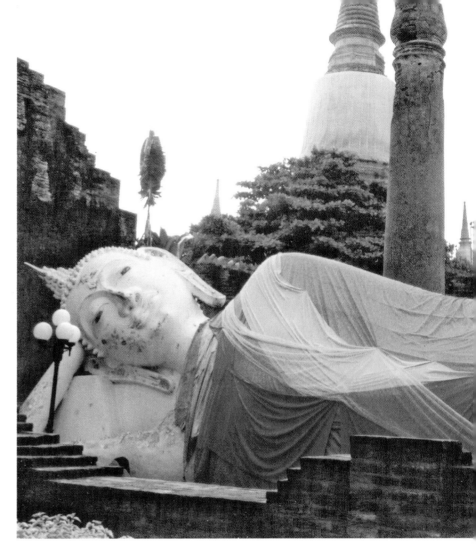

a sense of humor and an ability to deal with life in a sunny, happy manner. Often we are in a position of power. In contrast, we who choose this bottle in the second position may have fear about the smallest details in life. We may not easily see the light within ourselves, but we may be more able to see it in others.

Sunlight is about consciousness. It is self-awareness, which can sometimes manifest in a negative way as self-consciousness or a knot of contraction within the solar plexus. As the knot begins to loosen and we let go of fear, we can undo the knot of contraction completely and the light can begin to shine. More confidence emerges as self-consciousness is released. Knowledge begins to dawn more brightly. To let go of the knowledge (yellow) may be the first step toward refining our wisdom (gold). The Sunlight bottle's separation of yellow and gold symbolizes the necessity of discriminating between knowledge and wisdom. Knowledge can be acquired; wisdom is inherent.

B4 is part of the Chakra Set and the Rescue Set. It should be applied in a wide band around the circumference of the body at the solar-plexus level.

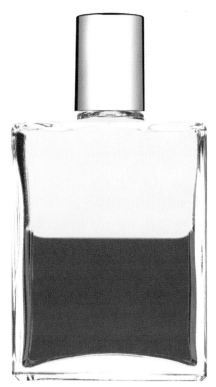

B5 Yellow/Red

Name: Sunrise/Sunset Bottle

Shakes Together As: Orange

Tarot Card: The Hierophant

Keynote: The opportunity to use the wisdom wisely in relation to the energies that we carry.

Sunrise/Sunset was the bottle that called to Vicky the most, and she referred to it as her "aura bottle." We can understand some of the issues she faced through considering the name of this bottle. Vicky endured many abusive situations throughout her life, which, in turn, produced emotional shocks. This led to stress in the solar plexus, exacerbating her preexisting genetic conditions and eventually affecting her pancreas and kidneys; she became diabetic in her mid-thirties. Sunrise/Sunset encompasses the beginning and ending of each day, and in each day we have the opportunity to deal with something anew. At the end of the day we do not really know just how well we have done with the possibilities presented to us within that twenty-four hours. In a way, each moment of our life is like that, as is each lifetime. B5 symbolizes making the most of and doing the best with what we chose for this incarnation.

As with all the color combinations, the "shakes together as" color (the color formed when the upper and lower fractions are combined) is significant in understanding the meaning of this bottle. Yellow/Red shakes together as orange, and thus the themes of orange symbolism are inherent in B5 (see "An Example: B5 and Aura-Soma," page 282).

B5 is allied with the base chakra and orange with the organs of reproduction. The base or root chakra is the source of our potential to reproduce. Within

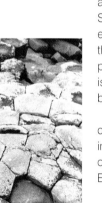

Above: Naturally occurring five-sided stones at the Giant's Causeway in Ireland.

Right: Five fruits on a table, representing the five elements of traditional Chinese medicine. Orangeville, Ontario, Canada.

Page 69: "Wig men" in the Highlands, Papua New Guinea.

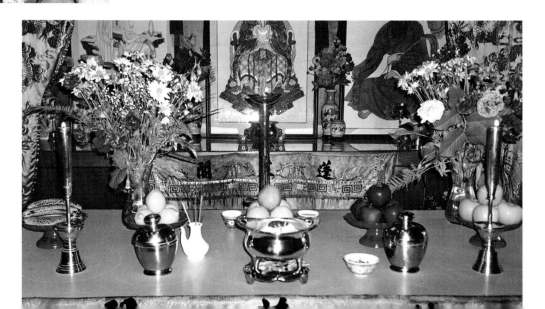

Related Bottles

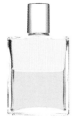

Related Color
B22

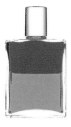

Related Reverse
B40

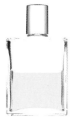

Closest Tint
B59

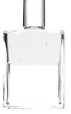

Reverse Tint
B61

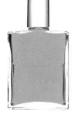

Shakes To
B26

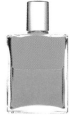

Return Journey
B83

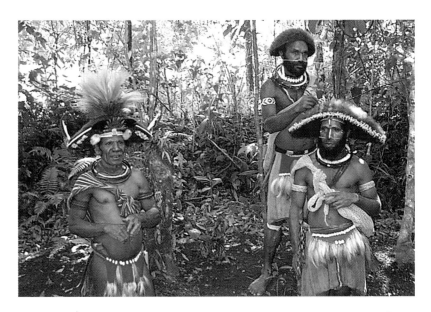

the base chakra is the possibility of awakening in relation to the kundalini force. This force is sometimes referred to as the source of light within the body. The light begins to emanate from the snake curled at the root. This potential lies dormant until the snake uncurls and light arises to join with all the chakras. The "sunrise" in this bottle's name indicates the beginning of a process of awakening the light within the root, or the initiation of creative forces journeying toward the crown.

Choosing this bottle suggests that we have joy and the knowledge (yellow) of how to wisely express our energy (red) in the world: we may be leaders; we may have a joyful though perhaps difficult path to fulfill our mission and purpose; we may have a generous soul and freely offer our qualities to others. We may have attracted difficult situations early in our life or may have been subjected to them. B5, in that it shakes to orange, could relate to emotional shocks. It also could describe us as overly dominating, even to those we care for most deeply.

Overall, B5 has effects similar to those of the Etheric Rescue bottle (B26). It may help us establish contact with ancient Tibetan and Chinese incarnations (see B40). It could possibly indicate abuse when it is chosen in the second or first position. Great care must be taken before making this kind of assessment. The aim of working through issues of abuse should never be vengeful or guilt apportioning. We recommend that anyone working with these issues should consult with an experienced therapist. The opportunity of a "rebirth" to a new point of view is inherent (see B22).

Those of us who select the B5 bottle as a soul bottle may find that we can identify with Vicky's own life story. B59 is the subtlest tint of both B5 and B22. The selection of B22 would suggest that we have gone through a spiritual rebirth to come into the life to fulfill our life purpose. The choice of B59 would mean that we have an ever increasing struggle with ourself in fulfilling our life's purpose in terms of how we judge ourself.

B5 is part of the Chakra Set. It is appropriate for application as low around the trunk as possible, around the entire lower abdomen, and upon the feet and legs.

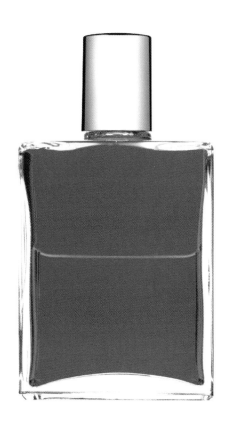

B6 Red/Red

Name: Energy Bottle
Shakes Together As: Red
Tarot Card: The Lovers
Keynote: Enthusiasm and love for life.

In Aura-Soma, red symbolizes energy. Red/Red is energy in a pure, powerful form, symbolizing the full drive within life. Hence red and B6 have an association with survival, with our basic instincts, individually and tribally, that impact our sexuality and our urge to reproduce. Our life force or creative energy can also lead us beyond the issues of survival toward awakening, and so red also represents kundalini, or the potential for awakening to the whole of our physicality.

Red has two effects: one encourages detachment and the other pushes away, rejects, and says no to things. Detachment helps us develop the ability to become less identified with things. Through experiencing the impulse to reject or push away, we can develop detachment and nonreactivity. Detachment releases energy that, in turn, becomes available to help us identify less.

Red/Red, like the lovers in the tarot, connotes unification, or the principles of male and female coming together. This union across many levels of existence expresses why red may be considered the fundamental life energy. Red is grounding and earthing and brings us into our physical body where consciousness resides when we are in physicality.

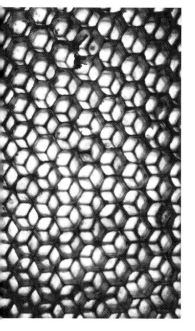

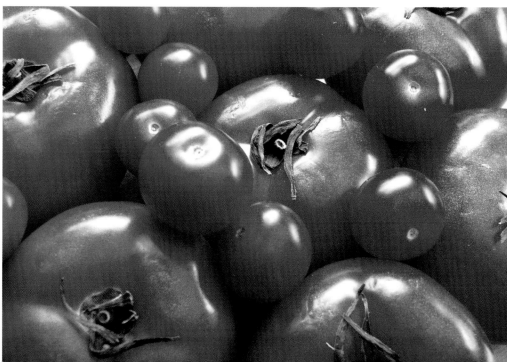

Related Bottles

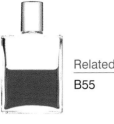

Related Colors
B55

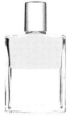

B71

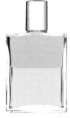

Closest Tints
B23

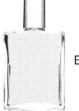

B52

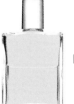

B81

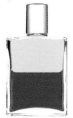

Return Journey
B84

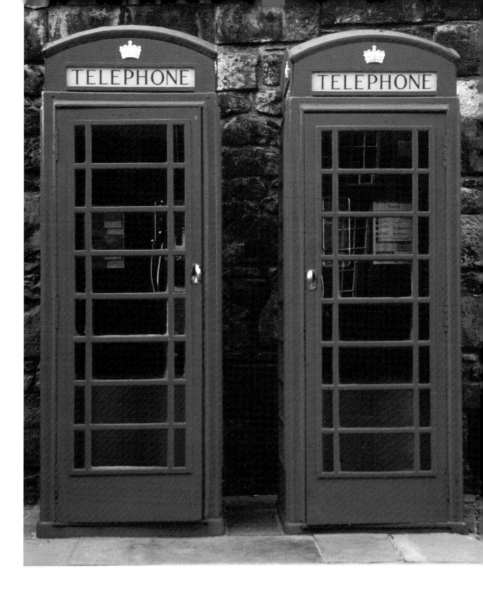

B6 indicates that we have vast energy and a zest for life, or perhaps it is time for a new beginning. B6 is a powerful bottle, one that carries the energy for awakening and the skill of complete detachment that permits a clear view of ourselves and others. Elsewhere, B6 may indicate resentment, frustration, and even anger or a lack of vitality and a need for energy. We may feel that our life energy is flowing away into things that are not helpful or useful, yet we may feel that we are not able to control or stop that flow.

B6 is part of the extended Chakra Set and, like B5 where red is first evident in the sequence, is linked to the base or root chakra. This combination can be applied everywhere below the hip area and is especially appropriate on the soles of the feet. It can be used whenever there is a lack of energy, and it is especially appropriate after serious operations or at times of extreme fatigue. If used too late in the afternoon or evening, it could be very energizing and result in difficulty sleeping.

Above: Affectionately speaking, side-by-side phone booths in Edinburgh, Scotland.
Page 70, left: Six-sided beehive form.
Page 70, right: Red, organic, sun-ripened tomatoes in Long Island, New York.

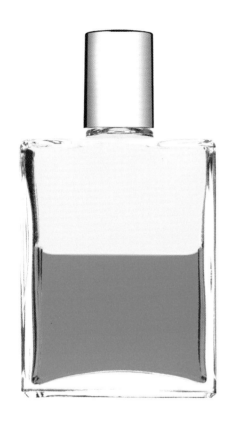

B7 Yellow/Green

Name: Garden of Gethsemene

Shakes Together As: Olive Green

Tarot Card: The Chariot

Keynote: Trust in the process of life, the hope in how things may unfold.

The name of B7 came through John Walker, who was head of the Radionic Association in the United Kingdom in the 1980s and had, at that time, connected with Vicky's work. John selected B7 during a consultation. He told Vicky that it reminded him of the Garden of Gethsemene. Vicky's spontaneous reply was that not only was it a reminder, but that it was what the bottle represented. This name has remained with this color combination ever since.

The Garden of Gethsemene is concerned with the final test of faith. According to Christian teaching, Jesus, who had already been recognized as a teacher, began to feel anguish in the Garden of Gethsemene. Although he had the knowledge and awareness that he and the Father were One, he still questioned whether he was alone with his predicament or whether his Father would be with him until the end.[7-a] In a more prosaic sense, the final test of faith is significant in relation to the opportunities of our life, and whether we can trust what lies within the depths of ourselves.

The more we make space within ourselves, the more the joy of knowledge and certainty can arise within our conscious mind. Trust within the depths of ourselves and knowledge within our conscious mind bring a sense of hope to the difficulties or obstacles we meet in our life experiences, allowing us to re-evaluate them in relation to a new beginning or a new opportunity that life may hold.

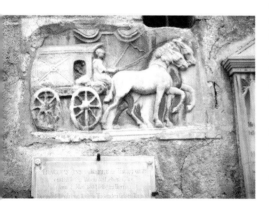

Above: Carving of a Roman postal cart on the wall of a medieval church built at the time of the Black Death, late 14th century, Austria.

Right: Chariot on road near the Danube River in Spits-an-der-Donau, Austria.

Page 73: Castle of Montségur in Ariège, Midi-Pyrénées, France. Final resistance place of the heretical sect, the Cathars. In March 1244 the 205 Cathar defenders finally surrendered and were burned en masse rather than renounce their beliefs.

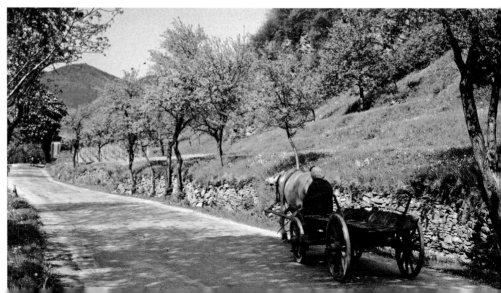

Related Bottles

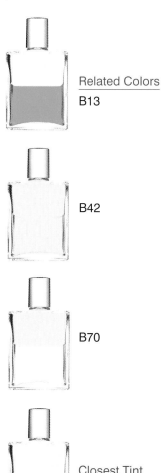

Related Colors
B13

B42

B70

Closest Tint
B74

Shakes To
B91

Return Journey
B85

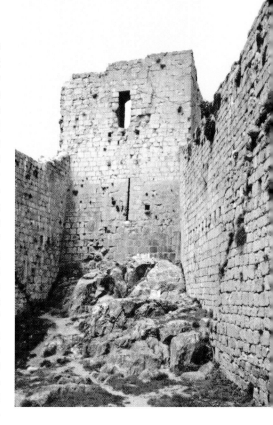

Nevertheless, doubt can also be a good companion. Failing to doubt and entering into situations unwisely can prove troublesome. If doubt is present in appropriate situations, we may become more aware of and more astute about the situation into which we are entering. The yellow, in one way, could suggest the knowledge of what existed in Christ's situation; it could also suggest that an element of fear existed in relation to the path ahead. We have a tendency to view the "negative emotions" from a negative point of view, rather than seeing the energy contained within the emotions. If we examine fear in ourselves and remove the label of judgment, then the energy, when understood, may have a purpose beyond the conceptualization of the label itself. Green is the way, the truth, and the possibility of making the right decision in orienting ourselves toward the right direction.

When the Dalai Lama left Lhasa for the last time, he said he felt a mixture of anxiety and absolute anticipation of the freedom that was to come.[7-b] His words suggest that within our own anxieties and anticipations, there may be help for each of us. B7, Yellow/Green, could speak to that situation.

B7 is also concerned with the possibility of betrayal. In one sense, the only person who could betray us is ourselves. Such self-betrayal connects to not trusting the process of life. The more we trust the process of life, the more our destiny is likely to unfold. Sometimes it is fear that functions as energy to help us across the difficulties ahead. Choosing this bottle could imply that we are troubled by fears and anxieties and we may not be able to make appropriate decisions or find our direction in life. B7 is almost always a test of faith.

Both B7 and B74 may help us to connect with incarnational experiences related to the Cathars. Also known as the Albigensians, the Cathars flourished in the 12th and 13th centuries in the Languedoc region of France.[7-c]

Part of our awakening may be in how we feel at home within ourselves, regardless of external conditions or circumstances. This sense of being at home could be with us wherever we are. This bottle suggests that we have the knowledge (yellow) of how to make space (green) for ourselves, and that we have an ability to share our knowledge, expressing ourselves in a kind and gentle way. This is a capacity to create a homey feeling, even though we may be continually on the move.

This combination should be applied around the circumference of the body to encompass the heart and solar-plexus areas.

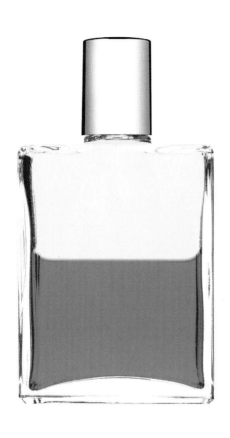

B8 Yellow/Blue

Name: **Anubis**

Shakes Together As: **Green**

Tarot Card: **Justice**

Keynote: **The communication of knowledge, the joy of peace.**

This bottle is very significant in Aura-Soma. The Egyptian god Anubis guards the threshold to the otherworld.[8-a] The Egyptian belief was that Anubis not only guarded the threshold but also measured the weight of the heart of those who wished to pass. He measured the weight of the heart against the balancing number of feathers to determine how much merit a person had gained. The means and direction to the next world were then given, according to the degree of merit. The fewer feathers needed to counterbalance our heart, the more we are able to retain for our wings. Our wings metaphorically relate to the lightness of our being.

The way this all relates to the color combination Yellow/Blue is that when we disturb the peace (blue) within our selves, we then tend to be in judgment of ourselves. When we enter into judgment (yellow), we quickly may lose any peace we may have. As this combination shakes to a green color, we can see

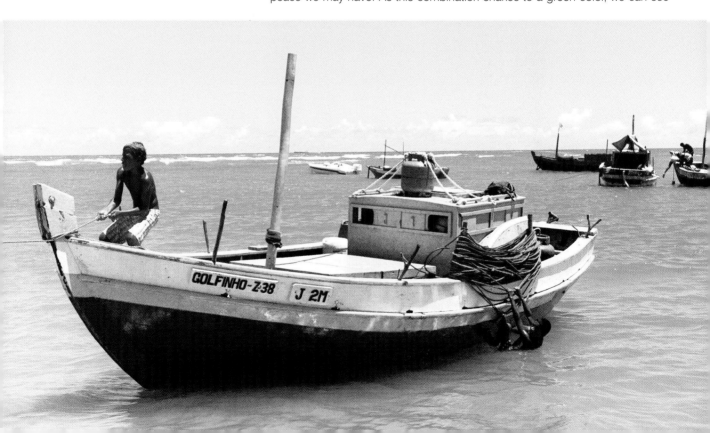

Related Bottles

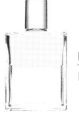

Reverse Tint
B94

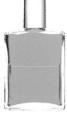

Shakes To
B10

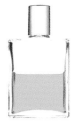

Return Journey
B86

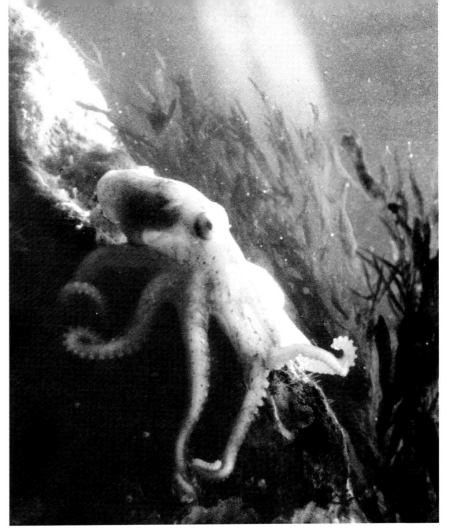

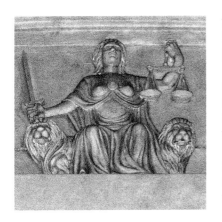

Above: Scales of justice. A relief on an outside wall of the Venetian Hotel in Las Vegas, Nevada.
Top right: Eight-armed octopus peers brightly through the blue waters of the Pacific.
Left: Fishing boat off the coast of Brazil in Salvador, Bahia.

that the judgments we make of ourselves and others can tend to accumulate in the heart (green). B8 may help resolve feelings of guilt from previous lives, particularly those that took place in the Middle East.

The tarot card associated with B8 is Justice, in this case a justice that relates to connecting the root with the heart. By skillful use of the sword of discrimination we can find the balance between these two centers. Anubis has to do with judgment and with what is being judged. Through finding peace (blue) within our selves, we can overcome our judgments and fears (yellow). .

Anubis is related to the dog. In English *dog* spelled backward is *God*. In one direction the letters imply the destructive, operative, and generative principle and in the other, the generative, operative, and destructive. Using discernment skillfully will determine how we experience these forces.

Fears and anxieties may result from the lack of feeling nurtured. Choosing this bottle may suggest that we have difficulty expressing deep issues, thus creating a lack of joy, even when things are going well. This bottle may indicate that we have a joy for life, great knowledge (yellow), and a sense of inner peace (blue). We may be looking for our appropriate direction (green), and by relying on the peace that lies within, we are able to find that direction and communicate (blue) it clearly and joyfully to others. The more we learn to trust the communication that comes from the depths of our selves, the more joy and knowledge can come.

B8 should be applied around the heart and root areas, encompassing the entire trunk and the pelvic area.

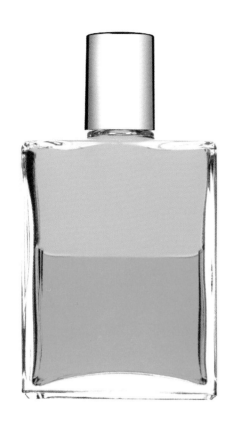

B9 Turquoise/Green

Name: Heart within the Heart/Crystal Cave
Shakes Together As: Deep Turquoise
Tarot Card: The Hermit
Keynote: The beginning of the journey. The process of individuation.

B9's primary name resulted from an Aura-Soma therapist who frequently came to Vicky for consultations. This therapist, years before, had experienced a marriage breakup, but she had not yet really let go of her husband. However, she had begun to take the journey within her own heart in a different way, and she was now prepared to let go. She felt no need to look for a substitute relationship or to resurrect the previous relationship. B9 was born in synchronicity with her process, and Vicky said that this combination represented the heart within the heart. Here turquoise appears for the first time in the bottle sequence, rather than as a potential combination of two colors being shaken together (B3). In B9, turquoise, which was hidden in B3, is supported by the green of the heart center proper. As with B3, this bottle may help establish connections with Atlantean incarnations.

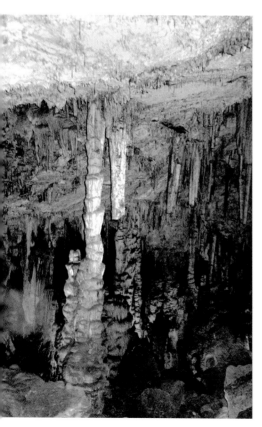

While B3 is the combination linked to the heart chakra, B9 represents another level of the heart chakra and the process of the Ananda Khanda unfolding. The Ananda Khanda is the energy center on the right side of the chest. Contact with the Ananda Khanda comes as we connect with the magenta energy coming down from the soul star, or the eighth chakra, above. This process in turn is dependent upon a connection with the earth star, a solid grounding that allows the pink energy to arise from under and move to touch the golden energy in the hara (belly). Only through this two-way process is turquoise awakened. The Ananda Khanda initiates the process of individuation, the journey within, which offers us the possibility of facing our shadow, of facing our inner world in a new way.

B9 also is known as the Crystal Cave. As we go within to the Ananda Khanda, we touch the crystal cave. Here are all the crystal patterns that hold our identities in place. We respond the way we respond, and we react the way we react, principally because of our conditioned patterns. It is within the crystal cave that we encounter the crystallization of those patterns of conditioning. Part of our journey toward individuation involves integrating different aspects of our selves, which requires us to assimilate that which lies within the crystal cave. Every aspect of our personality evolution that has been influenced by conditioned patterns, whether of this life or another (from teachers, friends, family, parents, authority figures, other role models), leading to our self-image, exists within the crystal cave. When we come to the point of development where we begin to explore the crystal cave, we begin to digest some of those conditioned

Related Bottles

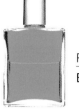

Related Colors
B10

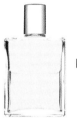

B42

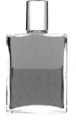

B88

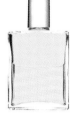

Closest Tint
B101

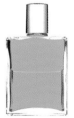

Shakes To
B43

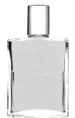

Return Journey
B87

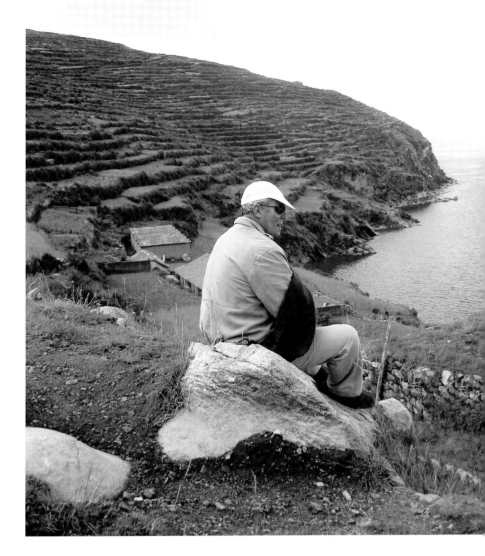

patterns we use to define who we truly are. We describe this as the process of individuation.

Individuation allows our real creativity to emerge. It is revealed that creativity follows the breaking up of the crystallized patterns of our conditioning, which in turn leads us to a new understanding of who and what we are. This process requires an inner peace, as indicated by the blue hidden in both the upper and the lower fractions of this combination. Thus, B9 can indicate that we are very creative and able to make space for ourselves to be creative (turquoise) and to do what we need to do, both for ourselves and for others. We may have evolved our feelings (green) and can express clearly and easily what lies upon our heart. In other interpretations, B9 may indicate that we are experiencing repression and guilt, which create problems in our knowing (yellow) what we are supposed to do, perhaps because our priorities are not sorted out. It can imply receiving or feeling jealousy and envy.

Apply the contents of this bottle across the entire chest area and around to the back, including over the spinal column.

Above: Mike Booth on Isla de la Luna, Lake Titicaca, Bolivia.
Left: Dictaean Cave, the birthplace of Zeus in Crete, Greece.

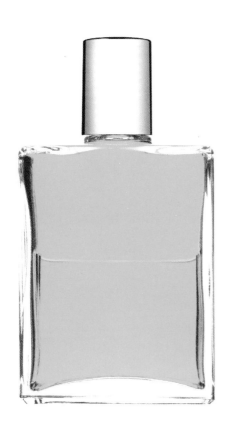

B10 Green/Green

Name: Go Hug a Tree
Shakes Together As: Green
Tarot Card: The Wheel of Fortune
Keynote: As you plant, so shall you reap.

Every morning of the seven years Vicky and Mike Booth spent together, they would go for a walk in order to help her maintain the remainder of her functional heart muscle. At some point during the walk, she would ask him to help her locate a tree so that she could commune with it. Communing with a tree was a way for Vicky to move quickly into another state of consciousness and was something she enjoyed daily.[10-a]

Vicky enjoyed this practice partially to be in touch with nature, with the force of existence that lies behind our busy lives, and partially to experience, via the tree, a stillness that is less apparent in human life. A tree views existence and its situation of life from the same perspective no matter how old it is, as the tree does not move around the planet as we do. If we tune in to a tree, we have the

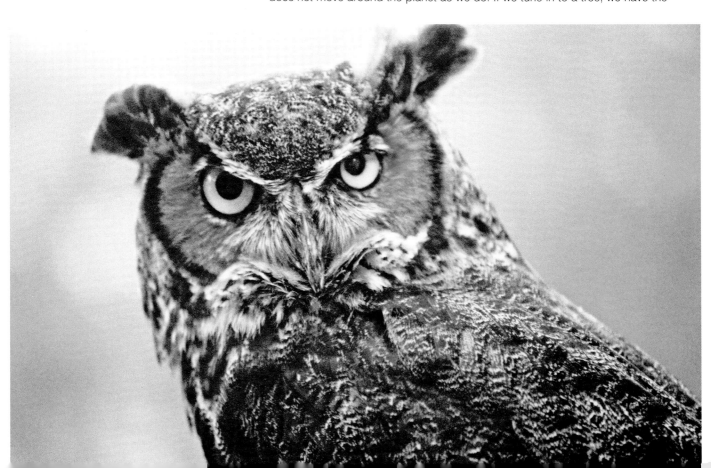

Related Bottles

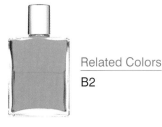

Related Colors
B2

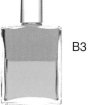

B3

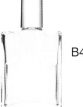

B42

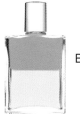

B63

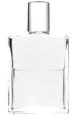

Closest Tint
B53

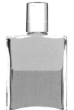

Return Journey
B88

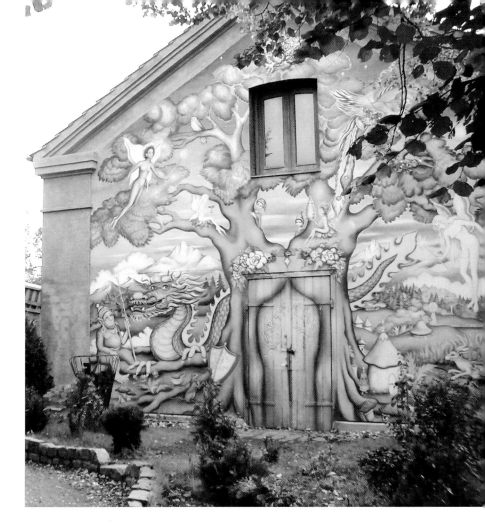

possibility of becoming aware of the rain forests being destroyed as well as of a new tree being planted somewhere upon the earth. To come into contact with a tree is to connect with the consciousness of trees.

The tree is a symbol of the spiral of time. When we tune in to the tree, we receive that spiral effect; indeed, in the rings and the spaces between the rings information is recorded concerning the passing of every year. B10 is about spirals; truth, direction, and space are all key concepts for this combination. The spiral connection reminds us that the tarot name for this bottle, the Wheel of Fortune, refers to cycles of time and the patterns of cause and effect.

Go Hug a Tree is a part of the extended Chakra Set. This bottle is often chosen by ecologists and naturalists and those of us who are lovers of nature. It used to be called Decision Maker, and indeed, choosing it indicates that we may be decision makers with an understanding of and empathy toward others. We may have the ability to see a situation from different angles, grasp other perspectives presented to us, and choose a clear direction. However, B10 may suggest that we are resistant to change and may need to let go of fears and learn to give before expecting to receive.

Apply the contents of this bottle around the entire chest area to form a band that includes the spinal column.

Above: Tree of Life. This mural stands at the entrance to Christiania's artist commune in Copenhagen, Denmark, where artists, activists, and intellectuals have lived on 800 acres of land, governing themselves by consensus since 1970.

Left: Great horned owl in Milton, Massachusetts, capable of turning his head 270 degrees and of seeing well in the dark.

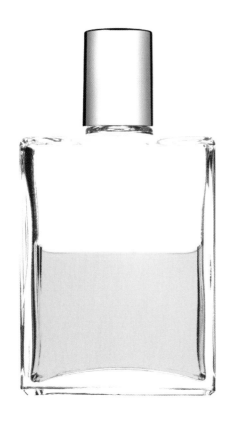

B11 Clear/Pink

Name: The Essene Bottle 1
Shakes Together As: Pale Pink
Tarot Card: Strength
Keynote: Taking responsibility for our thoughts and feelings.

B11 contains clear over pink, the first time these colors appear in the Equilibrium system. As such, B11 marks a new sequence, the birth of what is called the New Aeon Child Set. It is also a member of the Rescue Set and is known as the Love Rescue bottle.

The Essenes were one of the last groups of people (prior to our time) to work with color. They used color for the growth and expansion of consciousness and for healing. The Essenes were persecuted and ostracized by all other faiths of their time.[11-a] Both Mary, the mother of Jesus, and Elizabeth, his aunt, were Essenes, and Jesus himself may have been born in an Essene community.[11-b] Essene teachings are reflected in the Tree of Life, communion with angels, the Sevenfold Peace, and the Dead Sea Scrolls.[11-c]

B11, Clear/Pink, is a more intense version of B55, Clear/Red, known as the Christ bottle. Pink is the illumination of the red, bringing light to the red issues of survival and existence. The Essenes believed that the angelic realm needed to be brought into every aspect of life—into food, meditation, teaching, gardening, and so on. B11 represents both the suffering, the persecution, and the well of unshed tears and the angelic connection within every aspect of life.

Developing self-acceptance encourages the potential for clarity in the conscious mind. The pink encourages us to bring warmth, tenderness, and compassion to the deepest parts of ourselves. As we accept what we find within the shadow of ourselves, we may find it easier to bring more light into our conscious mind. This Essene bottle describes shining the light on the is-ness of acceptance, particularly the acceptance of self.

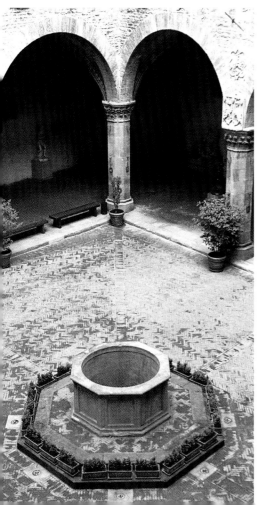

The Chain of Flowers symbolizes the illumination of the chakras, which are like flowers. Light represented by the clear fraction is brought to the energy centers. Through understanding suffering, we come to a point of acceptance. If these qualities are brought within the depths of the self, our being becomes illumined: the flowers become more full of light, and they blossom to become a chain of flowers.

The Chain of Flowers can also be the chain that leads to us being caught, or chained, to desire. It is one thing to see a shop full of cakes and appreciate them. If we then proceed to eat them all, we will inevitably suffer the consequences. Each of us must work with this concept and consider how the Chain of Flowers pertains to our own life.

B11 has much to do with the release of spiritual pride and the invoking of unconditional love. It may help a woman who wishes to conceive. Choosing it may

Related Bottles

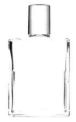

Related Color
B54

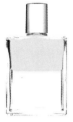

Reverse
B71

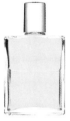

Closest Tint
B52

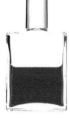

Closest Hue
B55

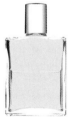

Shakes To
B52

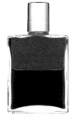

Return Journey
B89

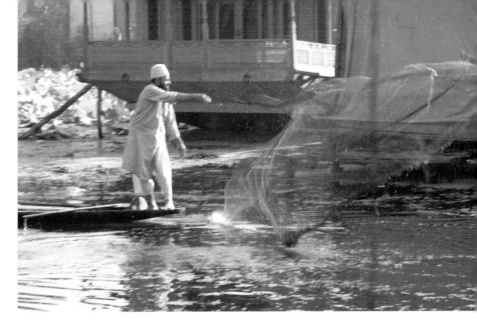

indicate that we have clarity of mind and are able to give love, warmth, and caring to others and to our selves, that we shine light on the love we have within. We may function as mediators. B11 can also suggest that we have the gift of unconditional self-acceptance. It can illuminate the need for us to learn to receive love as well as our innate ability to give love, to be a mediator, to be humble in self-acceptance, and to overcome self-doubt. B11 can clear the way when other Aura-Soma substances are not yet effective. It also facilitates contact with Essene incarnations.

The contents of this bottle can be applied around the throat and the entire trunk, including the hips, the lower abdomen, the lower back, and the lower spinal column.

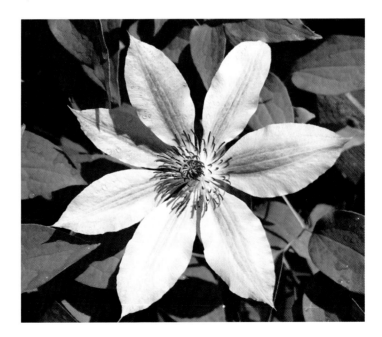

Top: Light catches the red net of a man from Shikara float on Dal Lake, Kashmir. Fishing is a source of livelihood for many people around the Srinagar's lakes.
Bottom: Clematis in Ripton, Vermont.
Left: Plaza del Bargello in Florence, Italy.
Note: The image on page 287 is also a visual expression of this bottle.

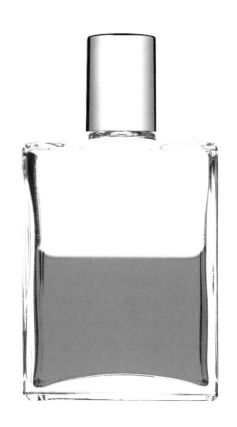

B12 Clear/Blue

Name: Peace in the New Aeon
Shakes Together As: Pale Blue
Tarot Card: The Hanged Man
Keynote: An initiation; shining the light on nurturing, faith, and peace.

In Aura-Soma, blue energy represents peace, and thus the blue in the base fraction of this combination indicates the possibility of peace within the depths of ourselves, with clarity above.

When a color is presented in its paler aspect, the qualities of that color are intensified. When B12 is shaken, the pale blue that appears is like the pale blue in B50, El Morya, whose key phrase is "Thy will, not my will, be done." If we are truly able to follow "Thy will," we are more likely to be at peace in ourselves, whatever the circumstances, and more able to fulfill a higher purpose.

B12 has also been referred to as a bottle of initiation. This is interesting when we consider its tarot title, the Hanged Man, which represents one who has been through a process of initiation but has not fully integrated the experience and therefore feels "upside down" in the world. Through the integration of light, the Hanged Man may become known as the Redeemer. An integration of the consequences of going through an initiatory process helps us come to a greater sense of peace, or the possibility of "Peace in the New Aeon."

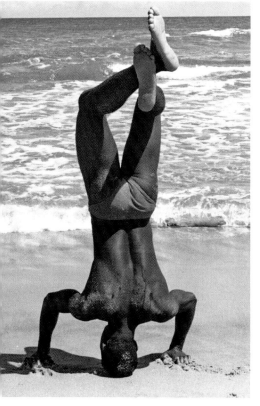

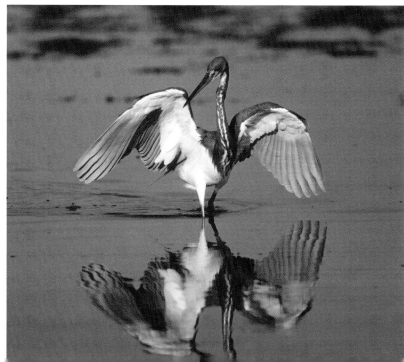

Related Bottles

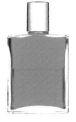

Related Colors
B2

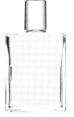

B50

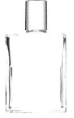

B54

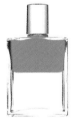

Reverse
B60

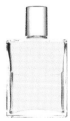

Closest Tint and
Shakes To
B50

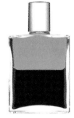

Return Journey
B90

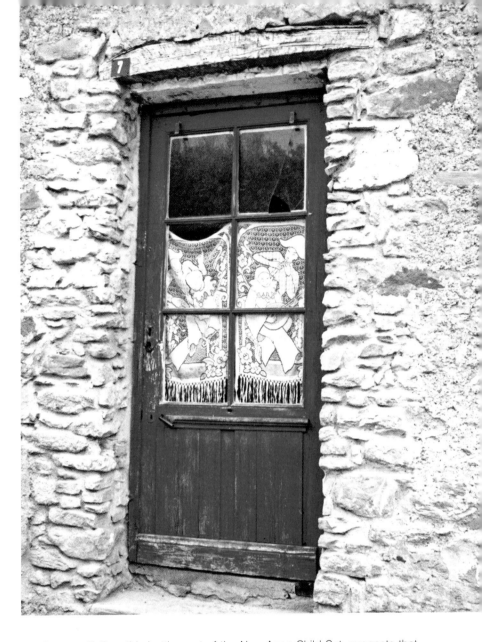

In consultation, this bottle, part of the New Aeon Child Set, suggests that we have both creativity and clarity of thought, that we have nurturing qualities (blue), and that we are able to communicate our feelings to others when in an atmosphere of trust. We feel inspired and can speak about our inspiration and intuitive insights. We are able to listen to our own feelings and find peace. Conversely, it may imply that we lack peace and may not allow our tears (clear) to flow. We may have difficulty with the masculine side of our inner self, and perhaps therefore we may not respond well to authority.

Apply the contents of this bottle around the entire neck.

Above: Doorway near Minerve, a Cathar stronghold in Midi-Pyrénées, France.
Page 82, left: Man doing a handstand, training in the Brazilian martial art of Capoeira, a foot-fighting technique disguised as gymnastics, which was historically how slaves prepared for a rebellion from slavery. Salvador, Bahia, Brazil.
Page 82, right: Tri-colored heron at the J.N. "Ding" Darling National Wildlife Refuge on Sanibel Island, Florida.

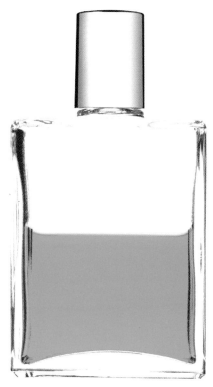

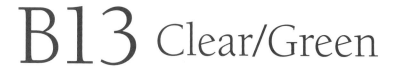

B13 Clear/Green

Name: Change in the New Aeon
Shakes Together As: Pale Green
Tarot Card: Death
Keynote: Illuminating of the emotional side of life.

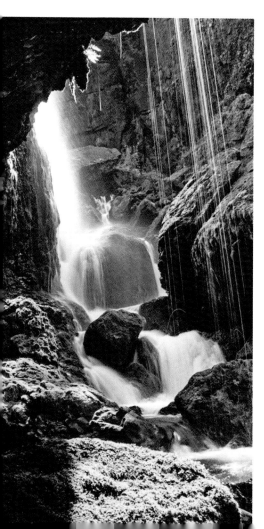

Green is associated with direction, decision making, making the space to find oneself, and the understanding of time and space. When a person chooses a bottle where green appears in the base fraction, that means these qualities represent a person's intrinsic nature. Such an understanding implies the possibility of being in the "here and now," from where change and new direction can occur.

In B13, another member of the New Aeon Child Set, light is shone on the green. Shaking B13 gives the pale green of B53, Hilarion, whose key phrase is "The Way, the Truth, and the Light." As light is brought to the heart, transition comes about; we experience a change of state from one thing to another. By making the space for our selves, more light can come to our heart.

For change to occur, we have to die to what has been, so something new can be born. B13's tarot association is Death, and at times we might view this bottle as a difficult one. In reality B13, like the tarot card itself, suggests new beginnings. This bottle supports metamorphosis; the transformative effect of clear and green helps us overcome "spiritual materialism." Although progress in these matters always depends on grace from above, this oil supports the process of understanding. It can be reassuring to remember that with every ending there is a new beginning.

Death is a powerful symbol for change, an obvious shift from one state to another. In this new millennium, perhaps change will be the way of the heart. In the past, humanity seems to have overemphasized issues relating to the first three energy centers (the root, sacral, and solar-plexus chakras). The energy of green, linked to the fourth energy center, the heart chakra, presents the opportunity for energy to come into the heart, wherein lies the feeling, emotional part of our nature.

Through B13, we purify and shine light (the clear fraction) on that green aspect, dying to what has been in the heart so that new light may shine on it. Maybe change will occur. The green suggests that we should have hope in relation to the changes that may occur, as we die to who or what we have been in the past. This bottle may be of help with rebirthing. It can symbolize that we are at a crossroads in life, which gives us an opportunity to see things clearly in a

Related Bottles

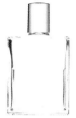

Related Color
B54

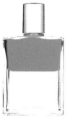

Reverse
B64

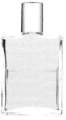

Shakes To
B53

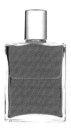

Return Journey
B91

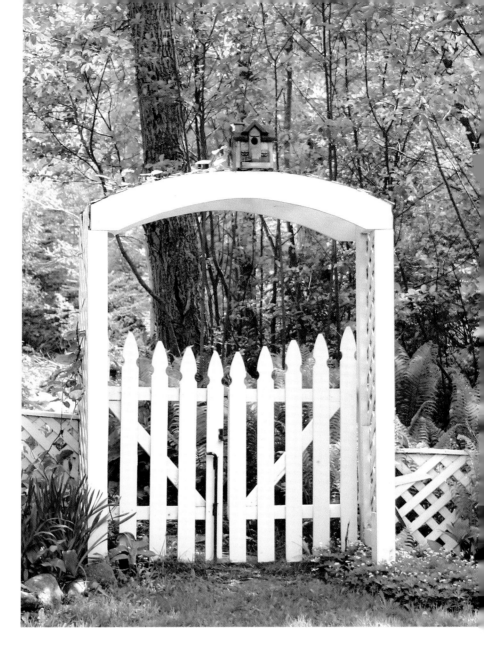

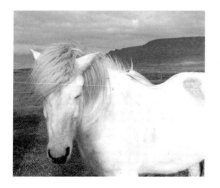

Above: Icelandic white horse, Iceland.
Top right: White gateway in Ripton, Vermont.
Page 84: The Falls of Lana above Lake Dunmore in
    Salisbury, Vermont.

balanced (green) and harmonious way. Hidden in this bottle are blue and yellow, helping in communicating joy and knowledge.

Paradoxically, change is the only constant. It is a time to face our circumstances and make decisions on the direction in which to move, to let go of the past, set new goals, and plan for the right time to implement them.

Apply the contents of this bottle around the entire heart area, in a band that extends around the back to include the spinal column.

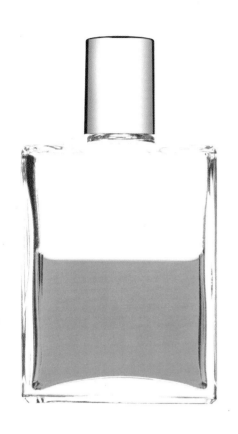

B14 Clear/Gold

Name: Wisdom in the New Aeon
Shakes Together As: Clear Bubbles Rimmed with Gold
Tarot Card: Temperance
Keynote: Getting in touch with wisdom so that clarity may unfold.

This bottle's colors represent the shining of light on the golden area within the self. The golden area houses what, in Aura-Soma, is called the true aura, the memory of the first cell, and the incarnational star (see "The Subtle Anatomy," page 23). Here we may touch our true essence.

The more we get in touch with the gold within ourselves, the more likely it is that we can find the clarity we need in our conscious mind to be able to let go of suffering and to find light within. However, before we can contact the gold, we must let go of the fears and difficulties that surround our identity and personality. Our inner wisdom can be a source of strength and encouragement in the process of letting go. We may then come to know ourselves more fully, and we can present our wisdom in the world when we find a way to rely on, or to be encouraged by, this inner wisdom. B14 may help heal wounds and scars from previous incarnations. For children, it may alleviate fears and anxiety related to starting school or taking examinations. B14 shows us the wisdom (gold) and clarity (clear) we need to discover who we really are, our "inner self," helping

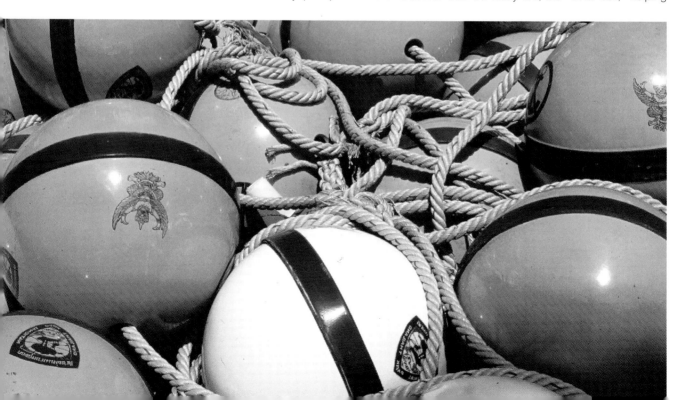

Related Bottles

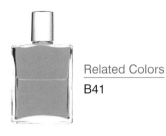

Related Colors
B41

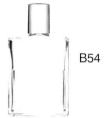

B54

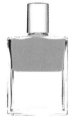

Reverse
B73

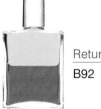

Return Journey
B92

us find freedom through recognizing our inner wisdom. To believe in ourselves brings deep happiness.

There is a distinction between knowledge and wisdom. Knowledge is what we acquire from books, teachers, media, and so on. Wisdom comes from within and is already existing inside us. We are trained and conditioned to search for knowledge outside our selves, unaware of the wealth of wisdom waiting to be contacted within. In B14, the wisdom lies beneath the light, waiting for the opportunity to express itself in the world.

Possibly in the New Aeon there will be different opportunities to gain in wisdom other than through suffering. Clear/Gold, a member of the New Aeon Child Set, reminds us of the intimate connection between suffering and the understanding of suffering (clear) and discovery of the wisdom lying within (gold). B14 offers the opportunity to move through self-doubt and address any anxieties, fears, or frustrations. It may suggest that we need to release painful memories and old wounds, to allow a healing process to commence.

Apply B14 in a wide band around the circumference of the body in the entire area of the solar plexus.

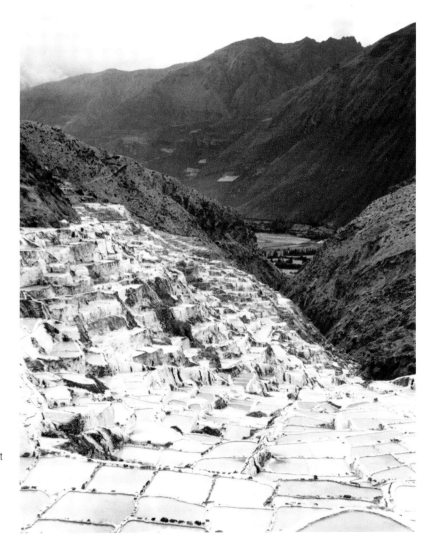

Left: Buoys on boat dock on Phi Phi Island, near Bangkok, Thailand. The dock is adjacent to the Viking cave Tham Phraya Nak, a source of swift nests used for bird's nest soup—the longevity soup fit for an emperor.

Right: Incan salt drying ponds, Maras Salt Mines, Machu Picchu, Peru

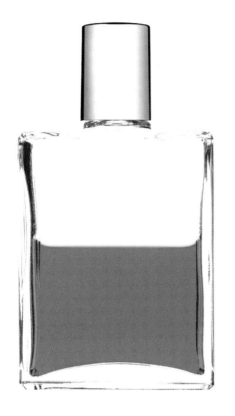

B15 Clear/Violet

Name: Service in the New Aeon
Shakes Together As: Pale Violet/Lilac
Tarot Card: The Devil
Keynote: Elevation of the self through purification.

In the man-made forests of the gothic cathedrals the Green Man is pent, the old pagan wildness tamed in frozen stone. . . . The Green Man derives in part from the horned god of the Celts, then it must have been a cause of supreme satisfaction to the Church Fathers to see the image they regarded as "devilish" caught and pinned on the roof-bosses of their own stone forests.[15-a]

As we look deeply within and begin to face the shadow of ourselves, we find clarity in relation to the spirituality within ourselves. We might become open to the transformation that comes as we become aware of the service that we are to perform in the world. B15 supports this process. In the Jungian sense of the term "shadow," healing involves releasing what lies in the subconscious. On occasion, Vicky referred to it as Healing in the New Aeon. It is a part of the New Aeon Child Set.

In the tarot, the Devil is traditionally depicted as a beast. The beast shows what we may experience when we neither recognize nor release the beast within ourselves. There has been a tendency, certainly over the past two thousand years, to deny the beast within and to project it outward, seeing it in "the other"; this can lead to conflict, both inner and outer. It is part of a problem: if we assimilate and accept the "beast," the problems that the beast represents would not present themselves. We might not as easily fall prey to the chains of those projections and demons of the psyche. Healing comes from the acceptance and integration of this aspect within ourselves.

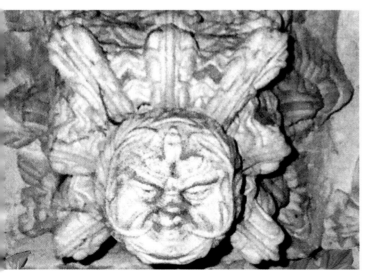

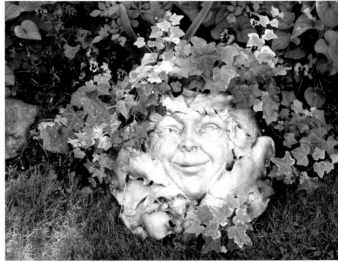

Related Bottles

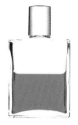

Related Colors
B12

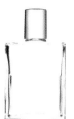

B54

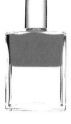

Reverse
B48

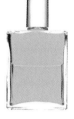

Shakes To
B56

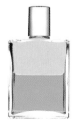

Return Journey
B93

Above: Gothic cathedral in Othery, England.
Page 88, left: Stone carving of Green Man with foliage at Rosslyn Chapel in Scotland.
Page 88, right: Pottery sculpture of Pan with Ivy in Ripton, Vermont.

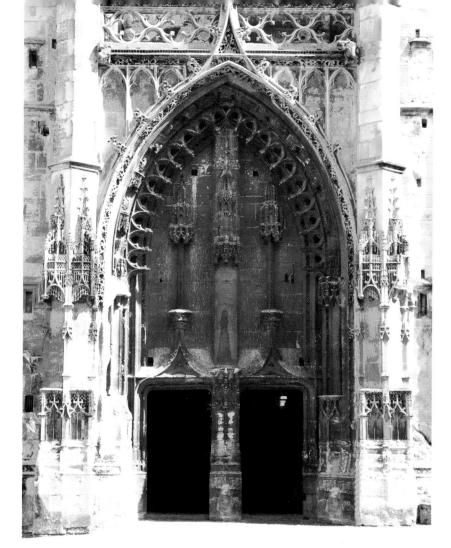

Unfortunately, this beastly aspect, that which we may deny within our selves, is the most difficult to heal. To see ourselves clearly, we need to move away from denial; this is part of the healing. Letting go of the suffering, represented by the clear fraction, brings the possibility of cleansing the denial; this in turn enables us to recognize the beast within ourselves. When we allow light to flood our conscious mind, the light of understanding supports healing within the depth of ourselves.

B15 may be appropriate for women in labor, as it can ease the intensity of contractions, and it could help bring about a quite conscious birth experience for the mother.

Choosing B15 may suggest that we have a clear vision to see who we really are and to connect with our service or, as healers (violet), to have the clarity of mind to allow our gifts to evolve. This clarity illuminates the shadows within. In turn, this selection may suggest that we are in need of healing and that we wish to be in control, both of ourselves and our circumstances. B15 may tell us to stop looking at situations from a purely materialistic perspective.

The contents of this bottle should be applied along the hairline around the entire head.

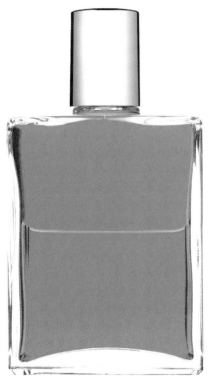

B16 Violet/Violet

Name: The Violet Robe

Shakes Together As: **Violet**

Tarot Card: **The Tower**

Keynote: Awakening to our true self and service. A complete re-evaluation.

Vicky used to perceive many things about people who were drawn to work with color, including that some "wore" robes of blue or violet. Taking on a robe has a tremendous tradition and history to it. A violet robe is sometimes referred to as a robe of initiation. It is a symbol of and preparation for a transformation yet to come.

B16 is linked to the Tower in the tarot. The path of the Tower joins together two pillars of the Tree of Life,[16-a] the light and the dark, mercy and severity. Violet/Violet represents metanoia, a complete change, a transformation that leads in the direction of a change of being. This change takes place not just in the way we think about things, but in every aspect of the mind. Everything we believed, thought, and felt is transformed. Similarly, wearing the Violet Robe represents a new level of spirituality, suggesting that the previous form of spiritual existence has fallen away and a new being has come about. Violet implies a deep transformational experience.

To paraphrase a Zen saying, "In the beginning the trees are trees, the rivers are rivers, and the mountains are mountains. As you go along the path, the

Right: Sailing on Lake Champlain. Oftentimes, sunset is the best time to see through the clouds. Despite a miserably cloudy day, the sun breached what few cuts in the cloud there were just enough to prove to everyone that it was still there.

Below: The Magere Brug Drawbridge in Amsterdam where a drawbridge has spanned the River Amstel since 1672. Illuminated with thousands of lights at night, originally it was known as the Skinny Bridge because it was barely wide enough for two people to pass.

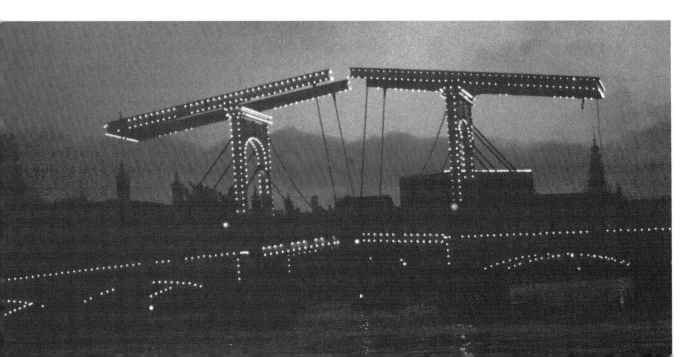

Related Bottles

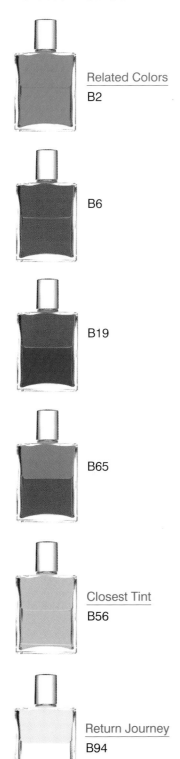

Related Colors
B2

B6

B19

B65

Closest Tint
B56

Return Journey
B94

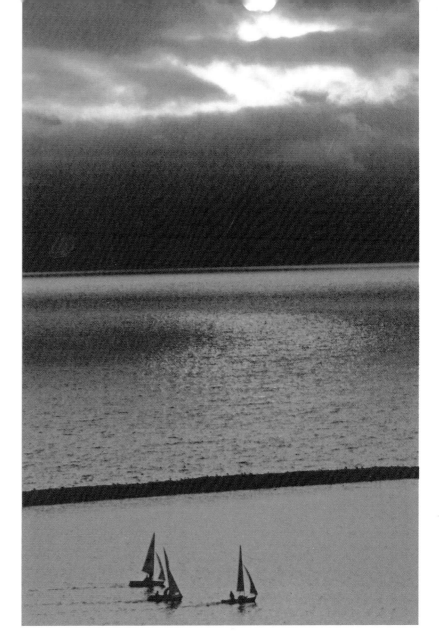

mountains are no longer mountains, the trees are no longer trees, and the rivers are no longer rivers. You go along the path a little further and the trees are the trees again, the mountains are the mountains again, the rivers are the rivers again, but the difference is that we no longer believe it."

The Violet Robe has to do with the development of spiritual understanding, initiated through psychological transformation. B16 suggests that we are experiencing a change that leads to a new direction: the search for true peace. This bottle may help us become aware of who we really are, why we are here, and what we are for, and it may indicate or alleviate self-destructive tendencies. It may indicate that we need to come to terms with grief, whether it is about ourselves or the loss of a loved one, especially when we tend to be confrontational or quarrelsome due to hidden anger. B16 can provide the drive and determination that we need when things are falling apart.

B16 is part of the extended Chakra Set and is connected to the crown chakra. Apply the contents of the bottle along the entire hairline.

B17 Green/Violet

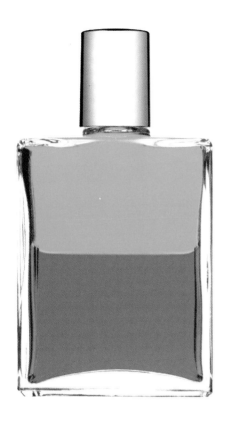

Name: **Troubadour 1/The Hope Bottle**

Shakes Together As: **Dark Green**

Tarot Card: **The Star**

Keynote: **A new beginning for spirituality, to get in touch with the star.**

I want to stay faithful, guard your honor,
Seek peace, obey
Fear, serve and honor you,
Until death,
Peerless Lady.[17-a]

The troubadours were performers who traveled through much of Europe during the twelfth to fourteenth centuries. Their beliefs in Christian mysticism were often opposed to the teaching of the Church. The Fourth Crusade, known as the Albigensian-Waldensian Crusade (1208–1213), was directed against the spreading of "heresy" in southern France, including that of the troubadours.[17-b] The troubadours, despite the Church's persecution, tried to spread their messages through song, dance, mystery plays, and drama—in effect, through creative means. They expressed their truth (green) in the service of others (violet). The persecution they experienced at the hands of the Church is an implicit part of B17. This bottle may aid us in contacting incarnations between the twelfth and sixteenth centuries, such as among the Cathars and Knights Templar.[17-c]

B17 is thought of as an "upside down" bottle because the heart (green) is above the head (violet), which in the human body is not possible.

Another name for B17 is Hope, and its tarot symbolism is the Star. The star principle and the three stars (the earth star, the incarnational star, and the soul star) are very important in Aura-Soma (see "The Subtle Anatomy," page 23). B17 offers us a beacon of hope for the future and a hint about the process of transformation of the heart: the hope is for the dawning of the Aquarian aeon, and the

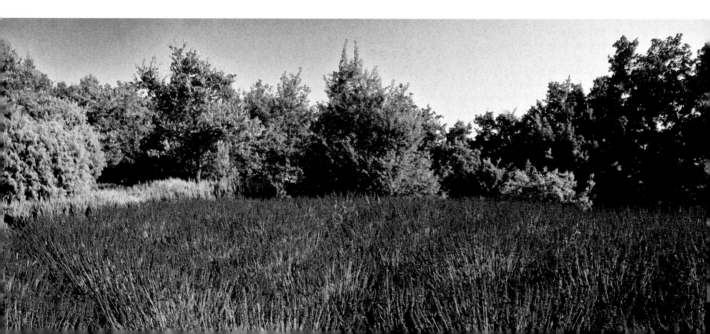

Related Bottles

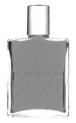

Related Colors
B2

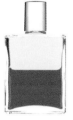

B5

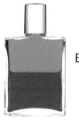

B30

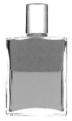

Reverse
B38

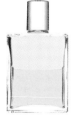

Closest Tint
B58

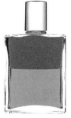

Return Journey
B95

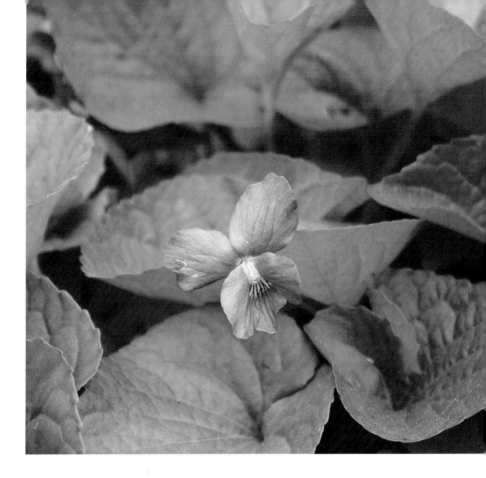

transformation of the heart is a spiritual one. For the past two thousand years we have been moving through the Piscean aeon.[17-d] We, humanity, are now in the process of change as we move toward the beginning of the Aquarian aeon. B17 can imply that we have found space (green) in which to show our feelings and express our selves, or that we have an inspirational creativity and can join our feminine intuition with our spirituality. It may provide hope to those of us who need to let go of fear and anxiety. This bottle can show that we have a need for healing, especially following an emotional upset or disappointment related to matters of the heart; it also highlights our challenges with self-doubt, stubbornness, and an inability to trust or a fear of trusting ourselves or others.

Many bottles relate to B17, B24, B38, and B49 suggesting that these bottles have many levels of meaning.

Apply this combination around the entire chest area in a wide band including the back, covering the spinal column. With problems of a spiritual or mental nature, also apply it along the hairline.

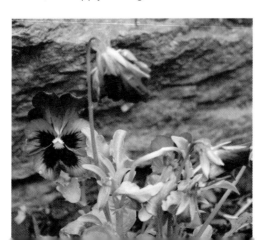

Above: Violet in Ripton, Vermont.
Left: A shy pansy in rock crevice in Ripton, Vermont.
Page 92: Sweet lavender field, in full bloom in June, providing the never-to-be-forgotten beautiful aroma of Provence, France, the region in which the troubadour movement arose and flourished. Here the troubadours and minstrals composed and performed songs and lyric poems of love and devotion.

93

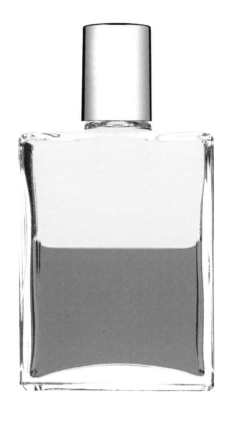

B18 Yellow/Violet

Name: Egyptian Bottle 1/Turning Tide
Shakes Together As: Deep Gold
Tarot Card: The Moon
Keynote: Refining the knowledge that we may get in touch with why we are here and what we are for.

In the Piscean aeon, the belief was that the priesthood held the keys to the door of our being. With the advent of the Aquarian aeon, the emphasis is changing to a sharing modality in which we all hold the keys. Those doing the sharing are helping to offer the keys to all the people who are able and willing to receive them, so that each may unlock his or her own door. This is a completely different belief system, based on equanimity, equality, and humanitarian independence.

Yellow and violet are complementary color opposites and represent mental and spiritual qualities. As we travel upon the journey of our lives, we have the opportunity to get to know ourselves more thoroughly. We become more whole and get in touch with the purpose of our existence.

B18 may be part of a healing for the patterns left from the Egyptian epoch (circa 3500 BC to AD 500[18-a]; see B39) and for issues related to the solar plexus. The Egyptian epoch occurred within the Piscean era, and this color combination relates very much to that energy. Curiously, B17, the bottle of the Aquarian aeon,

Page 95, top: Sunset viewed through a wheat field, on the border between Minnesota and South Dakota. An hour later a massive storm developed spawning tornadoes and severe lightning.
Page 95, bottom: Boar on river rock in Pittsfield, Vermont.
Below: The Harvest Moon, late September, overlooking Frenchman Bay in Acadia National Park, Maine.

Related Bottles

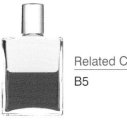

Related Colors
B5

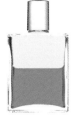

B8

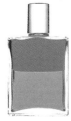

Related Reverse
B39

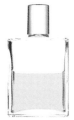

Closest Tint
B59

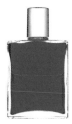

Return Journey
B96

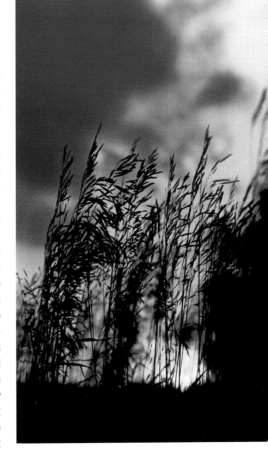

is next to B18 in the unfolding order of the Equilibrium. This arrangement has greater meaning when we consider the other name of the bottle, Turning Tide. B18 marks the current time, when humanity is between one era and another. The Piscean era has not completely ended, and the Aquarian aeon has not fully come into being; in a sense, we are at the point of a turning tide.

The tarot card associated with B18 is the Moon, associating the bottle with tides in another way. The moon influences the tides on earth. As water-based beings, we are subject to the power of the moon and the turning of tides. This concept can help us in understanding our own emotional cycles, and whether we identify with those or remain more centered. Yellow belongs to the solar plexus and violet to the head. Perhaps as we overcome our thinking and come to a great sense of joy, our own tides will turn.

B18 may help us connect to incarnational experiences related to moon worship and to lives in ancient Egypt. It may fit those of us who have a broad knowledge as well as a spirituality and a healing ability. It also reveals knowledge about how to find the appropriate healing for others. In turn, it may be chosen by those of us who suffer greatly from hidden fears and anxieties, who may let our imagination run wild. Fears are created by such internalization of thought, and we may not be able to think clearly.

Apply this combination at the hairline and in a band around the circumference of the body in the area of the solar plexus.

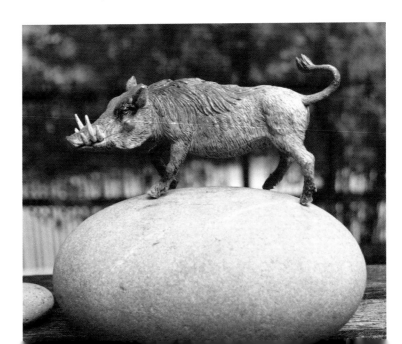

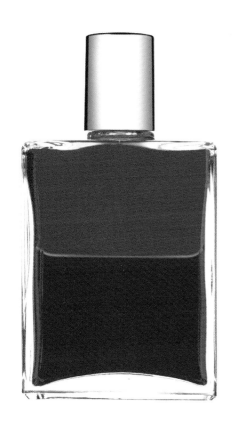

B19 Red/Purple

Name: Living in the Material World

Shakes Together As: Magenta

Tarot Card: The Sun

Keynote: The renewal of our bodies takes place when we change our thinking to build up new energy.

B19, Living in the Material World, has to do with coming to terms with life in the material sense, possibly after living in a spiritual community or doing a spiritual practice. Those of us who are well balanced and who have much energy, who can see into spiritual matters, and can serve through offering healing gifts may feel called to B19.

Red/Purple could help to deal with abusive situations, poltergeist phenomena, or other undesired past or present interferences or entities. If used too late in the day, it may be overenergizing; on the other hand, it might be helpful in cases of extreme fatigue.

Red above the purple may indicate an "upside-down" situation. If we are "upside down" and also living in the material world, we could be in danger of putting the whole of the material side of life above the spiritual, or we may be inclined to put the values of materiality above spirituality. Thus, B19 can suggest that in order to feel free, we need to let go of frustration, resentment, and anger.

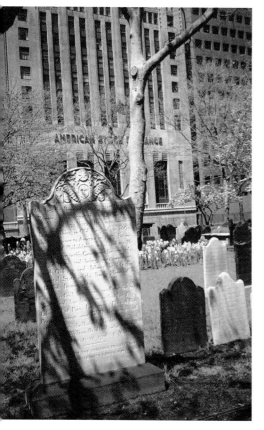

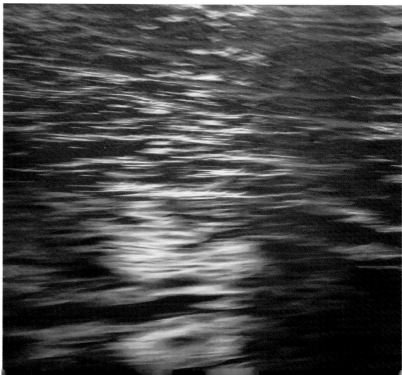

Related Bottles

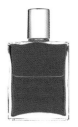

Related Colors
B6

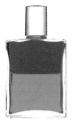

B29

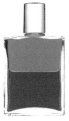

Reverse
B65

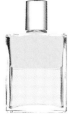

Closest Tint
B57

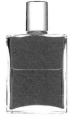

Shakes To
B67

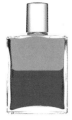

Return Journey
B97

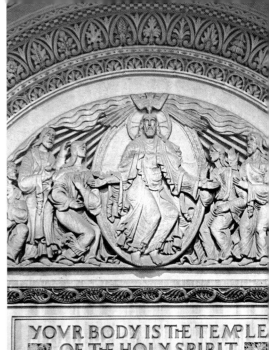

YOVR BODY IS THE TEMPLE OF THE HOLY SPIRIT

The passion within could instead be used for the good of the self. As each of us has chosen to come into incarnation, we have agreed to come to terms with the material world. We also are thus given the opportunity to spiritualize the process of living in the world. Our attitude can be the key to this. Often we live life through fear and anxiety; we may become focused on ourselves and on having to succeed at all costs, rather than on sharing the experience of life in a most meaningful manner. B19 reminds us of the opportunity to awaken to the spirituality that lies within, to come to terms with our survival issues so that we can live in the material world in a different, more spiritually based way.

Red/Purple can be awakening to spirit. Finding the discipline and focus necessary in the conscious mind to be able to heal that which needs to be healed within the depth of ourselves opens the door for us to move on with our service in the world and to live in harmony with the material world.

For mental or spiritual matters, apply the contents of this bottle along the hairline. B19 also can go around the entire lower abdomen and lower back area.

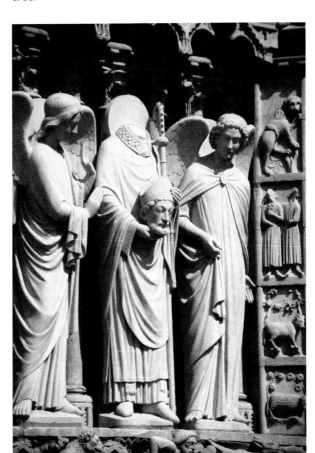

Above: The message of Saint Paul of Tarsus, on Saint Bartholomew's Church in New York City, a church committed to unconditional welcome for the seeker.
Left: Saint Denis holding his head, Notre Dame de Paris, France.
Page 96, left: Trinity Church graveyard, the site of one of the oldest churches in America, with New York Stock Exchange in background, New York City. For eight months, Trinity Church was a center for volunteer relief efforts after the 9/11 attack on the Twin Towers.
Page 96, right: Sunset on water, Long Island Sound.

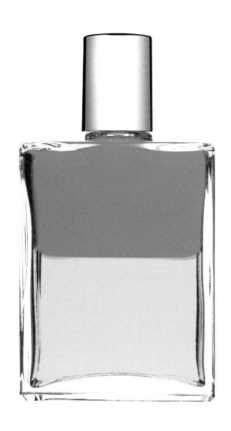

B20 Blue/Pink

Name of the Bottle: Star Child
Shakes Together As: Light Violet
Tarot Card: Judgment
Keynote: The communication of unconditional love. Peace in the conscious mind, self-acceptance within the depths of the self.

Note: The image on the acknowledgments page at the beginning of this book is also a visual expression of this bottle.

B20, Blue/Pink, is the Star Child bottle. It and B11, Clear/Pink, the Love Rescue bottle, are two members of the Rescue Set that do not have a deep magenta base. The Star Child, Vicky felt, might be a more appropriate Rescue bottle for children, as they had not yet developed to physical maturity, than would the Physical Rescue (B1). B20 may be helpful for children in ways similar to how the Physical Rescue bottle may be helpful for adults. But even as adults, we too may have a need to heal, to rescue, the child within us. This color combination offers a gentle four-way internal balance of the male (blue) and female (pink) within, that which is above us, and that which is beneath us. It contains the warmth and love of a child, with a child's potential for forgiveness. It can support us as we address issues connected with our childhood and with our own inner child. It is

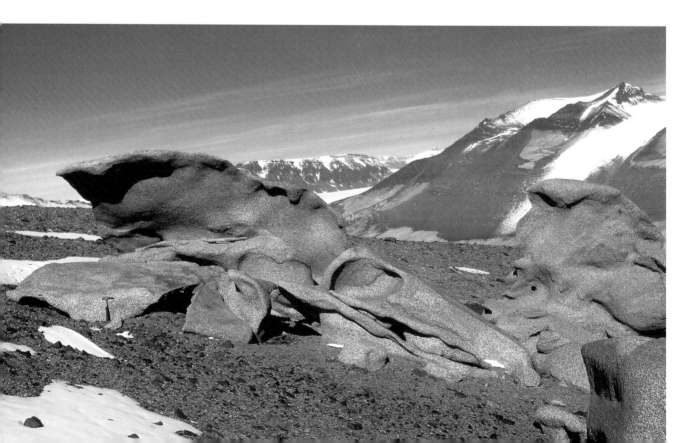

Related Bottles

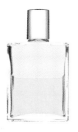

Closest Tint
B58

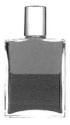

Closest Hue
B30

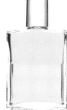

Reverse Tint
B57

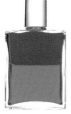

Reverse Hue
B29

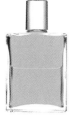

Shakes To
B56

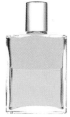

Return Journey
B98

also part of the New Aeon Child Set and part of the Chakra Set, associated with the crown chakra.

Blue/Pink presents the possibility of transmuting negativity and of reconciling the paradoxes that exist in the pink and the blue, internally balancing the male and female energies. Vicky would say that as humans, the only right we have is not to be negative. We have a choice about whether, through gossip, action, or whatever, we contribute to negative energies.[20-a] The color lilac, which results from shaking the blue and pink together, suggests the possibility of transmuting that sort of negative energy. The lilac is an alchemical transmutation within the self. B20 is especially useful in polarity work.

The Star Child poses the potentiality that part of our ancestry as human beings comes from the stars. To bring the earthly part (pink, which is red with light) together with the heavenly part (blue) is to acknowledge and fulfill our destiny.

In consultation, B20 may refer to those of us who have the peace (blue) to communicate our caring and love (pink) to ourselves and others. We might be compassionate communicators who know that love is a great transformer (the light violet B20 is shaken to), who embody unconditional self-acceptance and express nurturing. We may also need to resolve difficulties from our childhood, to forgive and accept ourselves, or to be more assertive.

This bottle can be applied anywhere on the body. With teething babies, apply to the jaw and around the entire neck (but be sure to use it only externally).

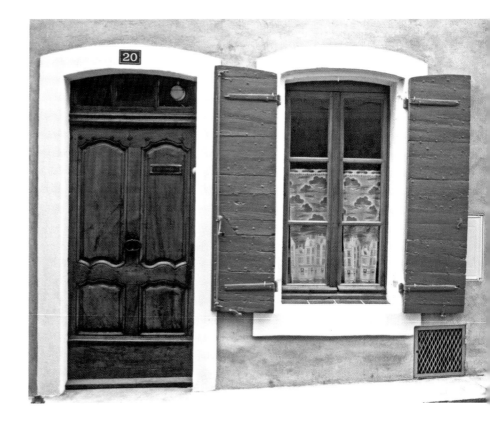

Above: Open window in Vaucluse region, France.
Left: Primal forces in Antarctica. Wind erosion in Bull Pass, where rocks are shaped by catabatic winds moving from the high atmospheric pressures over the Polar Plateau to lower pressure in the Dry Valleys.

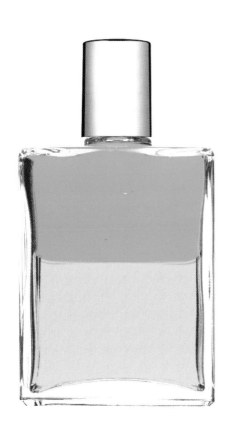

B21 Green/Pink

Name: New Beginning for Love
Shakes Together As: Green
Tarot Card: The World
Keynote: The emergence of freedom through self-acceptance.

B21, New Beginning for Love, shows us the green of the heart center and the pink of caring and warmth. Pink can express itself only through the green heart area. The energy presented in this color combination is like the beginning of spring, when the first new green shoots come into being, showing us new life and the bounty of the earth, the red of earth illumined to pink. We may start afresh with caring for ourselves so that love may flow through our hearts, renewed; as we love ourselves anew, we may experience giving and receiving love in a new way. Through increasing our self-acceptance (pink), we are more likely to come to the heart. This means making space for what we need to do for ourselves. If we do this, amid our hurry and the busy-ness of life, we can make a big difference to the whole of the way we live our lives.

B21 is a variation of B20, with the addition of yellow in the upper fraction,

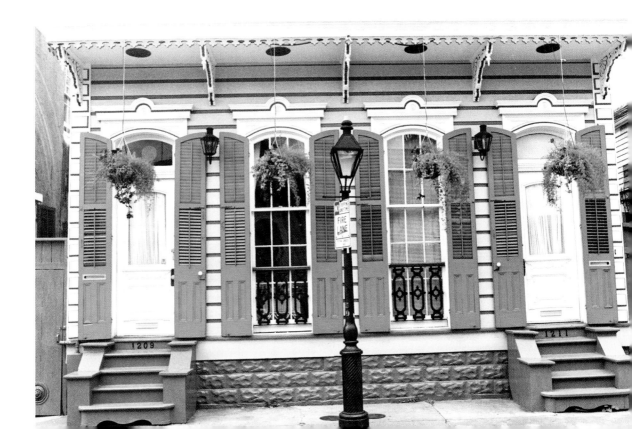

Related Bottles

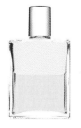

Closest Tint
B99

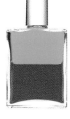

Closest Hue
B28

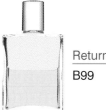

Return Journey
B99

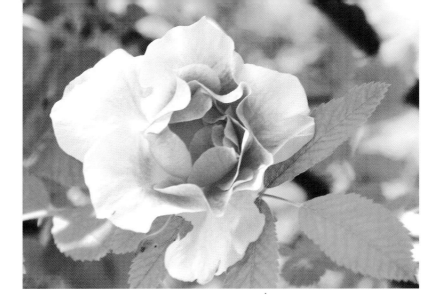

implying a knowledge (yellow) of the inner child (B20). Hidden within B21 is Blue/Pink (B20, Star Child) and Yellow/Pink (B22, Rebirth). Green/Pink is central to that sequence and suggests that the rebirth of the inner child comes in the context of a "new beginning for love." At the same time, these color combinations are very grounding, intensifying the red root in the pink, helping us connect with our root. When we allow ourselves to trust, we will find the love we have.

B20 may suggest that we have the space (green) to give love and warmth to others and that we can see many sides of situations. It may also suggest that we have a love of nature. Alternatively, B21 sometimes indicates our need to let go of pride and vanity in order to move forward. Then it is easier to learn the lessons life presents. We may need to accept ourselves and be less resistant to change. With self-acceptance, we may find a new heartfelt direction.

Apply B21 around the entire heart area.

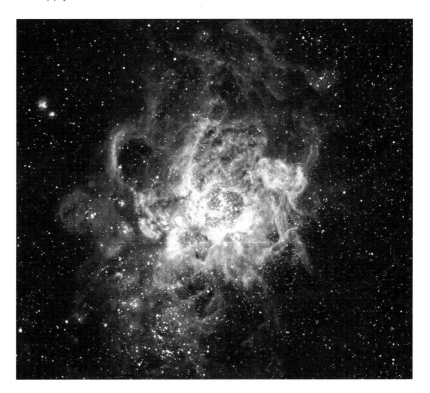

Top right: Rose in Ripton, Vermont.
Right: Birth of a star nebula.
Left: House in New Orleans, Louisiana.

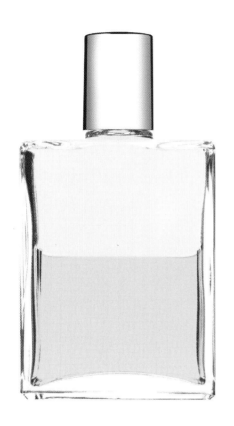

B22 Yellow/Pink

Name: The Rebirther's Bottle/Awakening

Shakes Together As: Pale Coral

Tarot Card: Return Journey of the Fool—The Awakened Fool, Fool's Mastership

Keynote: A new beginning for joy and self-acceptance.

During the early years of Aura-Soma, many people who came for consultations were practitioners of rebirthing. Rebirthing uses breathing techniques to help people remember their birthing experience, and to go through some of the energetics of the birth experience. Vicky noticed how frequently these people chose this color combination, and it became known as the Rebirther's bottle.

In the tarot designation, B22 is called the Fool's Mastership. Here the Fool attains the understanding he needs to become more realized and more awakened. This in itself is a rebirth. Jesus said that unless we become reborn in spirit, we cannot be reborn in the physical.[22-a] B22 speaks about many aspects of rebirth and awakening.

Right: English daisies and echinacea in Ripton, Vermont.
Below: Emergence: a monarch butterfly in Massachusetts.

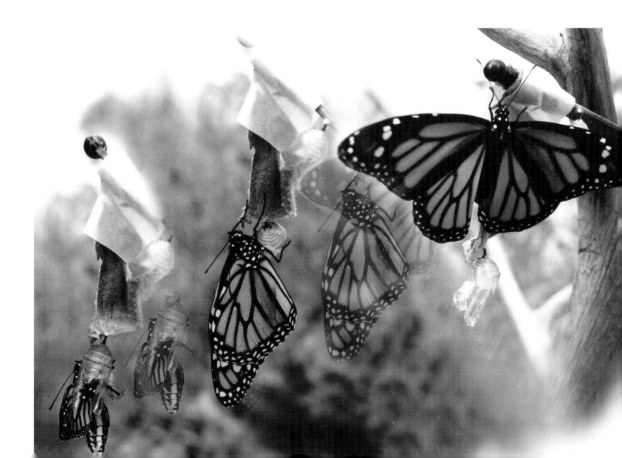

Related Bottles

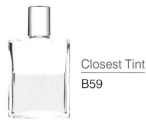

Closest Tint
B59

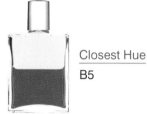

Closest Hue
B5

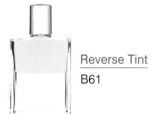

Reverse Tint
B61

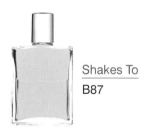

Shakes To
B87

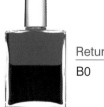

Return Journey
B0

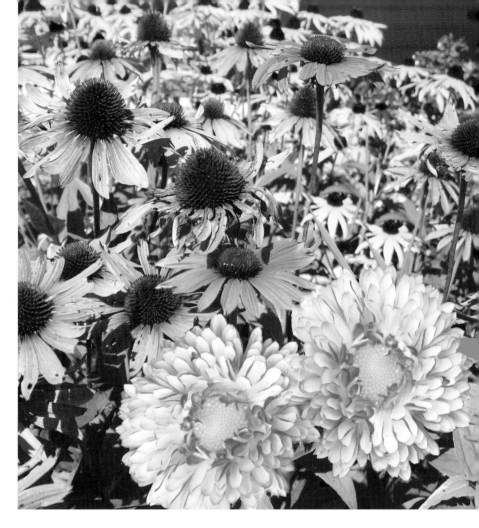

The Fool begins his journey with B0, the journey toward himself. As he develops himself through offering what he has learned—his knowledge—he becomes reborn, awakened, B22. The Fool of B0 travels through the paths on the kabbalistic Tree of Life, developing himself through meeting the challenges symbolized by the major arcana, until his journey arrives at B22. Here we see that the rebirth in spirit, the awakening of the Fool to be in touch with the wholeness of himself, presages the possibility and potential within B0. Thus, in rebirthing, B22 may help the client and therapist attune to the process. (B59 expresses similar issues, but more intensely.)

Yellow/Pink, when shaken, becomes a coral color. In Aura-Soma, this color is associated with the "New Man," the potential for awakening for all. Selecting this bottle implies that we have the knowledge to accept who we are without conditions, that we have the ability to love ourselves unconditionally. To reach this state, we need to find joy and to let go of fears and anxieties. That process allows love to come through. B22 may suggest that we need to get to know ourselves completely, becoming open to true love.

Apply B22 in a wide band around the whole body, at the level of the solar plexus.

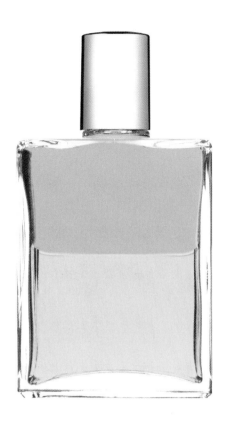

B23 Rose Pink/Pink

Name: Love and Light
Shakes Together As: Pink
Tarot Card: King of Wands
Keynote: Compassion and self-acceptance. The more we find the compassion in the process of seeing ourselves, the more we can accept of ourselves.

In Aura-Soma, pink suggests the energy of love. Pink is an intense form of red; the light coming into red amplifies it, so that all concepts connected to red are intensified in pink. In one sense, the source of light for the world is the sun, which sustains the organic film upon the earth. As the sun rises and sets each day, so the red/pink energy rises and falls. B23, Love and Light, signifies that light may come through caring, warmth, concentration, and the full acceptance of self.

B23 signifies a threshold within the system: in the tarot, it marks the start of the minor arcana and the end of the major arcana. B23 is the King of Wands; the wands represent the fire element, and the king is the principal of that element. The love that is shown by both the pale pink and the rose pink is the fire element in its positive expression. And reflecting the dual aspects of B23, Love and Light, fire has been used throughout humankind's history to illuminate.

Until the birth of B104, B23 was the only Equilibrium bottle to contain rose pink. Rose pink and pink blend passion and compassion. Compassion could be translated as a true feeling, beyond our thinking. Rose Pink/Pink may help us to get in touch with our true feelings. We are able to penetrate the layers of our

Right: Roseate Spoonbill, a large wading bird that feeds in shallow water, at the J.N. "Ding" Darling National Wildlife Refuge on Sanibel Island, Florida.
Below: Paddling a shikara to and from market on the Dal Lake waterways, which are abundant with lotus gardens. Dal Lake is in the Kashmiri Valley and is known as the land of milk and honey.
Note: The image on page 23 is also visual expression of this bottle.

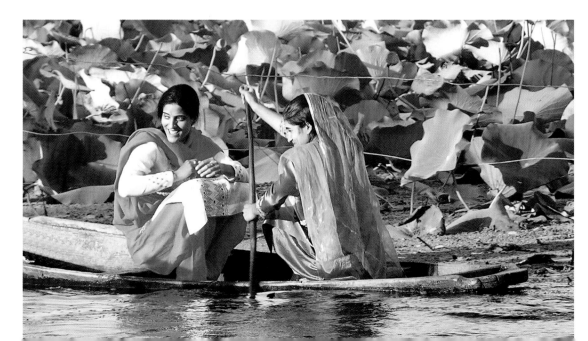

Related Bottles

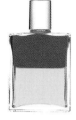

Related Colors
B80

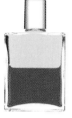

B84

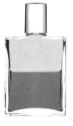

B104

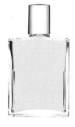

Closest Tints
B52

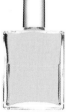

B81

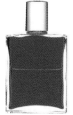

Closest Hue
B6

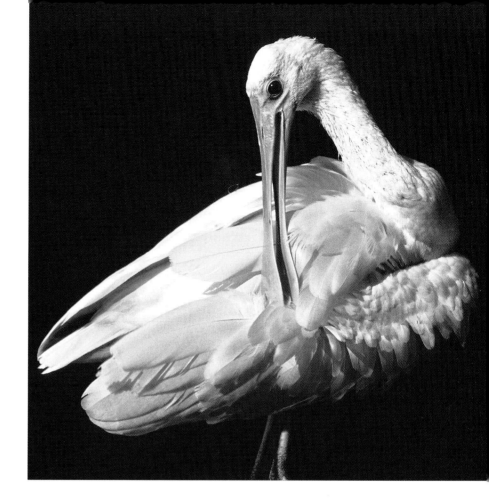

reactivity to understand our true feelings. B23 connects to the human expression of love: how we might care and feel kindness, compassion, and warmth toward one another and ourselves. If we cultivate these qualities, we have a greater possibility of self-acceptance, which can bring more lightness into our being. At times, we may find it easier to find reasons to care for somebody else, rather than ourselves. Even our motivation to become compassionate is frequently directed toward something external. To most fully develop the gifts of love and light, we must also find compassion for ourselves.

Choosing B23 indicates that we give love, warmth, and compassion. It also asks us to accept who we are with love and thus find inspiration and infinite wisdom within. These colors are an awakening combination that shed love and light on the darkest corners of the mind.

B23 may also suggest that we have feelings of not being loved because of fear, suspicion, and the frustrations of unfulfilled love. We may have a tendency toward intolerance, domination, and determination.

Apply B23 around the entire lower abdomen and lower back, including the spinal column. During difficult emotional situations, apply it around the whole heart area. In cases of spiritual and mental problems, apply it along the hairline.

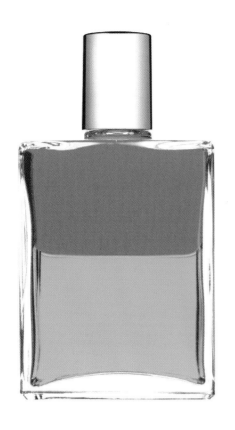

B24 Violet/ Turquoise

Name: A New Message

Shakes Together As: Blue-Violet

Tarot Card: Queen of Wands

Keynote: A communication from the feeling side of the being. A communication inspired from Spirit. A transformative communication from the heart.

B24 was previously known as the Messenger. The violet energy in the upper fraction is in the service of the communication that lies within the turquoise, the creative, heartfelt communication. Understanding the relationship between these two colors gives a sense of the meaning of the name New Message.

The turquoise energy is connected to what Carl Jung described as the collective unconscious, that stream of consciousness that is available to all and that holds relevant information for everyone. The collective unconscious is, to some degree, synonymous with, or parallel to, the process of individuation, the journey inward. On that inner journey we connect with something that is greater than our individual self, something also of the collective, of universal consciousness. Jung realized that as his clients became individuated, synchronistically their drawings expressed more universal symbolism. The personal journey is a journey from alienation through inner contemplation and self-development to more integration.

Page 107, top: Fingal's Cave in the Western Isles of Scotland. This natural cathedral inspired John Keats, Jules Verne, Mendelssohn's "Hebrides Overture," and many others.

Page 107, bottom: Whispering messages: statue in Musee d'Orsay, Paris.

Below: Goetheanum, a center for scientific study of the spiritual nature of humanity and the universe, inspired by Rudolf Steiner, Dornach, Switzerland.

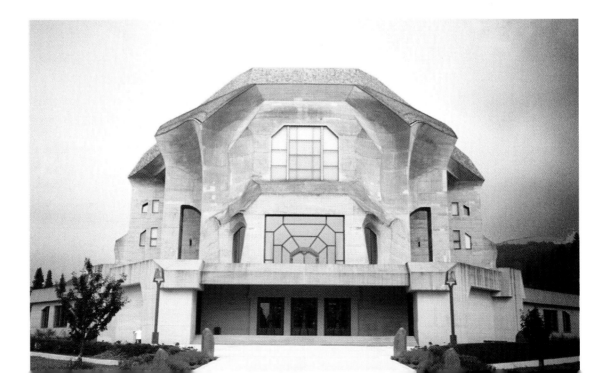

Related Bottles

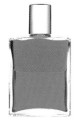

Related Colors
B37

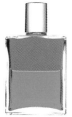

B38

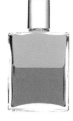

Reverse
B49

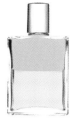

Closest Tint
B44

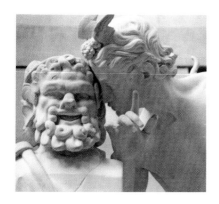

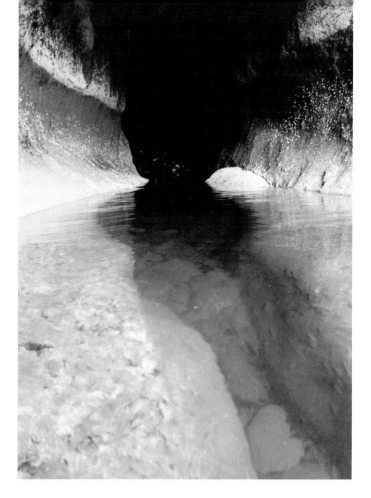

The contents of B24 have much to do with the energies of the planet Venus and thus with matters concerning our emotional life. The New Message of B24 comes from this universal/collective consciousness and may be received by it as well. If we are able to connect with the turquoise energy and offer it in service (violet) to the world, the availability of that which the turquoise carries and represents increases, and a spiritualization of the collective can take place. This is the New Message, the messenger for a new time. Such a messenger has warmth and caring in his or her heart, is able to communicate this to others, and is harmonious and peaceful and heals through service. This spiritual person has the potential to awaken others so that they may remember to give love to themselves.

The New Message arises in answer to the question "Who am I?"—a question in the Ananda Khanda. The New Message asks us to be in touch with the creative communication of our hearts through the feeling side of our beings, and to use that energy within the depths of ourselves to transform our thinking. In Turquoise/Violet, the creativity of turquoise is offered in service to bring the New Message, the new point of view, creatively into the world. This bottle may be appropriate for those of us who have challenges with communication or with expressing our feelings, who may be suspicious, or who may have difficulty in coming to terms with grief and the grieving process.

Apply the contents of this bottle around the heart area and across the back, over the spinal column. In cases of problems with speech or communication, apply around the throat.

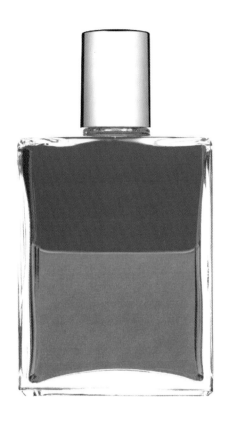

B25 Purple/ Magenta

Name: Florence Nightingale Bottle

Shakes Together As: Purple

Tarot Card: Knight of Wands

Keynote: A mystic. One who is inspired by the inspiration fed in from above. A pioneering spirit in the service of others.

Page 109, top: Summer blossoms in Middlebury, Vermont.
Page 109, bottom: Beauty in the fall in Manchester, Vermont.
Below: Setting sun on ocean in the Galapagos Islands.

Florence Nightingale (1820–1910), through her understanding of nursing, her quality of service, and her spiritual vision, helped change the way nursing is practiced in many countries.[25-a] In her attention to cleanliness and through her care for patients and fellow nurses, she expressed unconditional "love in the little things." This is magenta in its light-full form, as compared to the deep magenta in the base of the Rescue Set bottles. The violet of healing energy and service is in the top fraction in B25. Florence Nightingale is known as the Lady of the Lamp. Many images of her depict her carrying an oil lantern so that she might see her way to come to those in need, whether in a hospital or on the battlefield.

In the first stage of the mystic's spiritual development, there is an awakening of the self to the divine consciousness, to the direct, immediate presence of God. This event is nearly always abrupt and well marked—a "road to Damascus" experience. It triggers a complete shift of consciousness to a higher level. Florence Nightingale's awakening, late in her sixteenth year, was just such

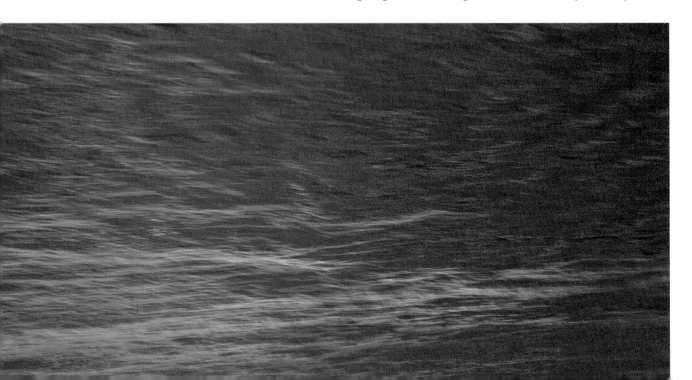

Related Bottles

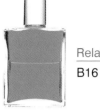

Related Colors
B16

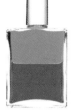

B65

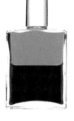

B78

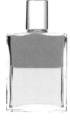

Closest Tint
B36

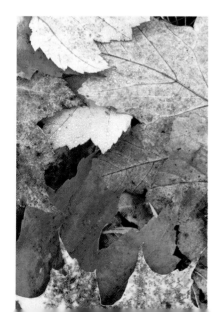

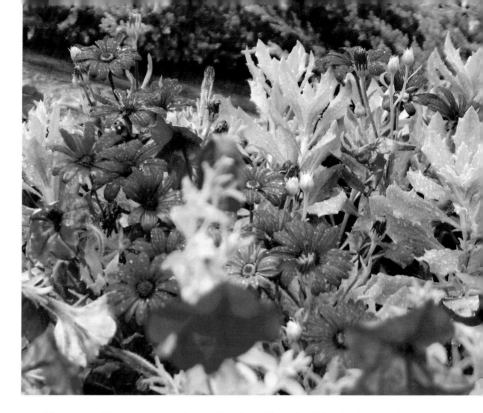

a striking event. She experienced a sudden inner "knowing" that is characteristic of the mystic's calling.[25-b] Often, the moment of awakening is preceded by a period of restlessness, uncertainty, or any activity to which he or she is drawn that readies the person for this encounter with the divine—such as Florence's selfless immersion in nursing during the influenza epidemic of 1837.

Thus, this bottle can indicate that we are called, like Nightingale, to service in healing, expressing deep caring and an ability to see the whole picture. We may have great perseverance and will complete what we have started. If we allow it, magenta energy can come through us. This is love from above, from the soul star, the eighth chakra, our connection to the "source," expressed as putting love into all the details and incidental moments of life. This quality of attention and caring can alleviate the suffering of the dis-eased. B25 symbolizes all of this: service, healing, and love from a divine source put into attentive care.

When we choose this bottle in the second position, often we have been through a major illness, whether mental, physical, or emotional, or we are in the process of recovery, of convalescing, after a major state of dis-ease. When we have been through a trauma or a major dis-ease, we undergo a recovery period during which, although we have improved, our body is still rallying its resources. B25 can symbolize the process of those energies being gathered. We may still need to have caution, as our immune system is vulnerable. B25 may be effective in cases of myalgic encephalomyelitis,[25-c] an illness with symptoms of extreme lethargy and fatigue, headaches, and muscle pain.

Purple/Magenta encourages us to take sufficient care to effect a full recovery. Caregivers, nurses, or medics actively involved in caring for someone recovering from such a serious illness may also be attracted to this color combination. Issues brought forth for attention by B25 may be great disappointments, convalescence, and the need for love. B25 may suggest that we are impulsive or insensitive and may be compensating for feelings of guilt.

Apply B25 along the hairline.

109

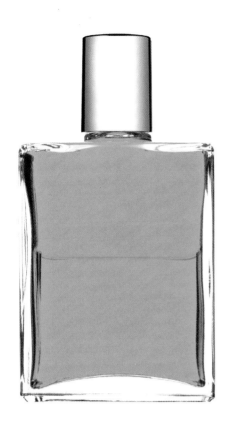

B26 Orange/Orange

Name: Etheric Rescue/Humpty Dumpty Bottle

Shakes Together As: Orange

Tarot Card: Page of Wands

Keynote: The healing of the timeline. Helps us to pull together discrepancies to find a balance toward synchronicity.

B26 is one of the most popular bottles. The egg shape is one of the few forms entirely harmonious to human consciousness. The egg represents the etheric field, the field of developed consciousness in relation to the etheric body. The etheric body is the orange band that goes beyond the bio-energetic field of the physical body.

When we are born, the shape surrounding our physical being is similar to that of a mushroom or tree. As we grow physically and our consciousness unfolds, we have the opportunity for the subtle bodies, which surround the physical body, to develop. Out of that tree or mushroomlike form, the luminous egg-shaped etheric body evolves and becomes more luminous.

Humpty Dumpty of the traditional nursery rhyme has the body of an egg. The most common version of the rhyme begins with this:

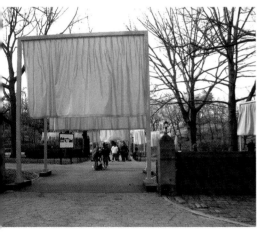

> *Humpty Dumpty sat on a wall.*
> *Humpty Dumpty had a great fall.*
> *All the King's horses and all the King's men*
> *Couldn't put Humpty together again.*

The horses symbolize the emotional body.[26-a] The emotions and somebody in authority, such as the king, have a major repair job to do in relation to the consciousness of the egg. However, neither through emotions nor through authority could they put Humpty Dumpty together. Only through other forces may the state of the egg be brought back into wholeness.

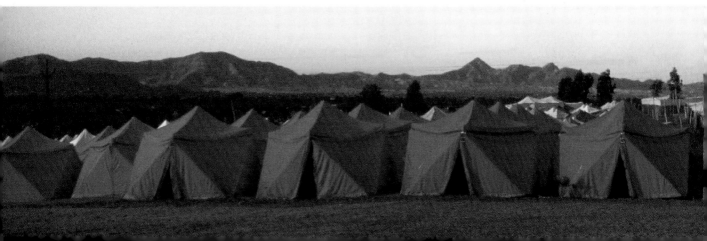

Related Bottles

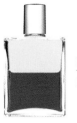

Related Colors
B5

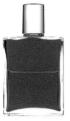

B6

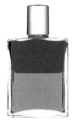

B40

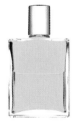

Closest Tint
B87

Right: Humpty Dumpty.
Page 110, top: Gates in Central Park created by Christo and Jeanne-Claude as a public work of art in New York City. There were 7,500 gates installed along the walkways of the park for just two weeks in February 2004. The temporary nature of the project endows their work with a feeling of urgency to be seen.
Page 110, bottom: Tents at Pushkar Camel Fair in India. Each November, during the full moon, the small town of Pushkar comes alive with thousands of people and camels. Primarily a spiritual event, the fair becomes circuslike with camel and horse races, camel beauty contests, and dancing women dressed in brightly colored saris. People who come with their camels stay with them, sleeping on the ground or in wagons. On the night of the full moon the air is filled with the voices of hundreds of women chanting and praying.
Note: The image on page 270 is also a visual expression of this bottle.

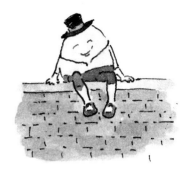

In Aura-Soma, the Humpty Dumpty bottle, as Vicky called it, has a significance relating the whole of human consciousness development to understanding the subtle fields and how the development of these fields manifests as an egg.

As Etheric Rescue, the bottle has similar implications. If we have been through a trauma, Etheric Rescue can help us put our parts back together. In the event of trauma, the true aura, which lies in the golden area within the center of the self, moves toward the etheric gap located on the left side of the body, between the bottom of the left rib and the pelvis. Using B26 may assist us in returning the true aura to the golden area.

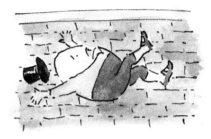

Within the life of any soul there are many memories related to the death experience. Some of those deaths may have been traumatic or had shocks associated with them. Traumas can take us out of our alignment with our time-line and may, in turn, diminish our potential to be all that we can be, to be out of synchronic-ity. Choosing this bottle may indicate that we have a need to let go of the past. Unresolved shock can lead to indecision and difficulty with relationships, resulting in feelings of being tor-mented by fear or burning with anger. B26 helps clear up the timeline and bring back synchronic-ity after traumas of the past, whether they are of this lifetime or from previous incarnational experiences. It can bring our attention to the present and future.

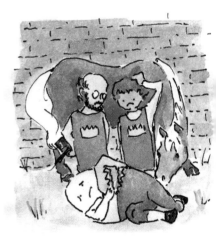

B26 is part of the Chakra Set, relating to the second chakra, the sacral center. It is applied in a very specific way: First, apply it around the entire abdomen and also from the left earlobe to the left shoulder in a small band downward. Then, beginning under the left arm, apply it in a wider band down the whole left side of the trunk, to the ankle. In cases of thyroid problems, apply it around the throat. In cases of muscle tension, massage it onto the affected areas. In situations of extreme holding on—in any circumstance, from constipation to holding on to past relation-ships, fear, or jealousy—apply around the lower abdomen. For animals, apply only around the abdomen.

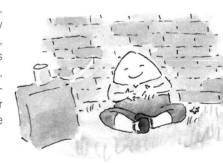

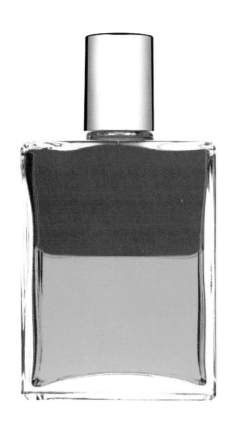

B27 Red/Green

Name: **Robin Hood**

Shakes Together As: **Red**

Tarot Card: **Ten of Wands**

Keynote: **A balance between the head and the heart, and the root and the heart, where we find the relationship of the male and female within ourselves.**

Red and green, the colors that compose the fractions of B27 and B28, were the original colors of the Tao. The ancient Chinese, followers of the Tao, instead of choosing blue and yellow, perhaps the obvious primaries, to distinguish the polarized world in terms of color, chose red and green. In the *ku* symbol, the traditional symbol of the Tao, light and dark are shaped as tadpoles, in the form of a 69. Always the light appears as a circle within the dark tadpole, and the dark appears as a circle within the light tadpole, confirming the yin within the yang and the yang within the yin as part of the essential understanding of the Tao. Light and dark, as expressed by red and green, are both formed through combining blue and yellow. The addition of light in the appropriate density can bring them together as red; the addition of pigment brings them together as green. Conceptually a very revealing understanding can emerge through the contemplation of this issue.

Red above green is also indicative of associations to the material side of life. According to legend, Robin Hood was born Robin of Loxley, a nobleman of the twelfth century.[27-a] He returned from the Crusades, the "Holy War," to find that new governors and laws had taken his land while he had been away. The rich noblemen and those in power were stealing from and harming the people

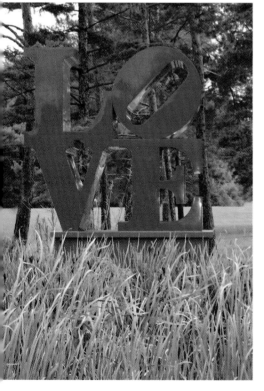

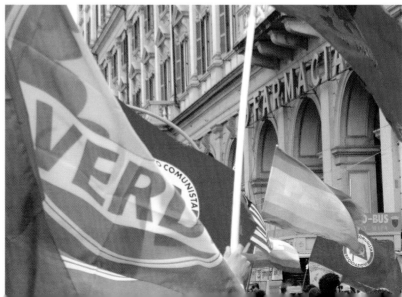

Related Bottles

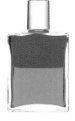

Related Color
B29

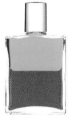

Reverse
B28

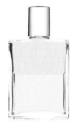

Closest Tint
B57

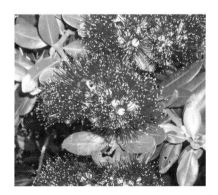

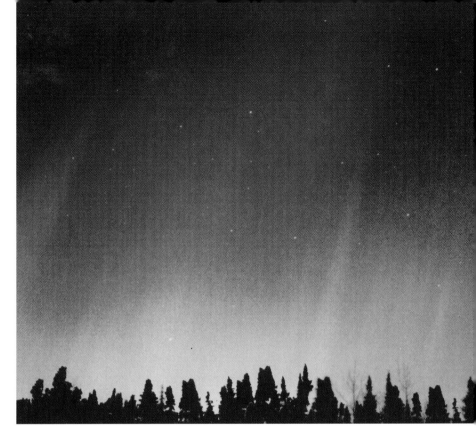

Above: Metrosideros, a tree from a range of species inherited by New Zealand from Gondwana approximately 200 million years ago.

Page 113, top: A rare and magical gift from the sun. This stunning display of northern lights with great patches of red is caused by intense sun flares and solar wind. Photographed at Cleary Summit (elevation 4134 feet) 20 miles outside of Fairbanks, Alaska.

Page 112, left: Love sculpture at Middlebury College in Middlebury, Vermont.

Page 112, right: Protest for freedom and justice in Rome, Italy, June 5, 2004.

of the land. Recognizing these difficult conditions, Robin Hood energetically embarked on setting things right. He became an outlaw, living in the woods with others who sympathized with his cause. Robin's group was sometimes referred to as the Men in Green. Red/Green tells the story of connection with the material side of life: survival through the red, and the search for truth and justice in the green.

Robin Hood had lost everything. Yet through that material loss, he found a new way of life. Thus, this bottle indicates that we have perseverance, determination, energy, and an enthusiasm for life. We are truthful, are able to make the right decisions, and have the energy to put our feelings into action.

Through Robin Hood's experience of loss, the whole situation was turned upside down. As we can see from the colors in this bottle, the upside-down quality is reflected in the inverted position of the red (the root chakra) over the green (the heart chakra). The juxtaposition of the fractions also gives us an insight into the meaning of the bottle: the material indications in the upper fraction (red) are above the holding of the truth (green).

For women, this bottle may indicate that we have problems relating to men, or it may indicate a separation or divorce. For men or women, B27 may help us handle transexuality, the experience of feeling like a woman in a man's body, or vice versa. B27 may highlight issues of experiencing responsibility as a burden, and consequently feelings of resentment or frustration or a desire of wanting to be in another's space. It may indicate that we do not allow ourselves to feel but may actually be very angry at heart, though we do not acknowledge this even to ourselves.

Apply the contents of this bottle around the entire trunk.

Please also read the explanation of B28, Maid Marion, as the meanings of B27 and B28 pertain to each other.

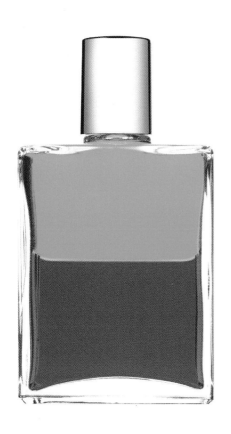

B28 Green/Red

Name: Maid Marion

Shakes Together As: Red

Tarot Card: Nine of Wands

Keynote: Awakening of the heart. A balance between the female and the male, the intuitive and the analytical.

Maid Marion was the companion and beloved of Robin Hood. B28, Green/Red, Maid Marion, is sometimes chosen by a woman who has been stereotyped as "a doormat." When she realizes that she is being used in this way, the woman decides to separate from the situation. She realizes, at a psychological level, that her situation may have to do with the conditioned factors of the male/female relationship within her self. In other words, if her mother always behaved so that she would be in the position of wiping her husband's feet, that is, if he had been continuously in the position of dominance, then the woman's father was not in a position of receptivity. In terms of conditioning, it is likely that the woman, as a child, went through experiences that emphasized the left side of the brain and the right side of the body. The male side of the self would be dominant and

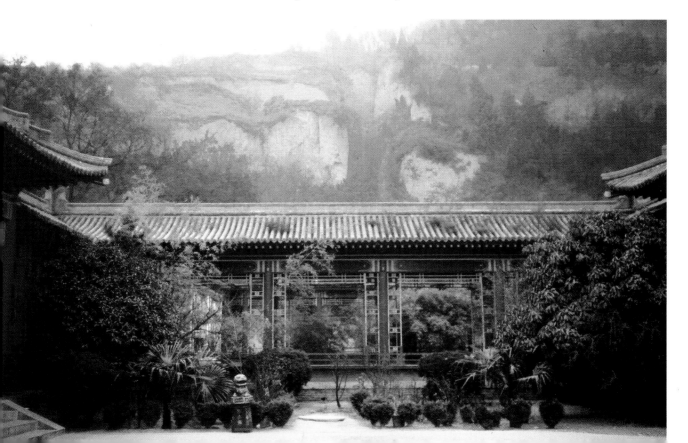

Related Bottles

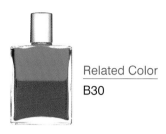

Related Color
B30

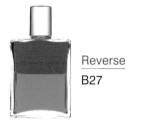

Reverse
B27

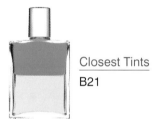

Closest Tints
B21

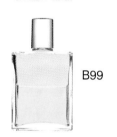

B99

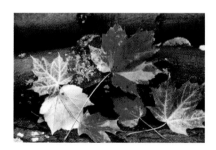

Above: Red and green leaves.
Left: Summer palace retreat near Beijing, China.
Right: Ivy growing at Dartington Hall in Totnes, Devon, England.

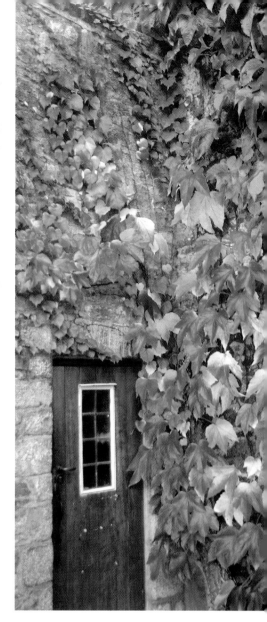

would use the feminine intuitive in a domineering way. Thus, the doormat is both an inner and an outer situation. This is a distressing concept, but one that applies to an attitude that some men and women have toward particular women. If a man chooses this bottle, it may suggest that he has problems with women.

In the story of Robin Hood and Maid Marion, the sheriff of Nottingham (a local governor) knew that Marion was associated with and cared for Robin; therefore, reputedly, the sheriff treated her badly, trying to use Marion to get what he wanted. Robin Hood had let go of his title, home, and land to live in the forest with a group of people who supported his work opposing the new laws of the land. Maid Marion also recognized the error of the new laws. She found it difficult to consider letting go of the life she lived, in a grand house with servants, to live the life of a peasant in the woods with Robin. Yet by remaining in her position, living a life of pretense, Marion could be effective in informing Robin of the strategies of the sheriff of Nottingham and King John.

Although confusion and difficulties are suggested by the Red/Green and Green/Red combinations, a wholeness and total balance is also contained within them.

Both B27 and B28 are concerned with gender issues and possible confusion with those issues. A pertinent issue is the balance or imbalance of male and female energies. We tend to have a preference for Red/Green or Green/Red when we are experiencing a divorce or separation and are reassessing the male/female relationship within ourselves.

A man choosing B28 may be reflective of how he experiences the validity and strength of his inner feminine self. A woman who realizes that she is being used in the wrong way and decides she is no longer willing to be a doormat often will choose B28, reflecting her feelings about her whole situation.

Choosing B28 reveals that we have found the space to channel our energy and are able to trust our intuition. B28 indicates that we are becoming true to ourselves and to others, bringing more joy and happiness. Alternatively, this bottle may point out that we do not trust our own judgment, due to misplaced trust in others or a lack of confidence as a result of not having made space to recognize what is true for ourselves.

Apply the contents of this bottle around the entire trunk.

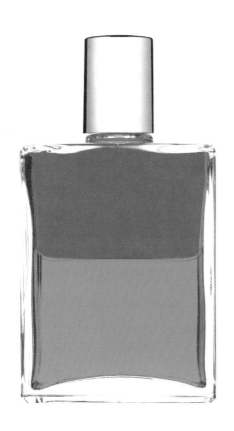

B29 Red/Blue

Name: **Get Up and Go**

Shakes Together As: **Violet**

Tarot Card: **Eight of Wands**

Keynote: **Living in the material world, a balance within the solar plexus between two extremes.**

B30, the Blue/Red, is the reverse of B29, having the same colors but in opposite positions. Both shake together as violet, which represents healing through service. In a way, B29 and B30 could be seen as opposites, but they also contain similar energies that are approached and manifested differently.

Get Up and Go has red energy in its upper fraction and blue beneath. It marks the availability of the energy needed to go and do something, to actually step ahead and materialize something from inspiration. B30, with the blue above and the red below, represents a tendency to wait for, think about, and be at peace with inspiration before doing something about it.

Right: Bridge in Concord, Massachusetts, where the first shot of the American Revolution was fired, commemorated in the poem "Concord Hymns" by Ralph Waldo Emerson. "By the rude bridge that arched the flood, / Their flag to April's breeze unfurled, / Here once the embattled farmers stood / And fired the shot heard round the world."

Page 117, top: A store on Dal Lake in Kashmir, where shopping is done by shakara.

Page 117, bottom: Making clay bricks on Flores Island near Tengaara, Indonesia.

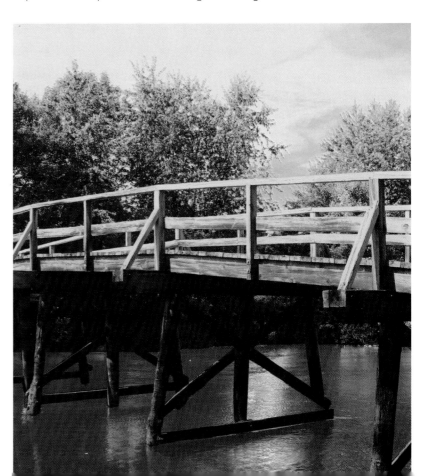

Related Bottles

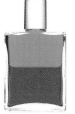

Reverse
B30

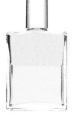

Closest Tint
B57

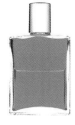

Shakes To
B16

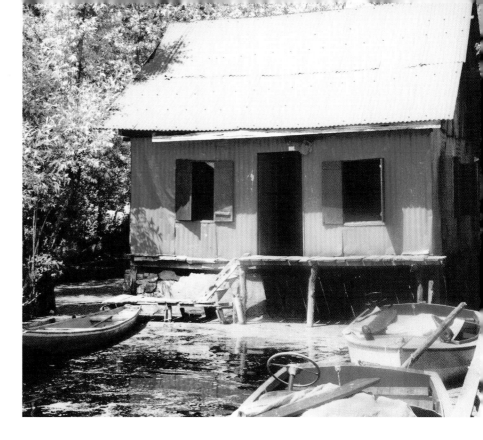

Choosing this color combination suggests that we could be high achievers, energetically motivated to be of service, successful, even materialistic, and that we have much energy for life and communicate this to the world. Our survival issues are tempered by a sense of inner peace. Alternatively, we may currently pursue material gain at the expense of peace within ourselves. In this case, B29 indicates the need to feel inner peace, to be no longer overshadowed by anger, frustration, resentment, and the material side of life.

B29 is helpful when we feel low on energy. Apply it around the entire trunk.

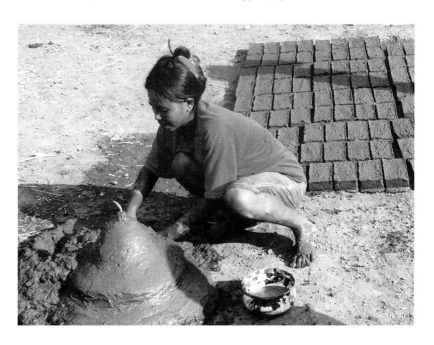

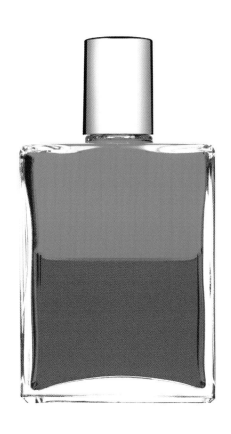

B30 Blue/Red

Name: **Bringing Heaven to Earth**

Shakes Together As: **Violet**

Tarot Card: **Seven of Wands**

Keynote: **Head in heaven, feet on the earth. Awakening to the communication of peace.**

B30 and B29 both shake together as violet, which represents healing in service. In B30, Blue/Red, the blue is the blue of heaven and the red is associated with earth. One of Vicky's favorite aphorisms was "Head in heaven, feet on earth, center flowing free" (see B65). The golden area of our bodies, between the red and the blue, is the central place within which lies the memory of the first cell, the true aura, the incarnational star. This golden area lies within the physical base between Heaven and Earth. The more attention we give to that place, the greater is the possibility to bring Heaven upon Earth. If the golden center is harmonious and relaxed, the conditions surrounding the center come together.

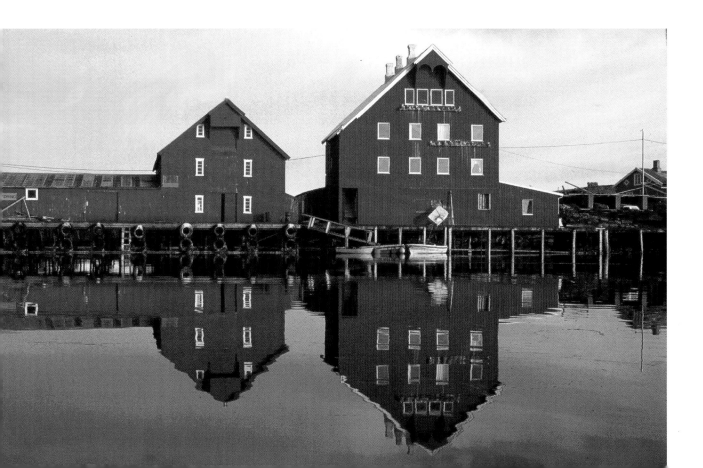

Related Bottles

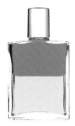

Closest Tints
B20

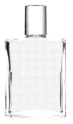

B58

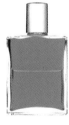

Shakes To
B16

The blue in the top fraction of B30 shows the clear mind, or peace in the conscious mind; the red represents grounding, or the strength derived from having our feet on the earth. When blue in the conscious mind combines with red in the subconscious to make violet, healing and transformation become possible. Heavenly possibilities are brought to earth. Thus, this bottle carries the energy to awaken us to the knowledge of who we are and the ability to communicate that. It suggests peace, examination of survival issues, and a potential for service to others. It may indicate that we have the inner strength to see things through.

B20, Star Child, is "hidden" in this bottle, implying that we may need to heal our inner child and release anger and frustration. We could fail to communicate well about our passionate feelings.

Apply B30 around the entire trunk of the body. In cases of headache and spiritual problems, apply it along the hairline, too.

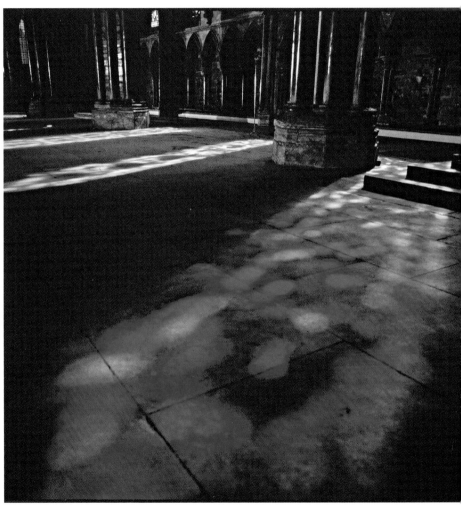

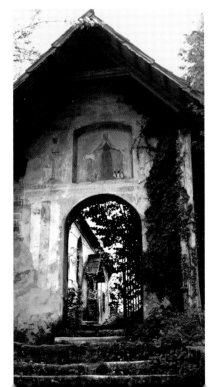

Above: Light shining through stained glass window in Lincoln Cathedral in Lincoln, England.
Left: Roadside shrine in Austria.
Page 118: House in Røst, Norway, land first settled by the Hyperboreans. Røst, a small island at the outer end of the Lofoten island group, is about 115 miles north of the Arctic Circle. The mild winters, cool summers, and relentless winds are ideal for the islanders' livelihood of exporting fish. The island's scenery is spectacular—flat marshes contrast with steep towering cliffs that serve as home to the largest colony of nesting birds in Norway.

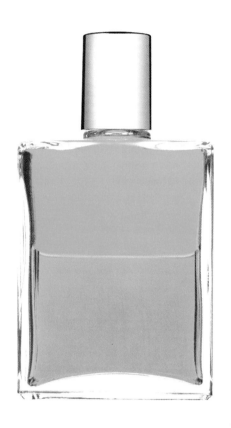

B31 Green/Gold

Name: The Fountain

Shakes Together As: Olive Green

Tarot Card: Six of Wands

Keynote: The wisdom of the heart. To make space for the deepest joy to spring from within the depths of the self.

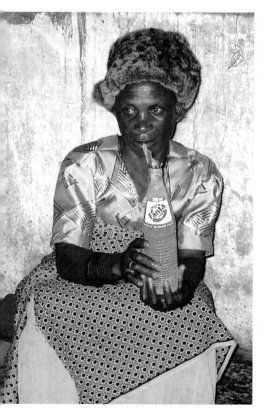

This combination addresses the three levels or aspects of our being. To understand this, let us consider a metaphor of three brains: the intellectual brain, the emotional brain, and the instinctual or moving brain. The intellectual brain is located above the neck and is where we take in ideas. The emotional brain is located around the diaphragm and is where we get the feeling of something. The instinctual brain resides in the pelvic area and is the place into which the feeling gets "fed." When this happens, we no longer have to think about or feel how to do something; it just happens. This is a little bit like the process of learning to ride a bicycle. Eventually, after all the stages have been processed, the skill or response becomes automatic. If we imagine the brains as bowls in their respective locations, it is easy to imagine the movement of energy between the ideas, feelings, and movements, flowing down like a fountain from one bowl to the next.

Every person has a natal and a developed chart of energy patterns that exist from a stellar point of view. Our soul and whole being are receptive to these patterns. In this concept of a fountain, the energy initially comes into the head and overflows from there into the feeling area. From there, the energy overflows into the instinctual area of our being. For a fountain to work effectively, it must have a source of power, which pushes energy upward so that it may then fall down. This is parallel to the understanding in Aura-Soma of the human subtle anatomy and the three stars. The energy source in a person is the golden energy of the incarnational star. The journey of that energy begins with the earth star, when the red energy at the root turns pink and makes its way toward the incarnational star of the person. When this journey of the pink commences, a similar energetic movement begins in the soul star and travels downward toward the emerald of the heart (see the subtle anatomy chart, page 24).

Together, the flow among the three bowls and the energetic movement that connects the three stars in a person create an image of the Green/Gold fountain. The golden area communicates with the emerald of the heart within the self. When the wisdom (gold) within has found space to be expressed through the heart (green), we feel joy and harmony. In this aspect, B31 can help us find a personal power spot, a place in nature, where we feel content and especially "connected."

Related Bottles

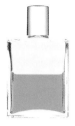

Related Color
B4

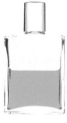

Related Reverse
B7

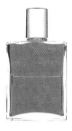

Shakes To
B91

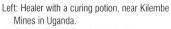

Left: Healer with a curing potion, near Kilembe
  Mines in Uganda.
Right: Islamic style fountain in Spain.

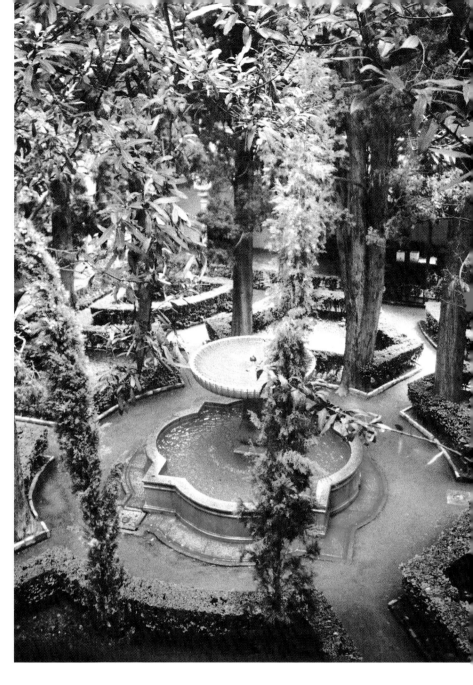

Green and gold also tie back to the Green Man and his association with vegetation myths and kingly sacrifice—the youth who dies and is reborn. The green of the Green Man gives way to the gold of transformation and rebirth.

B31 is supportive and perhaps calming when we face examinations. When we have found a balance between the truth of our heart and the wisdom of our belly, we are likely to be honest and have integrity. B31 may also suggest that because we cannot express our fears, we have difficulty in decision making. Jealousy, anxiety, and envy can prevent us from feeling energy and positive emotions.

Apply the contents of this bottle in a band around the body, between the heart and the area below the navel.

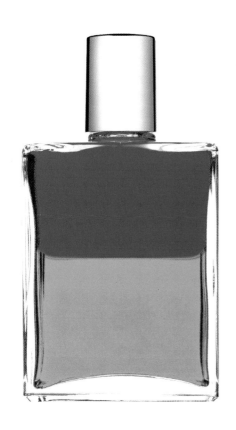

B32 Royal Blue/Gold

Name: **Sophia**

Shakes Together As: **Emerald Green**

Tarot Card: **Five of Wands**

Keynote: **Clarity in relation to the wisdom that lies within. A message from the stars.**

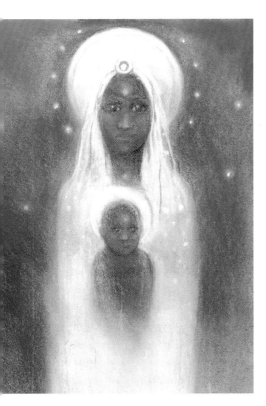

In traditional tarot imagery, such as that of the Rider-Waite Tarot, the Five of Wands depicts a group of people apparently in conflict with one another. Yet upon closer examination, the people are not fighting with one another but are, in fact, building a five-pointed star. Royal Blue and Gold are complementary opposites. Like the Five of Wands, although they may appear to be at odds with one another, they integrate into an expression of one's inner truth (when combined they create a beautiful green).

Sophia is the goddess of the stars; Rudolf Steiner speaks of Sophia in his theories of cosmic intelligence.[32-a] When we bring our attention into our belly, into the golden area within ourselves, we go into the dark night sky. In that dark, we see all the stars that exist. The galaxy we see at night is only a reflection of what is inside, and vice versa. There is a starry night inside each one of us and in the heavens above.

In this color combination, royal blue, the higher intuition, connects with the golden area within the self. When shaken, the colors blend to an emerald green, representative of the feeling side of life. The emerald issues are inherent. B32 may indicate our constructiveness, perhaps obscured by difficulties, or that we have a well of inner wisdom (gold) and can communicate it for others' benefit (royal blue), learning and gaining wisdom from experience.

To help the emerald to form, we may draw our breath into the belly, the golden area. When our attention and breath are brought to this area, we may bring more clarity to the sense doors (the royal blue), supporting the wisdom of the true aura in the golden area with clarity. Royal blue helps us express the clarity of our heart's truth (emerald).

Sophia relates to the deeper aspects of the feminine intuitive. The ability to observe and perceive intuitively helps reveal underlying patterns. Certain patterns within the royal blue, having to do with authority, intimidation, and manipulation, can contribute to anxiety in the conscious or subconscious mind. Emotional patterns and responses to these issues are brought to light when the royal blue and gold combine, yielding the emerald green. All of the higher mind functions are attributed to the sixth chakra, the royal blue. The combination of the penetrative insight of the royal blue and the wisdom of the gold may help us be aware of our own truth.

Related Bottles

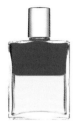

Related Colors
B47

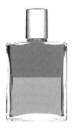

B72

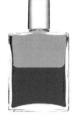

Reverse
B97

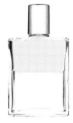

Closest Tint
B94

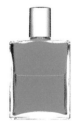

Shakes To
B10

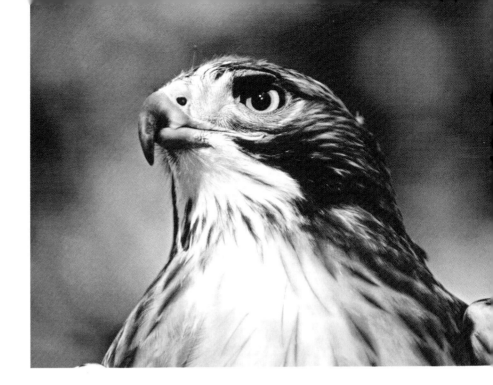

B32 helps touch into ancient memory, perhaps connecting us with Aztec, Mayan, or Toltec incarnations. We who choose this bottle in the first position may have been born with the umbilical cord around our neck, an experience that could reflect issues of a past life. Fear and anxieties we hold within can lead to difficulties with communication. B32 also may suggest that we suffer from bitterness, disillusionment, and intense jealousy.

Apply this combination around the circumference of the body anywhere between the head and the navel.

Left: *Mother and child* by Alma Midgehope. Inspired by the Black Madonnas of Southern France.
Top: Captive red-tailed hawk at the Blue Hill Trailside Museum in Milton, Massachusetts. Hawks have three fovia, which provide an incredible concentration of cones for clarity of vision.
Bottom: Utah Red Lands, above the Colorado River.

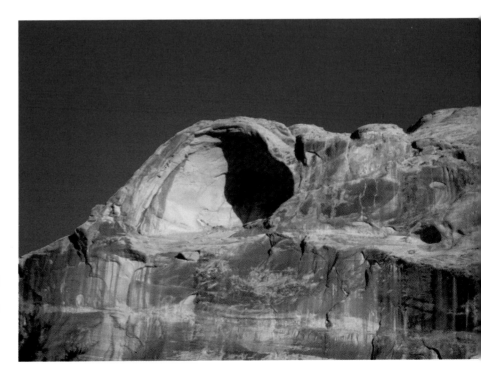

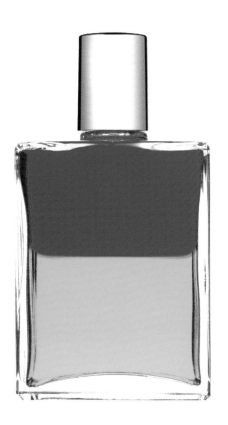

B33 Royal Blue/ Turquoise

Name: Dolphin Bottle/Peace with a Purpose

Shakes Together As: Blue

Tarot Card: Four of Wands

Keynote: Clarity and playfulness. Spontaneity and joy. A communication from the heart clearly expressed.

Page 125, top: Eye of peacock feather, symbolic of beatific vision and clear perception.
Page 125, bottom: Dolphin fresco at a Minoan temple in Knossos, Crete.
Below: Dolphin swimming in the open seas, Florida.

Buddha once said that there are three orders of beings on this planet that can reach enlightenment: dolphins, whales, and humans. Perhaps the order of this list implies that dolphins and whales have a greater chance of enlightenment than do humans. Perhaps dolphins and whales do not worry about survival, about food and shelter, in the same way humans do. Dolphins seem to be able to spend their time in playing, creating in their brain more neural connections. The survival issues humans struggle with seem to keep our neural connections to a minimum, as we are caught in repetitive thought patterns. If we could worry less about how and from where our food and shelter come, we could spend less time involved with survival issues. This perspective has to do with how this combination came to be known as the Dolphin bottle.

Royal blue and turquoise show a connection between the sixth chakra (higher intuition) and the Ananda Khanda (the process of individuation). This relationship releases inner creativity, allowing the ethic of play to develop. To be creative is to be playful, not serious. Playfulness encourages a sense of peacefulness within us.

B33's other name is Peace with a Purpose. The Blue/Blue of the Peace bottle, B2, is evident within this combination, and it has transited from the peace that passeth all understanding in B2 to peace with purpose in B33. Peace is a fundamental energy that can be used in a constructive way. We can all have a sincere intention toward peace, toward creating peace. Royal blue signifies the

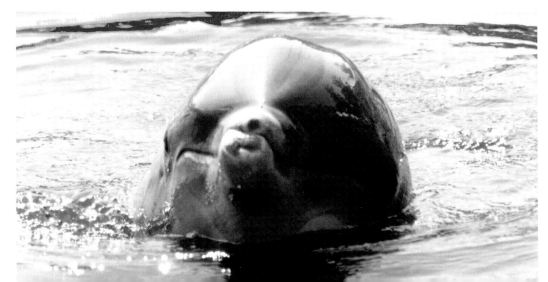

124

Related Bottles

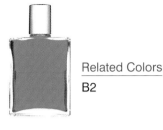

Related Colors
B2

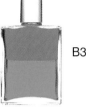

B3

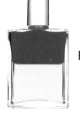

B47

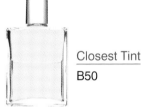

Closest Tint
B50

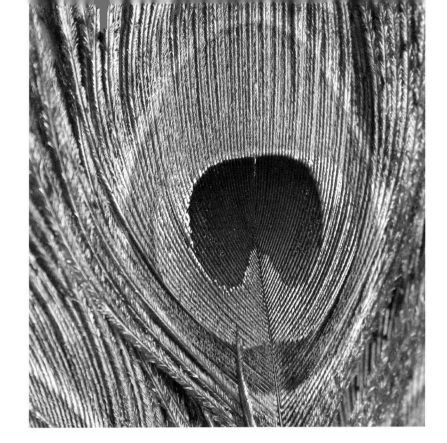

possibility of doing something practical toward creating peace, to put into action a belief that encourages peace rather than conflict. This element of practicality, of groundedness, may also be the secret of prayer or meditation. The red of grounding added to the blue of peace makes royal blue.

For example, if we practiced greater compassion toward others, we would experience a certain degree of inner peace. As this intention (royal blue) begins to grow, the peace (blue) within begins to have a purpose. Perhaps we become more creative (turquoise) in relation to our compassion as it precipitates changes with our self. Joy (yellow) added in just the right amount transforms blue to turquoise.

Choosing blue may may imply that we have or need inspiration (royal blue) and communicate inspiration with feeling to everyone (turquoise). B33 may call us to be or suggest that we are calm and peaceful souls who find pleasure in being creative. B33 can suggest that we have difficulties with the male/father model and with authority, or that we habitually play the martyr. It may be useful in polarity work.

With the presence of turquoise and the hidden colors of B3, B33 may help us establish contact with incarnations in Atlantis and Lemuria (a civilization thought to have existed at the same time as Atlantis).

Apply the contents of this bottle around the throat, neck, and jaw area; along the hairline and on the forehead; and in a band across the entire chest and back, including the spine. In cases of eye ailments, apply it near the eye sockets (only upon the bone structure around the eyes, not in the eyes).

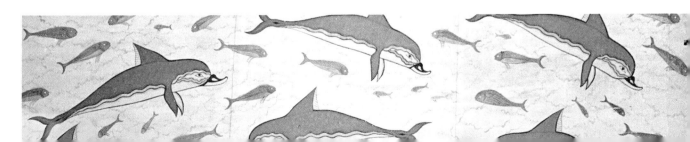

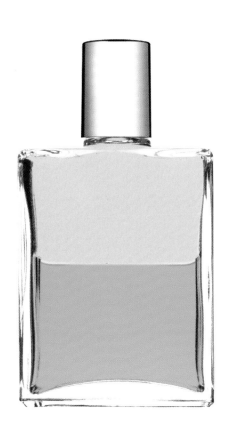

B34 Pink/Turquoise

Name: **The Birth of Venus**

Shakes Together As: **Violet with Sparkles of Pink**

Tarot Card: **Three of Wands**

Keynote: **Getting in touch with beauty and the beauty that lies in the emergence of self through acceptance of self from within the feeling side of the being.**

B34's name, Birth of Venus, refers to the painting by Botticelli of a beautiful woman emerging from a clamshell. Venus was born between the waves and the sky. Perhaps the birth of Venus is the result of water and air combining. B34 shows us the feminine pink energy appearing out of the turquoise ocean. Venusian energy is the energy of love, harmony, caring, and warmth, and it is birthed from the ocean. When visible, Venus is always seen near the sun, cycling between preceding it as the morning star and trailing it as the evening star. This cycle is representative of the constancy of beauty that comes with the ending of the night and the birth of a new day. Venus reminds us that when situations become a little difficult or dark, we still have a light to guide us, even when we feel there is nothing else.

Compassion (pink) and the communication of the heart (turquoise) come together in this bottle. Red, especially in its intense form of pink, can indicate an awakening. The Botticelli woman celebrates life. She is in the ocean of life, the turquoise creative aspect, the creative communication of the heart through

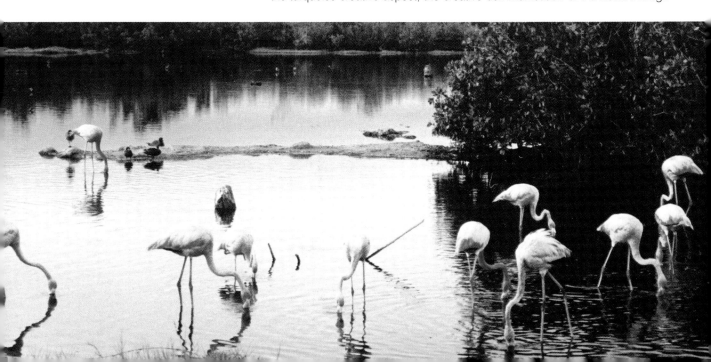

Related Bottles

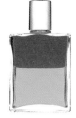

Related Color
B75

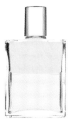

Closest Tint
B57

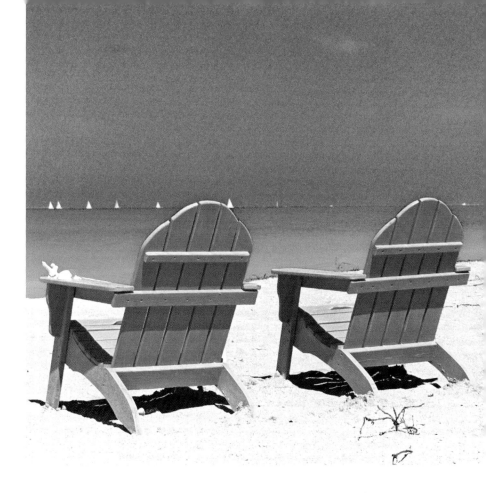

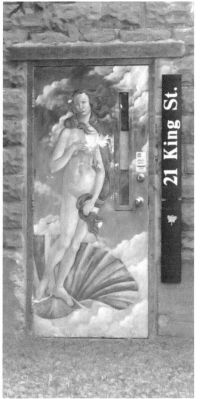

the feeling side of our being. The celebration is about waking up to the moment she finds herself in, immersed in the waters of the collective consciousness. B34 suggests that we wish to improve our circumstances: giving and receiving love produces change. Loving ourselves helps us communicate what is hidden in our heart. This aspect makes B34 useful for children who feel threatened; it also may help with dream work. Issues highlighted by this bottle include being influenced and manipulated by flattery and the need to deal with disappointments to help the mind and body heal. Letting go of past problems brings joy.

Venus is love being born in the waters of the collective. When the pink energy makes a connection with the turquoise, there is a possibility of the birth of something new and very beautiful. There is an innocent quality in this love, indicated in the painting by the woman's nakedness. Creative love brings the love of Venus.

Apply this combination around the heart and across the back, including the spinal column. In cases of menstrual problems, apply around the lower abdomen and lower back. For dream work, use along the hairline.

Above: Pink chairs, receptive and in waiting, on the beach in Captiva, Florida.
Left: Painted door in Burlington, Vermont, inspired by Botticelli's *Birth of Venus*.
Page 126: Flamingos on Santa Maria in the Galapagos Islands. Flamingos turn pink based on their diet, as when we nourish ourselves with thoughts of love, we radiate love.

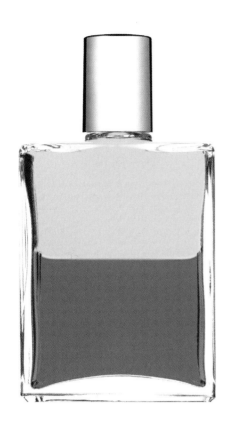

B35 Pink/Violet

Name: Loving Kindness

Shakes Together As: Lilac

Tarot Card: Two of Wands

Keynote: Transformative. Detachment. Unconditional love in the service of others. Love from above.

In this bottle, the caring and warmth of the pink relates to the violet. The traditional Buddhist meditations, which are called the loving kindness meditations, are intended to help us develop the flame of loving kindness equally, without discrimination, toward both that with which we have difficulties and that which we like. This practice helps clean our inner landscape. B35 is an expression of how to use warmth and caring (pink) in the context of feeling service and healing to enhance spirituality (violet).

Right: Interior of the Goetheanum, the Center for Anthroposophical Studies in Dornach, Switzerland.

Page 129, top: Pink light radiating behind Basilica of Our Lady of Pilar in La Recoleta in Buenos Aires, Argentina. Originally a refuge from a yellow fever epidemic, the Recoleta area is now one of the wealthiest neighborhoods in Buenos Aires. In the cemetery are magnificent and elaborate mausoleums and tombs of the most influential people in Argentina's history, including presidents, scientists, race car drivers, and Eva Peron.

Page 129, bottom: Gladiolas in Ripton, Vermont.

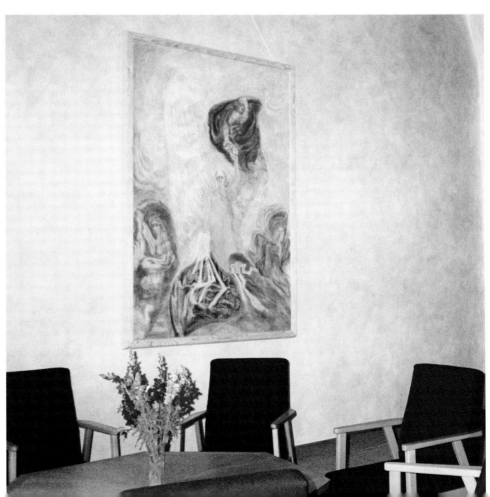

Related Bottles

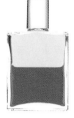

Related Color
B84

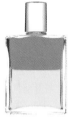

Reverse
B36

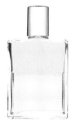

Closest Tint
B57

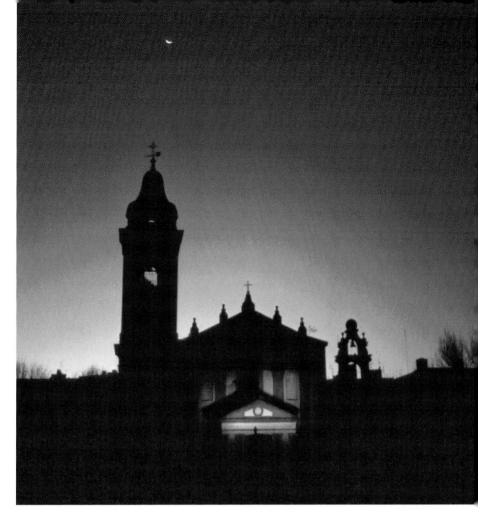

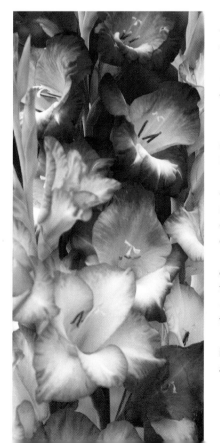

Ultimately, developing loving kindness is for our selves, but the intention of the meditation is to take on the suffering of others and to purify that suffering for the benefit of all beings. Thus, B35 shows that our spirituality (violet) brings us love (pink) to give to others, that we are self-confident and have the gift of healing. This color combination is an expression of that type of kindness and warmth that comes from the unfolding of the thousand-petaled lotus, which is immediately above the crown (violet) area. B35 presents the possibility of a deep level of transformation. This may apply to those of us who are suffering from depression or those of us who, because of our spiritual pride, can be dominated by ourselves or by others.

Unconditional love in the service of others, which is suggested by the colors of this bottle, begins with a little kindness. The meaning of the name Kindness is profound, especially when we consider that through kindness we may proceed to deeper levels of understanding of compassion and caring, toward both ourselves and others.

B35 and B36 are important in Aura-Soma both conceptually and energetically. They are linked with the Ace of Wands and the Two of Wands, which, in the kabbalistic Tree of Life, symbolize the fire world in the two highest sephirot (spheres receiving and emanating divine qualities): Kether and Chokmah. These two bottles represent an awakening through love to our purpose.

B35 may be helpful in situations when we suffer physically, for example, if we are in pain but no specific cause of the pain has been found. Apply anywhere.

129

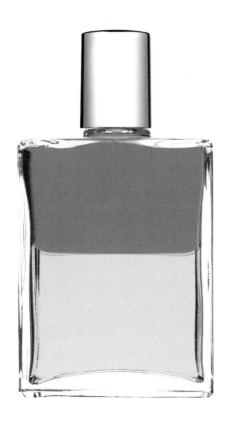

B36 Violet/Pink

Name: **Charity**

Shakes Together As: **Lilac**

Tarot Card: **Ace of Wands**

Keynote: **Caring, warmth, and kindness toward ourselves, extended into the world.**

B36, Charity, is the reverse presentation of B35. Charity is unconditional love (pink) in the service (violet) of others. If we accept ourselves (pink), even those aspects that we find most objectionable, a healing effect occurs in the conscious mind (violet).

Faith, hope, and charity are a trinity of virtues.[36-a] Charity is the feeling of wanting to give of ourselves to something we believe in and value. Often this is connected to an awareness of a higher purpose. Charity is the expression of the care we feel about something we believe in through our actions, through giving something precious, such as our time or energy. Charity comes through developing self-acceptance (pink). B36 shows us spirituality, healing, and transformation in the conscious mind and unconditional love and caring within us. The joining of these two impulses leads to charity. Charity is not a strategy but a natural consequence of the hand of compassion extending into our lives. Thus, B36 implies that we are compassionate. It suggests that we let go of the past

Page 131, top: Pomegranates, an important symbol to Solomon and the building of his temple, symbolize righteousness and fruitfulness. Pomegranates also are featured in the myth of Persephone. Persephone, goddess of innocence, was married off to Hades, ruler of the underworld, by her father, Zeus. When her mother, Demeter, goddess of the harvest, discovered this she was outraged and filled with sorrow, missing her daughter. By withholding her blessings from the earth, leaving the earth barren and drought-ridden, Demeter was able to negotiate for her daughter to be returned. However, while preparing to return to earth, Persephone ate seven seeds from a pomegranate. By eating from the fruit of the underworld, Persephone relinquished the right to return to earth for good. From then on she spent a portion of the year with her mother on earth and the rest of the year in the underworld. Greek mythology tells us that this is how the different seasons were established: When Persephone leaves the earth Demeter begins to grieve, bringing the cold, desolate winter and when she returns to earth she brings with her the awakening of spring.

Page 131, bottom: Clematis in Ripton, Vermont.

Right: Sunset on Ganges River in India. This river, sacred to the Hindus, represents divine consciousness flowing to earth and offers the possibility of spiritual evolution and immortality.

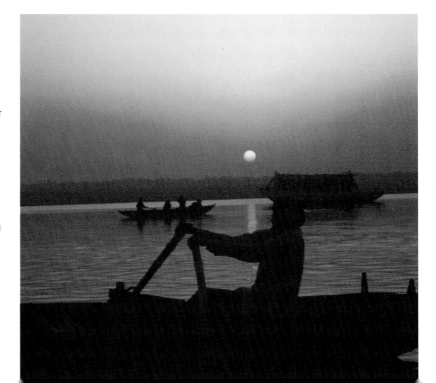

Related Bottles

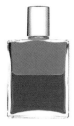

Related Color
B65

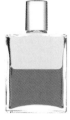

Reverse
B35

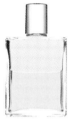

Closest Tints
B58

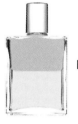

B66

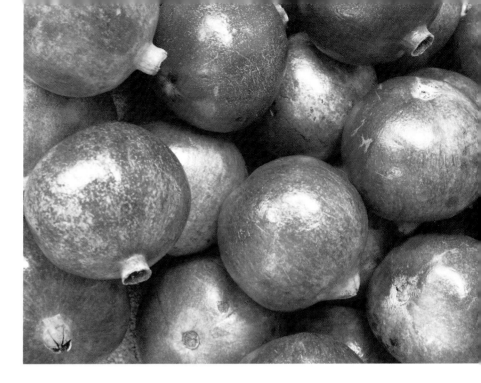

and expand the potential for new beginnings by putting our energy into new interests, projects, and inspirations.

B36 may be helpful when we are working with our inner child. In this situation, B36 can point to feelings of not being loved or to excessive worrying, especially about survival issues. We may think a great deal and tend not to allow our feelings to be communicated from our heart.

In this combination, energy appearing as pink, the intense form of red, flows through to violet, which we ascribe to the head area. Nevertheless, B36 may be applied everywhere on the body, as the colors cover the body from the root to the crown.

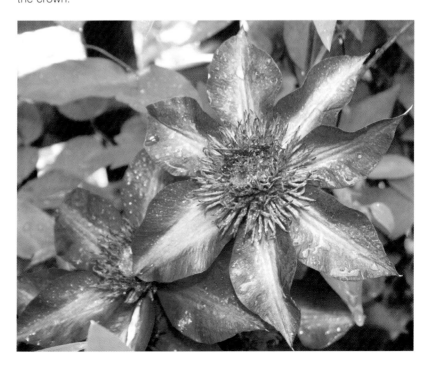

131

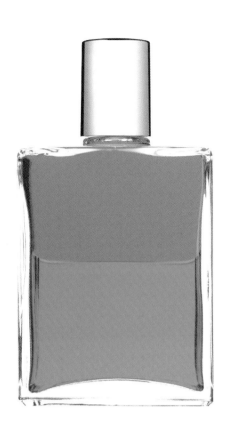

B37 Violet/Blue

Name: The Guardian Angel Comes to Earth

Shakes Together As: Royal Blue

Tarot Card: King of Cups

Keynote: Transformative communication. A nurturing and peaceful communication that may be of benefit to ourselves and others.

B37 was previously known as Peaceful Service. Its current name, the Guardian Angel Comes to Earth, emerged after the birth of B44, the Guardian Angel, quite a long time after B37 was born. Violet and blue are hues of pale violet (lilac) and pale blue, and so B37 is a deeper, more grounded version of B44.

Peace in our depths, in our subconscious/unconscious mind, can be a key to transformation in our conscious mind. The possibility of the guardian angel coming to Earth moves us to another level of our being. Violet/Blue contains B2, Blue/Blue, the Peace bottle. When the guardian angel comes to Earth, it brings a sense of peace that goes beyond our understanding. It is as if the angelic

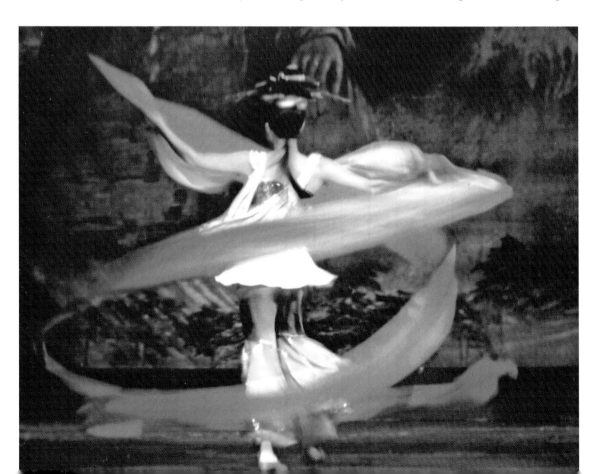

Related Bottles

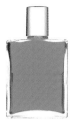

Related Colors
B2

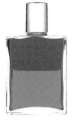

B29

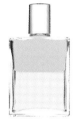

Closest Tint
B44

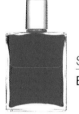

Shakes To
B96

Left: A dancer, performing in a Chinese theater in Kissimmee, Florida. The movement, enthusiasm, and sheer joy of the dance communicate a sense of how life is truly worth living.

Top: Little blue heron, a solitary wading bird, at Corkscrew Swamp Sanctuary, an 11,000 acre wildlife refuge in Naples, Florida. For the Native Americans a water bird is symbolic of the renewal of life, distant travel, wisdom, and far vision.

Bottom: Bachelor Buttons, symbolic of single blessedness, in Ripton, Vermont.

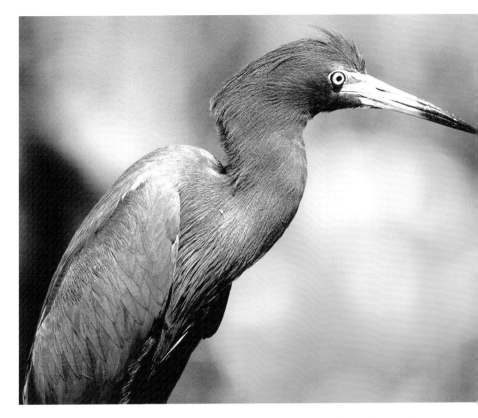

aspect of us were finding a space for integration with the rest of ourselves and then grounding this in our physicality. The Peace bottle hidden within this combination reminds us that peace (blue) is essential for our real transformation.

B37 may suggest that we have peaceful, healing communication abilities (violet). It may indicate the need for those abilities as well, therefore aiding us when we think that we have no inspiration or intuition. B37 can open us to the unexpected. It also can balance and stimulate the third eye and help develop our psychic abilities (symbolized by the royal blue, which this combination shakes to).

Apply B37 along the hairline and around the throat and neck area.

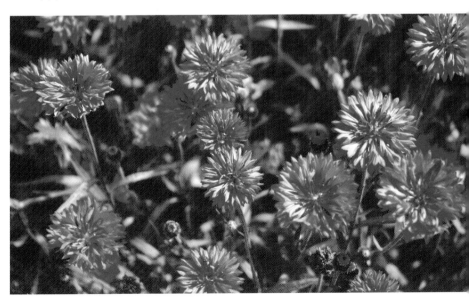

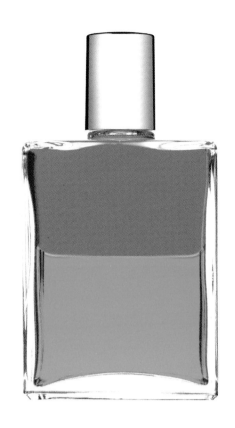

B38 Violet/Green

Name: Troubadour 2/Discernment
Shakes Together As: Deep Green
Tarot Card: Queen of Cups
Keynote: Letting go of the difficulties of the past so that the heart may be free to express its truth. Leads to transformation within the self.

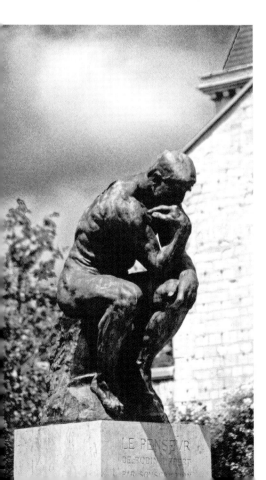

B38, Violet/Green, is the second of the Troubadour bottles. Here the colors correctly reflect the chakra alignment of the human body, in that the violet of the crown chakra is above the green of the heart chakra (see image of subtle anatomy on page 24). The same colors appear in B17, the first Troubadour bottle, but are there reversed.

B38 may help us connect to medieval incarnational experiences. Both B17 and B38 speak about persecution (see the explanation for B17). B38 may be an expression of the memory of persecution during the Inquisition or similar times. B38 is often reflective of our need to express truth (green) in the service (violet) of others and to find what is true in our heart in relation to our spirituality. This need requires a balance of our conscious and unconscious minds. B38 indicates that we may be intuitive and spiritual with maternal, nurturing qualities. Choosing B38 suggests that we are likely to compassionately nurture healing.

B38's name is Discernment. When the messages of our head and heart are able to collaborate, we express the qualities that can lead to discernment. Often, our heart says one thing and our head says another. To develop discernment, we need to find the truth that lies in our heart. Our mind needs to listen to our feelings, and our feelings must be free to be uncompromised by our thinking. Our thinking must understand the validity of what our heart says. Feelings of jealousy, envy, and lack of trust can prevent this; B38 can bring knowledge of those feelings or open the way to clearing scars of emotional wounds. The selection of Discernment suggests that we have attained a certain degree of knowledge.

Like B37, B38 has B2, the Peace bottle, hidden within it. Blue is the first primary color, and peace is a fundamental principle throughout our understanding of color. This allows B38 to aid us when we are disillusioned, in particular with relationships.

Apply B38 along the hairline, around the heart, and across the back, including the spinal column. In cases of bladder and kidney problems, apply where the pain is and around the abdomen.

Related Bottles

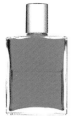

Related Colors
B2

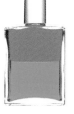

B3

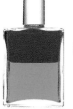

B27

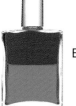

B29

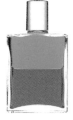

Reverse
B17

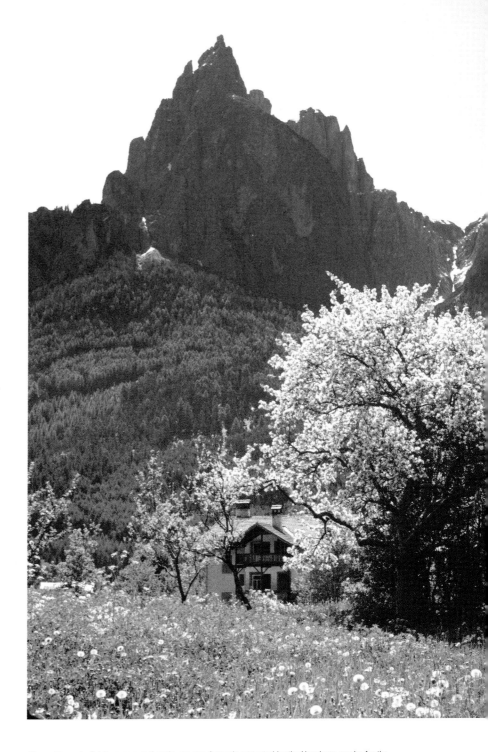

Above: House in Salzkammergut, Austria, an area formerly protected by the Hapsburg empire for the profitability of salt production.
Left: *The Thinker,* by Rodin, at Musée Rodin in Paris, France.

135

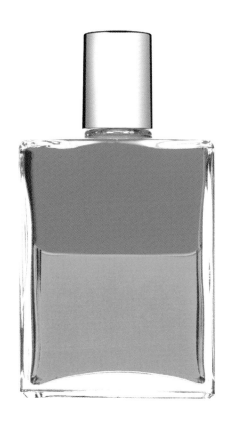

B39 Violet/Gold

Name: Egyptian Bottle 2/The Puppeteer

Shakes Together As: Reddish Orange

Tarot Card: Knight of Cups

Keynote: Transformative wisdom. A deep level of joy as a consequence of a transformative experience. Wisdom and service, compassion and understanding.

Right: Crisped trees, from the Yellowstone National Park forest fires of 1988, against a sunset and gathering storm clouds.

Below: Crocuses in Sturbridge, Massachussetts. Used since ancient times, crocuses are a highly valued source of the most exalted spice, saffron, and a yellow orange dye.

A puppeteer pulls the strings of a puppet. Each of us is like a puppet in relation to our conditioning. In a sense, our role models and authority figures and all that we have experienced within our genetic history, including at the cellular level, pull the strings of who we are now. Our reactions—our feelings, thoughts, and actions—are products of the strings that are being pulled. This is the situation addressed in B39.

The puppeteer manipulates us through the strings of conditioning into behaviors and habits that may not be for our greatest good. B39, the Puppeteer, represents the situation that allows the head (violet) to rule while denying the belly (gold). When this happens, we are not able to work through our conditioning. As we get in touch with the gold and understand our true aura, we can find healing in our conscious mind. Through this process we can stop being a puppet to our conditioned patterns.

If we are centered in the golden area of the belly, the possibility exists for transformation in our thinking. Our inner master (see page 55) can pull the necessary strings to use the self to be of service in the world. The violet of spiritual energy pulls the strings of the golden energy that lies deep within to reveal the true wisdom of the inner self.

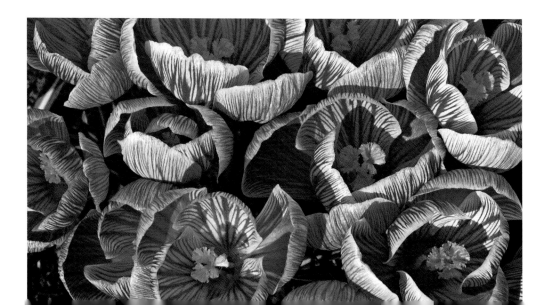

Related Bottles

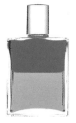

Related Colors
B32

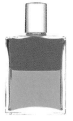

B40

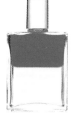

B47

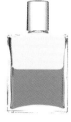

Related Reverse
B18

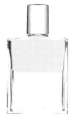

Closest Tint
B61

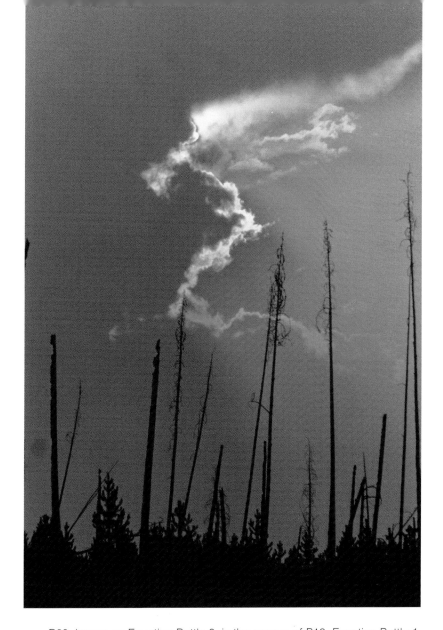

B39, known as Egyptian Bottle 2, is the reverse of B18, Egyptian Bottle 1. In B39, the gold in the base can be representative of anxiety in the depths of the self. We may pick this bottle because we wish to make amends for how we used or misused power in the past. B39 may help us connect to incarnational experiences in ancient Egypt. Incarnating in ancient Egypt would have presented two options: to incarnate as a slave or as a master, such as a scribe, pharaoh, or priest. If we lived then in a situation of privilege and power, we may carry feelings of guilt in the present or have a tendency to hold on to anxieties and fears from the past. So that the wisdom inherent in the gold may be expressed in a helpful way, anxiety in relation to the use of power in the past needs to be released. B39 thus opens us to healing abilities and to being in tune with our own process. B39 can suggest that we may be experiencing an inner transformation.

B39 may also indicate that our self-praise could lead to difficulties in making friends.

Apply this combination along the hairline and around the abdomen and back, including the spinal column.

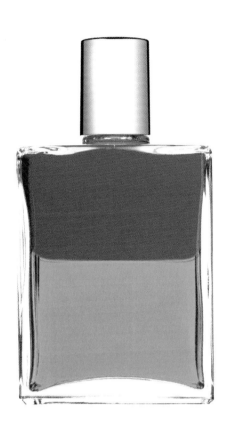

B40 Red/Gold

Name: The "I Am" Bottle

Shakes Together As: Coral

Tarot Card: Page of Cups

Keynote: The energy for wisdom. The energy that is the consequence of wisdom. A sense of expansion, enthusiasm, and growth.

B40, Red/Gold, has the name I Am because of Vicky's connection with a dentist. This dentist was a determined lady who had managed to tread her own way through a profession that (at the time) was dominated by men. When the dentist wrote about the Red/Gold combination, she referred to it as "I Am."

Red/Gold gives us a feeling of "I am." The significance of the "I am" is two-fold. One aspect is the positive, profound spiritual level that comes at the point when we find ourselves, the true nature of "I am," almost like a higher state of being. The second aspect is like that of a defiant child in the face of opposition, relating to the necessity of coordinating various tendencies within the self, like bringing the different "I's" together. "I am" can also be related to how we present ourselves rather than who we are.

Each of us may have reached a point at some time in our life when circumstances have dictated that we behave in a certain way, and we have complied with that externally. Internally, however, we may be doing or feeling the precise

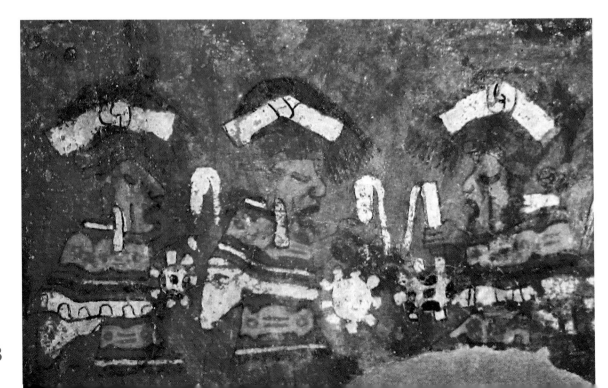

Related Bottles

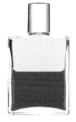

Related Reverse
B5

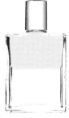

Closest Tints
B61

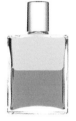

B76

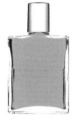

Shakes To
B105

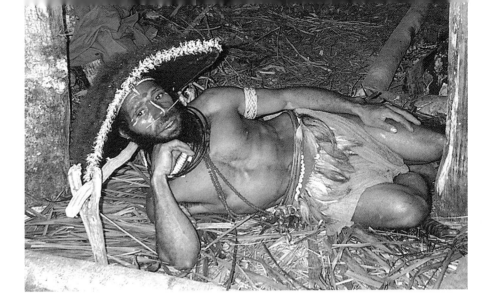

opposite of what we are expressing or displaying on the outside. This situation comes when we are determined to behave and act exactly as we want to, regardless of how people on the outside may require us to be. This is the case when we are fearful, anxious, angry, or frustrated. In these circumstances, we may be manipulated by our own insecurity and suffer from self-criticism. Red could represent frustration and anger in the conscious mind in relation to the gold within. Red could be termed righteous anger, but it is not necessarily the case.

Red is often expressed as energy and gold as wisdom. Perhaps the "I am" represents the varied expressions that result when we connect with our inner wisdom and energy is released. B40 suggests that we have positive energy and are centered and in touch with ourselves. We have the detachment (red) necessary to allow our inner wisdom (gold) to be expressed.

This combination shakes together as the hue of coral, which is connected to the energy of deep insight, the awakened insight into difficult situations.

Apply B40 around the circumference of the body between the base chakra and the solar-plexus chakra.

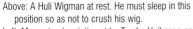

Above: A Huli Wigman at rest. He must sleep in this position so as not to crush his wig.
Left: Mayan tomb painting at La Tumba Huihazoo on the Puuc route in Mexico.
Right: Red Coat of a British soldier. During the American Revolution, the assertive appearance of the red coats in the natural landscape made the British extremely visible.

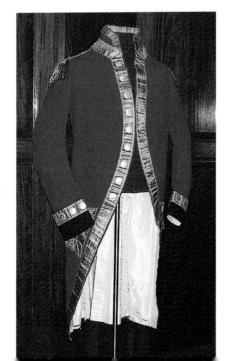

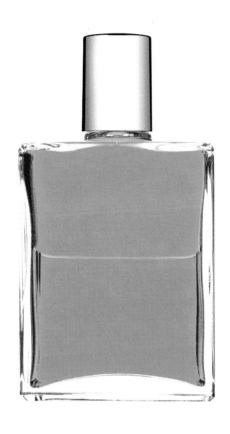

B41 Gold/Gold

Name: The Wisdom Bottle/El Dorado

Shakes Together As: Gold

Tarot Card: Ten of Cups

Keynote: As we fill the cup within ourselves, it is able to overflow within the world. Wisdom realized and shared.

El Dorado is a legendary place where vast, elusive treasure waits to be discovered. When the Spanish invaded South America in the 1500s, they often found cities empty of both people and treasure. The missing treasure and population was a mystery to them. Perhaps the peoples of the time and place had a wisdom, a preknowledge, that averted disaster and prevented the invasion from being truly successful.

B41, Gold/Gold, is about that mystery of a wealth that lies hidden within. The gold can be refined, but it is difficult to discover. Wisdom is elusive and can never be owned. It is possible to go to the golden area within us, to be within the true aura, and to connect with our incarnational star. But there is no permanence to that experience. It is possible only to continuously practice making our way to that golden area. However often we have been to that place before, being in

Below: Lion with cubs in Kenya, Africa.

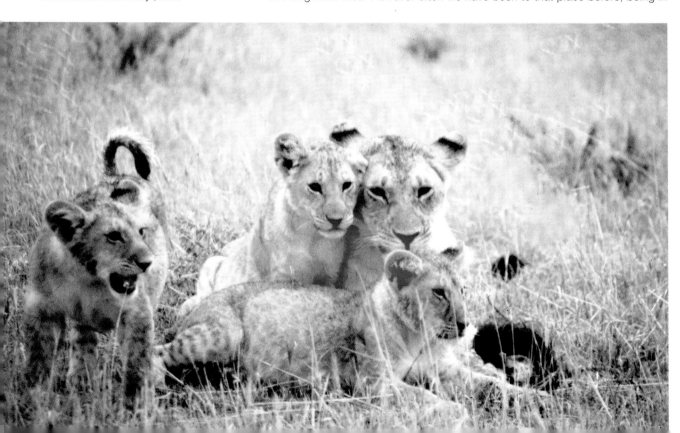

Related Bottles

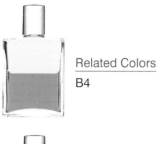

Related Colors
B4

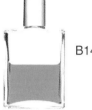

B14

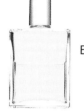

B42

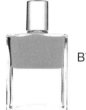

B73

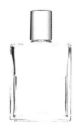

Closest Tint
B51

Above, right: Golden Buddha. Thai people pay their respects by placing three objects of offering in front of Buddha—a candle to symbolize the light of understanding; a lotus flower, special to Buddha and considered to be exalted; and incense sticks. If a person places gold leaf on a Buddha statue it is believed he or she will receive certain benefits. When placed on the mouth the giver will be blessed with good speech or sweet talk, on the head he or she will become wiser, and over the heart the giver will be ensured of a good heart in the sense of both health and kindness. The gold can also symbolize generosity.

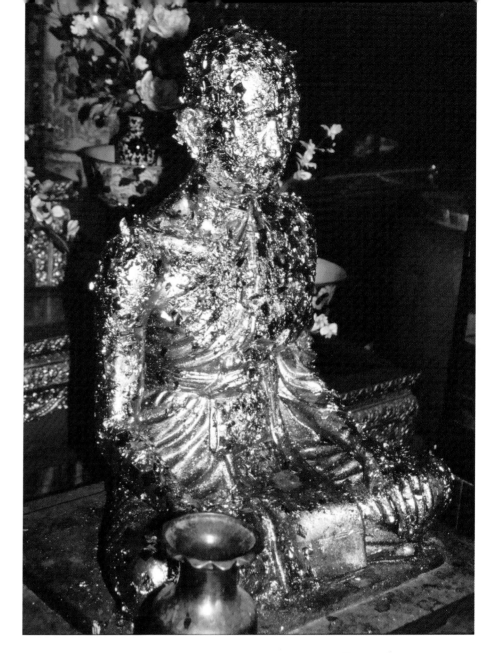

that place is an experience that cannot be owned or possessed. The experience is in the realms of the transpersonal. As soon as we are there, it is not ours. It is an amazing paradox. Just like those who search eternally for El Dorado, we cannot possess the inner wisdom.

B41 carries a feeling of joy and wisdom through positive thinking, expression, and action. B41 suggests that we have found the quintessence of our wisdom, the pot of gold at the end of the rainbow, by connecting with our center, the golden area of the body. When we need B41, we may be withdrawn, resulting in fear, anxiety, or confusion, or we may not be breathing deeply enough.

This bottle may dissolve blockages in the middle of the body and can help with assimilation. Apply the contents across the solar-plexus area and around the back, including the spinal column.

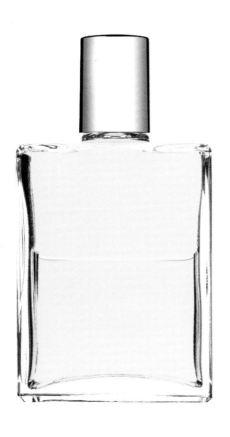

B42 Yellow/Yellow

Name: Harvest

Shakes Together As: Yellow

Tarot Card: Nine of Cups

Keynote: Self-consciousness, joy, happiness, intellectual clarity. The understanding of self.

B42, Yellow/Yellow, is called Harvest, reminding us of the season when seeds in their fullness are brought to fruition. Here is the yellow of joy and sunshine, the yellow of fully ripened grain. A harvest is tangible, provided that the seeds have been planted in the right way. We experience a good harvest when the weather and all external conditions are optimal for the seeds' growth. Analogously, if we plant the appropriate and helpful seeds within ourselves and those seeds come to fruition, it is time for celebration, and we can experience great joy. We who have found emotional happiness, joy, and fulfillment may be called to B42. We are self-aware and have found knowledge that stimulates our mind, or we may be intellectuals who emit contentment.

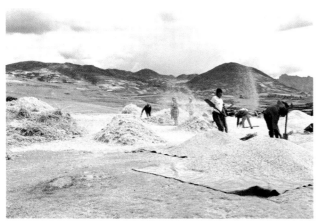

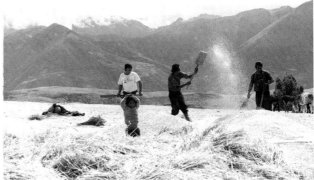

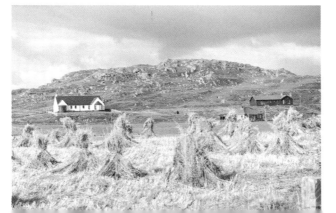

Related Bottles

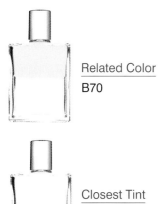

Related Color
B70

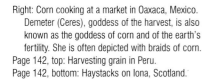

Closest Tint
B51

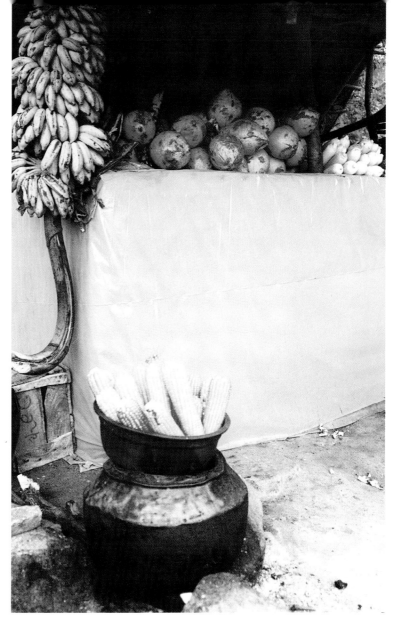

Right: Corn cooking at a market in Oaxaca, Mexico.
Demeter (Ceres), goddess of the harvest, is also
known as the goddess of corn and of the earth's
fertility. She is often depicted with braids of corn.
Page 142, top: Harvesting grain in Peru.
Page 142, bottom: Haystacks on Iona, Scotland.

At harvest time, we can reap only what we have sown. For example, if we plant cabbages, we can expect only cabbages to grow and to be harvested; if we plant roses, we may harvest roses. The harvest is always a consequence of what we have planted: "As you sow, so shall you reap." In that light, B42 can point to those of us who may be self-conscious or have negative feelings. We could be anxious about overeating or confused but trying to put on a happy face. B42 can be useful prior to examinations. It also can affect the astral body, helping us release our illusions.

Apply B42 around the solar-plexus area, particularly in cases of winter or seasonal depression (seasonal affective disorder).

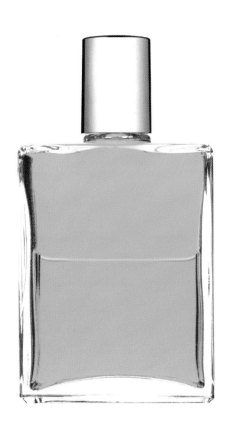

B43 Turquoise/ Turquoise

Name: Creativity

Shakes Together As: Turquoise

Tarot Card: Eight of Cups

Keynote: Creative communication through the feeling side of the being. The process of individuation unfolds.

Within Aura-Soma, turquoise is related to the creative communication of the heart through the feeling side of the being. It is the color of the Ananda Khanda, "the Bright," the little center on the right side of the chest just above the right nipple (see the illustration of subtle anatomy on page 24). Turquoise represents the process of individuation, the collective unconscious, and self-expression.

Vicky said that beginning in 1966, the turquoise and magenta colors became more visible within the rainbow. She understood this to be a sign marking the beginning of the diminishing of the old Piscean aeon and the commencement of the new Aquarian aeon. The amplification of these two colors is a confirmation of the covenant between then and now. (See also the descriptions of B45 and B75.) Turquoise is one of the colors of the Aquarian aeon. One of the principal Aquarian ideals is humanitarian independence, to which the process of individuation could lead. The nature of creativity is that as we become more individuated, we begin to express our creativity, whether in little or big things.

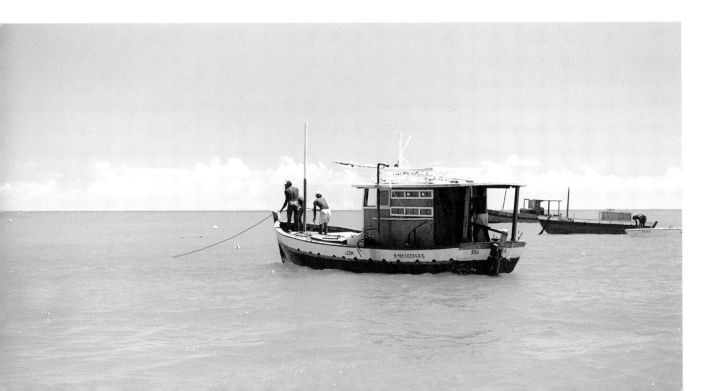

Related Bottles

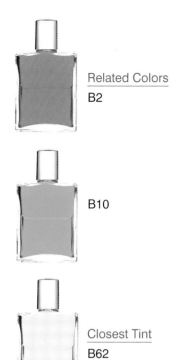

Related Colors
B2

B10

Closest Tint
B62

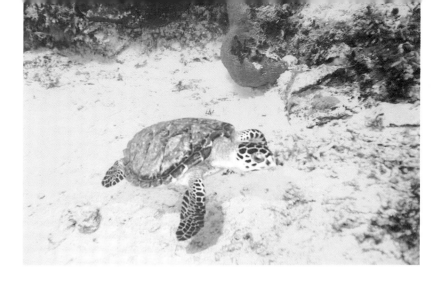

A secret to a fulfilled life is to value creativity expressed in simple things and in great things equally. Thus, B43 can tell us of a need to acknowledge inner fears or confusion that may be stopping the flow of creativity or preventing us from knowing what we want to do to fulfill our purpose.

The appeal of the creativity in the act of painting or of a painting can be very subjective. Yet there is the possibility of a painting touching the same feeling within each onlooker. Perhaps for there to be an objective form of art, the artist needs to be more individuated and thus in touch with the collective voice within him or herself. This concept is encompassed within the turquoise and the process of creativity. The awakening that arises from the stimulation of the Ananda Khanda marks the movement into our heart of the wisdom resulting from the mystical search into the eternal mysteries.

Apply B43 around the chest and across the back, including the spinal column.

Left: Fishing Boat off the coast of Salvador, Bahia, in Brazil.

Top: Turtle and coral reef at Palancar Gardens in Cozumel, Mexico. Turtles, thought to be the second incarnation of Vishnu, are symbolic of immortality. They represent the primal mother and the ability to unite heaven and earth.

Bottom: Two dolphins near Bimini Island in the Bahamas. Symbolic of music and the nine muses, dolphins are known for their intelligence and speed. Poseidon (Neptune), god of the sea, and Aphrodite (Venus), the woman of the sea, may both be represnted by a dolphin.

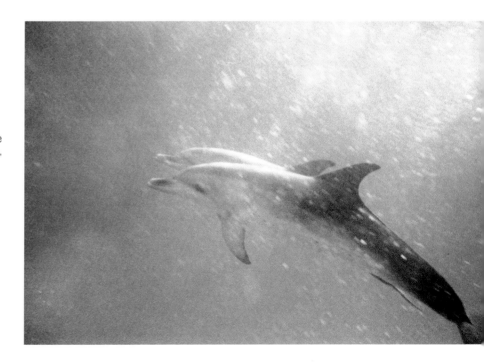

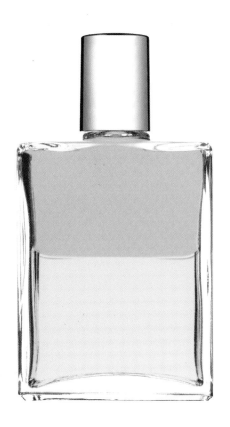

B44 Lilac/ Pale Blue

Name: The Guardian Angel

Shakes Together As: Lilac

Tarot Card: Seven of Cups

Keynote: The sense of a presence. Being in the moment whereby clarity comes in communication.

This was the first bottle that Vicky asked Mike Booth and his wife, Claudia, to birth. Prior to this time, Mike had not actually realized what went into the process of "birthing a bottle," although Mike had witnessed Vicky bringing new bottles into being many times. To this day, it is still incredibly difficult to convey what actually happens to allow a bottle to be born at a specific time. The birth involves many inner and outer conditions coming together until the time arrives when the colors need to be poured into the bottle that awaits them, and another component/being of the Aura-Soma Equilibrium range is born.

Before they began working with Aura-Soma, Claudia and Mike had been involved with work connected to angelic realms, particularly in using a visualization of a pale blue sphere with lilac flames surrounding the sphere. B44 is an expression of that work, and this is why the combination is named the Guardian Angel.

A guardian angel is a protective angel, a being who looks after us, preventing from coming in those things that are not wanted. It is another level of being, always with us and continually trying to inspire us to do our best. B44 therefore suggests inspiration in the heart and the trust to bring that inspiration into reality. B44 helps us discover our own divinity, the angel we are.

Page 147, top: Clouds in Sydney, Australia.

Page 147, bottom: *Cupid and Psyche,* by Antonio Canova, at the Louvre in Paris. Cupid reminds Psyche that love cannot live without trust. Finally Cupid's kiss awakens Psyche from a deep sleep.

Below: Region of the Marmolada in South Tyrol, Italy, an area fought over during World War I. Angels love high places.

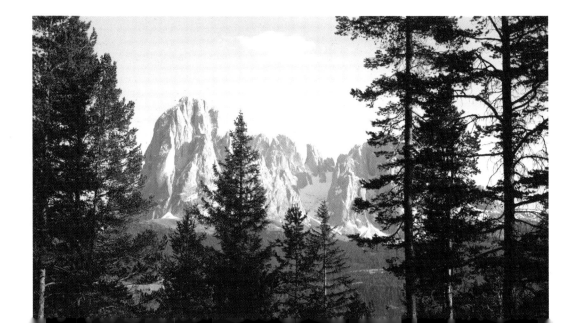

Related Bottles

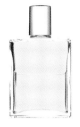

Closest Tints
B50

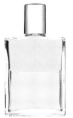

B57

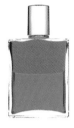

Closest Hue
B37

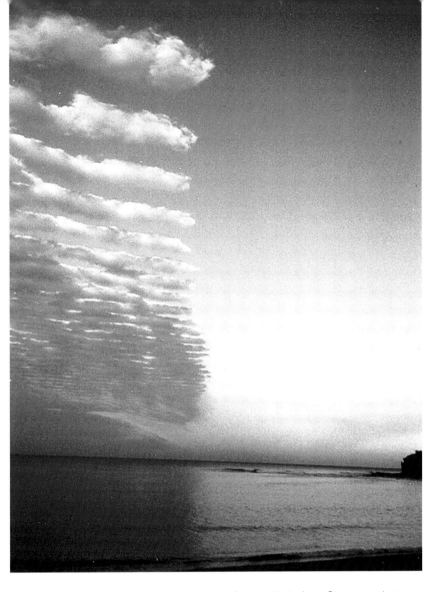

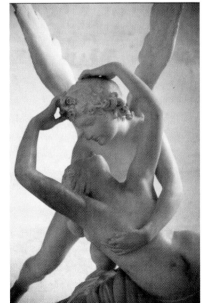

The meditation that we practice most frequently in Aura-Soma seminars involves visualizing a pale blue sphere surrounding the physical body. The color of the sphere is the same pale blue that is in the base fraction of B44. The upper fraction is the color of the lilac or violet flame surrounding the pale blue sphere. The pale blue offers absolute protection, while the lilac flame is constantly burning away negativity, transmuting it.[44-a] Negativity can be a consequence of identifying with negative emotions or with what is less than the best within us. We may want things to be a certain way but not know how to achieve those goals. We may suffer from illusion or self-deception, perhaps living too much in the past. We may find it difficult to express how we feel about what we are thinking.

The two colors together create the guardian angel (see also B37). As we bring the guardian angel closer, the guardian angel and ourselves may become more aligned. The combination gives strength to those people who may have had encounters with UFOs, extraterrestrials, or angels and who, as a result, feel threatened, confused, or insecure.

Apply B44 around the throat and along the hairline.

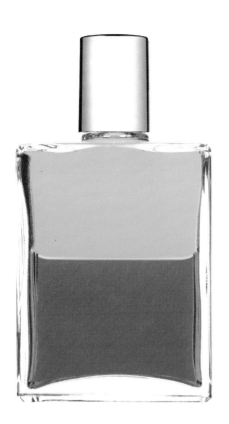

B45 Turquoise/Magenta

Name: **Breath of Love**

Shakes Together As: **Violet**

Tarot Card: **Six of Cups**

Keynote: The need to unfold the love from above in relation to the feeling side of the being. The gift of the coming and going of the breath, moment to moment.

Page 149, top: Flower opening in Barbados.
Page 149, bottom: Flowers along stone wall in Koh Samui, Thailand.
Below: Cottage in Derwent Valley, Tasmania, during a moment of respite.

When B45 was first born, it was called Dottie's bottle. This is because Dottie Hook, a longtime Aura-Soma associate, had arrived just as this bottle had been born. In addition, Dottie had bought a gift for Vicky and Margaret, a mobile that contained exactly the same colors as the new bottle. Mobiles are used as decorative objects and as energetic tools in feng shui. They hang from the ceiling and are moved by air. Coincidentally, this bottle has a connection with air, through the breath of love.

At a later date, during a workshop in France, Mike experienced a healing with a Tibetan monk who was staying at the same center where the workshop was being held. The monk had been shown how to transmit healing energy through the breath, and he used the technique, called the Breath of Love, to help people. From this experience the bottle acquired the name it now has, Breath of Love. Love in the little things (magenta) and the free flow of turquoise help bring conscious attention to the breath and direct it in the body. B45 thus

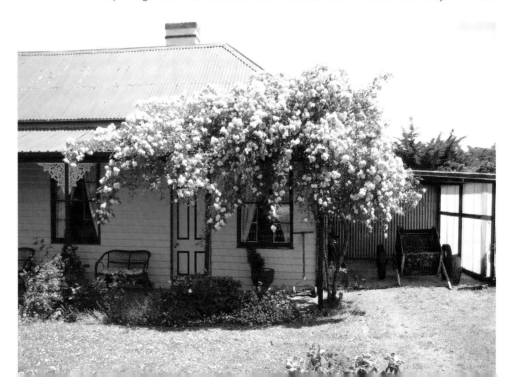

Related Bottles

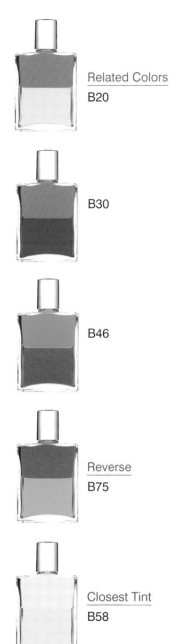

Related Colors
B20

B30

B46

Reverse
B75

Closest Tint
B58

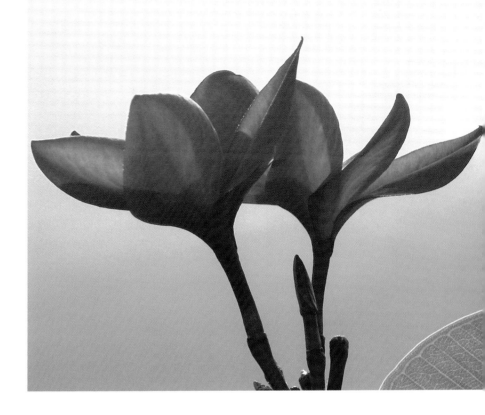

indicates that our qualities of loving kindness and compassion are to be shared with others. Creative expression—such as music, dance, and poetry—helps with healing all over the world.

In B45 is the intense form (compared to deep magenta) of the magenta energy—to be able to have and to give love through attention to little things—with the individuation and creativity of turquoise. The turquoise area on the body is in the location of the lungs, where the breath naturally comes. As we breathe in the love from above, it is directed to, and makes its first contact with, the Ananda Khanda, the turquoise center on the right side of the chest. This process opens the Ananda Khanda to move toward the emerald of the heart on its journey toward the golden area within the self. The breath of love is about the opening of the Ananda Khanda, the fourth and a half chakra (see "The Subtle Anatomy," page 23).

B45 assists us in overcoming our disappointments in love and in restoring our creative flow. This is necessary if we tend to take on other people's problems and may need to overcome pride. B45 points to a need to allow new love to enter and to let go of past memories that may stifle happiness.

B45 may be applied everywhere. When there is deep stress, apply it around the heart.

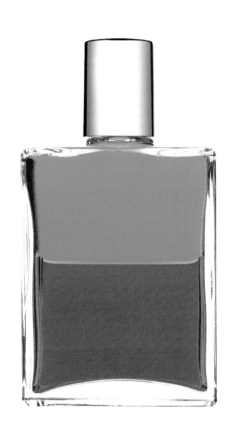

B46 Green/Magenta

Name: The Wanderer

Shakes Together As: Deep Jade Green

Tarot Card: Five of Cups

Keynote: Attention to details reveals a truth in the simplicity. Caring that is given the space to expand.

B46 pairs the green of the heart with the magenta energy. Green is in the conscious mind, the upper fraction. If we find our own space or our own direction, the love from above (magenta) can come into the depths of ourselves (the base fraction of the bottle). Magenta then starts to move underneath the emerald of the heart and begins to connect with the golden area (see "The Subtle Anatomy," page 23).

Many who are attracted to Aura-Soma are wanderers. We wander around the earth doing what we are called to do. Wanderers are at home wherever we are. This comfort can offer a sense of freedom. When we are seeking the truth, with love in the depths of ourselves, we can be at home in any situation. A nonattachment in relation to the feelings (green) offers a sense of freedom,

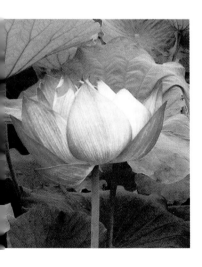

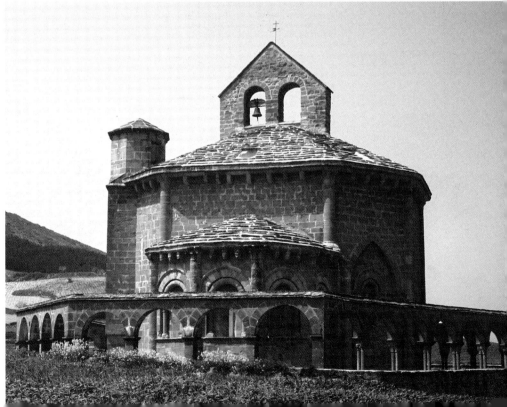

Related Bottles

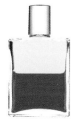

Related Colors
B5

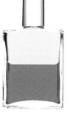

B8

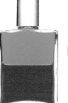

B28

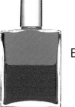

B30

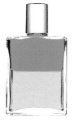

Closest Tints
B21

B99

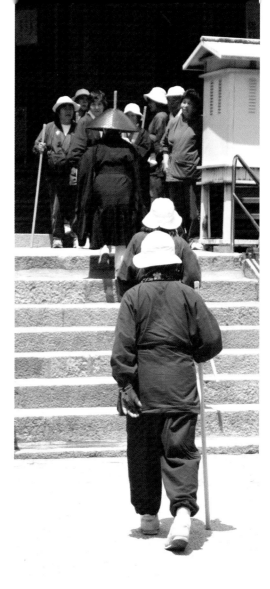

here linked to wisdom, as the magenta has begun to connect to the gold. Thus, B46 indicates that we have faith and trust, the qualities of divine love, and a creative power.

We could at times wander aimlessly, experiencing deep anxiety and lacking any sense of direction. We may have feelings of jealousy or envy. In this situation we have become disillusioned, unwilling to look at what rules our lives, reaffirming unhelpful patterns. This color combination could help us release from those rules, feelings, and patterns.

Apply B46 around the heart and across the back, including over the spinal column. In cases of menstrual problems, apply around the lower abdomen.

Above: Henro pilgrims walking the eighty-eight temple pilgrimage route established by Kobo Daishi Kukai in Shikoku, Japan.

Page 150, left: Lotus in pond. The lotus grows with its roots in the mud and its blossom in the sunlight, symbolic of our soul's progression from the primeval mud through the waters of emotional experiences to enlightenment. The pink lotus symbolizes the supreme being of Buddha.

Page 150, right: Chapel along El Camino de Santiago de Compostela, a pilgrimage route between the Holy Land and Compostela in Spain, a sacred site for thousands of years that is also known as the field of the stars. During the Middle Ages the Knights Templar offered protection along this route.

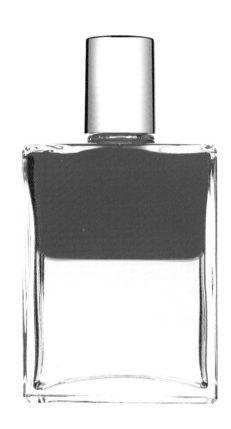

B47 Royal Blue/ Lemon Yellow

Name: The Old Soul Bottle

Shakes Together As: Emerald Green

Tarot Card: Four of Cups

Keynote: Intellectual clarity. The gift of understanding the emerald of the heart.

Vicky called B47 the Old Soul Bottle. In her view, old souls liked this color combination because they incarnate on a bright yellow ray, endeavoring to understand the mystery of everything that is.

Traditionally, in the tarot, the Four of Cups is the only card, other than the aces, to show a hand offering something from a cloud, from an unseen origin, from another level. This suggests a person with mystical knowledge who is open to the higher mind functions, to heavenly peace, and to inspirational creativity.

In the Rider-Waite Tarot, a cup is being offered to a person sitting underneath a tree. There are three cups on the ground. The cup represents the water element. What is being offered relates to a shift of faith or trust, both of which are attributes of the water element. Some things still remain in the realm of mystery.

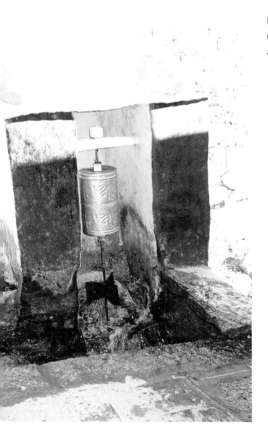

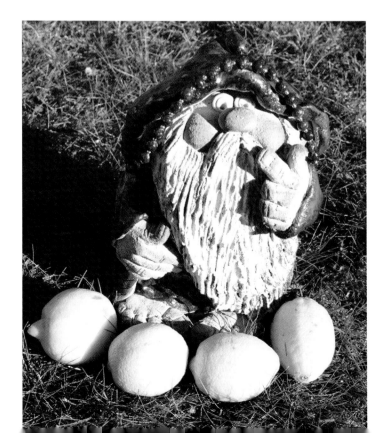

Related Bottles

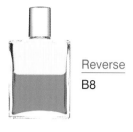

Reverse
B8

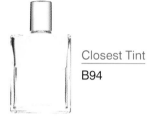

Closest Tint
B94

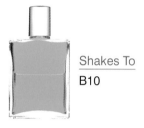

Shakes To
B10

Right: Cave 4 at Qumran, where Dead Sea Scrolls were found by two Bedouin shepherds in 1947.
Page 152, left: Prayer wheel at the Drepung Monastery in Lhasa, Tibet.
Page 152, right: Gnome from Scotland with lemons and lapis.

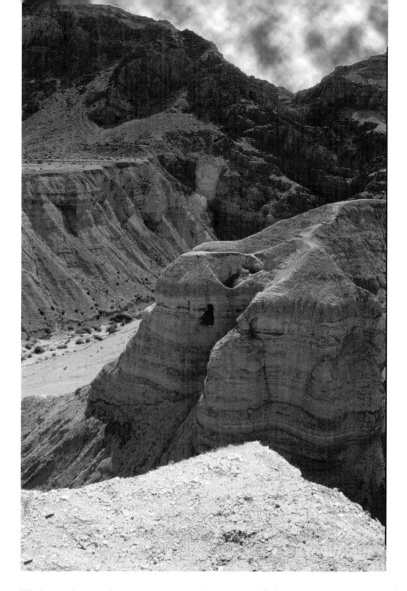

We know that we have an opportunity to trust a little more, yet more trust does not necessarily mean a change in our understanding. We may be part of something that unfolds in spite of us, rather than because of us. Perhaps we are not the key player in the scene but, rather, a part of the greater whole that is unfolding. In this imagery is a feeling similar to that manifested by Excalibur appearing mysteriously out of the lake to the Arthur who would be king.

B47 is the only bottle in the Equilibrium range that has lemon yellow in the base. Lemon yellow represents a sharp intellect, which can be bittersweet. It leads to the higher intuition (the royal blue in the upper fraction) and the possibility of clarity at the sense doors, which, in turn, may allow us to get in touch with clarity within the intellect. The royal blue and the lemon shake together as emerald green. The emerald green qualities may be expressed as a new possibility for humankind.

This bottle may help with boredom with intellectualization, hidden fears, or depression from internalizing too much.

Apply B47 around the body over the area of the solar plexus and the heart, as well as along the hairline.

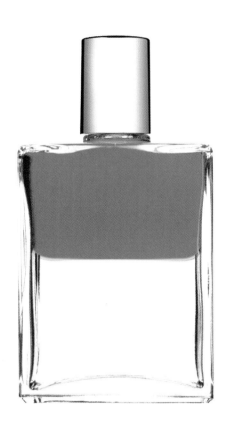

B48 Violet/Clear

Name: Wings of Change
Shakes Together As: Lilac
Tarot Card: Three of Cups
Keynote: An understanding of the light within the depths of the self. A transformation in the conscious mind.

In B48, Wings of Change, the clear in the base fraction is like the light of angel wings. The wings are so bright that they are difficult to see. The spirituality and healing of the violet is in the upper fraction, in the conscious mind. The wings are folding around the suffering (clear) that lies within, creating a safe place for the transformation (violet) in the conscious mind, for the light within to emerge. As the light from within shines, we experience the potential for finding our spirituality,

Violet and clear shake together to create lilac. This color of transmutation is the alchemy that brings a completely changed state. An alchemist changes base metal into gold. B48 is concerned with how we can turn the negative aspects of ourselves into positive ones. To find peace and healing in the conscious mind, we need to become more clear and shed repressed tears. Wings of Change carries us from one state to another. B48 may be chosen by those of us who have experienced much grief and suffering or even shock, often in connection with a death experience. The possibility for healing from that experience exists; transformation in the conscious mind and a healing of the suffering contained within us may occur.

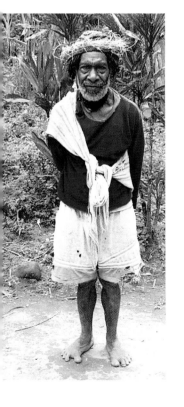

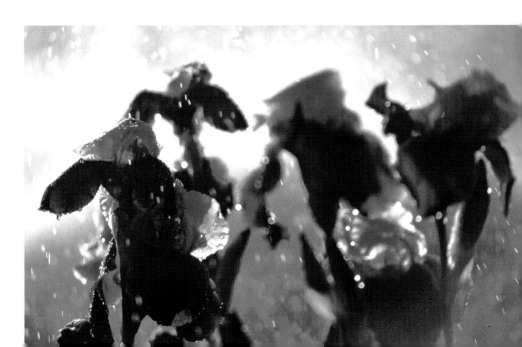

154

Related Bottles

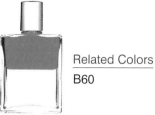

Related Colors
B60

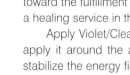

B69

Reverse
B15

Shakes To
B56

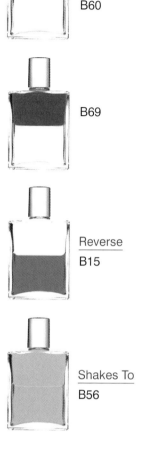

Right: Hacienda dating to 1613, a time of great struggles over sugar cane production, now a hotel in Morelos, Mexico.

Page 154, left: Farmer from the Highlands of Papua New Guinea.

Page 154, right: Irises "singing in the rain" in Bondville, Vermont.

Each of us has wings. If we are suffering greatly, our wings may not be in good health. The idea offered by the Wings of Change is that our wings may be restored to full health through relief from suffering. B48 can carry us forward toward the fulfillment of our service (violet) to the light. An orator who is fulfilling a healing service in the world may be drawn to B48.

Apply Violet/Clear along the hairline; for hormonal-related back problems, apply it around the abdomen. B48 may be useful after craniosacral work to stabilize the energy fields.

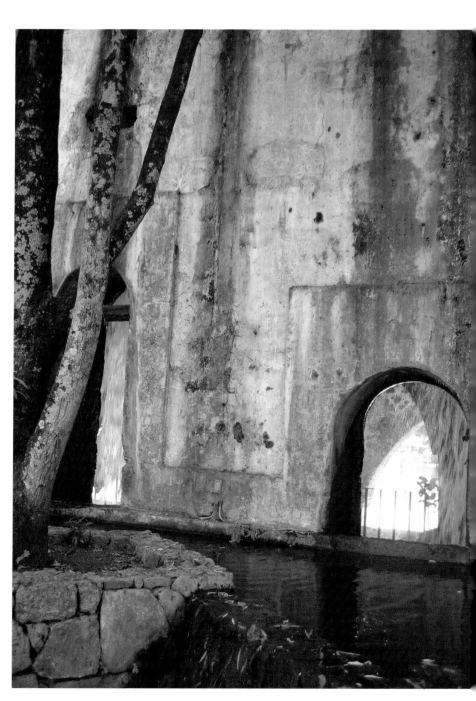

155

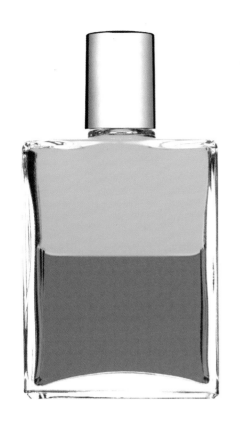

B49 Turquoise/Violet

Name: The New Messenger

Shakes Together As: Deep Violet Flecked with Turquoise

Tarot Card: Two of Cups

Keynote: Creative communication of the heart in the service of others.

B49 is another messenger: the New Messenger. It is related to B24, Violet/ Turquoise, the New Message. The potential exists for those called by B49 to bring joy and happiness to others, by expressing peace, harmony, and a sensitivity in communications. But the colors in B49 are upside down relative to the body's chakra centers (see "The Subtle Anatomy," page 23). Therefore, the healing qualities that are to be shared with love from the heart may be hidden.

Page 157: King Arthur's Court, Chalice Well Gardens, Glastonbury, England. Arthur, with his sword Excalibur, is known as the once and future King.
Right: Aurora outside of Fairbanks, Alaska.
Below: Winged Messenger at the Musee d'Orsay in Paris, France.

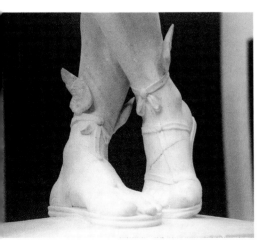

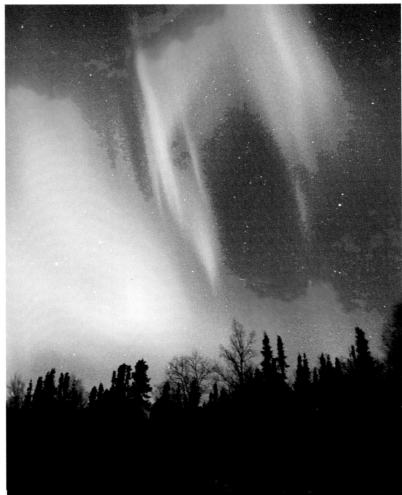

Related Bottles

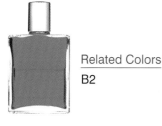

Related Colors
B2

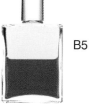

B5

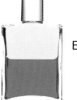

B8

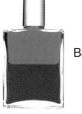

B30

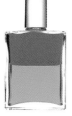

Reverse
B24

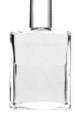

Closest Tint
B58

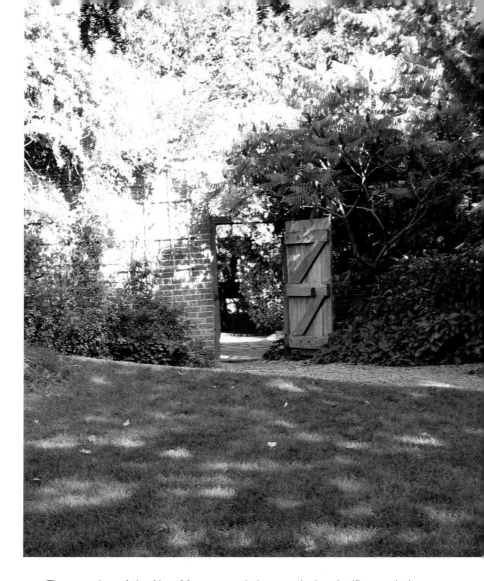

The meaning of the New Messenger derives particular significance in its position immediately prior to the revelation of the Master Set sequence, which starts with B50 and runs through B64. B49 heralds the entrance and cooperation of the Masters (see the description of the Masters on pages 38–39). B49 symbolizes an immensely positive message that informs us of the good that is to come.

The New Messenger marks a point in the development of Equilibrium. Choosing B49 can indicate that a message is available to us. Perhaps we have had difficulties with communication or our creativity has been stifled. We may need to heal our heart and find love or to let go of guilt after losing our way. In B49 is a message associated with a communication from a deep level of transformation that is waiting to come through into the feeling side of our selves; it marks an elasticity of our mind resulting from being in touch with our inner voice.

Apply B49 around the body over the chest area and along the hairline. In the case of speech problems, apply it around the throat and neck.

157

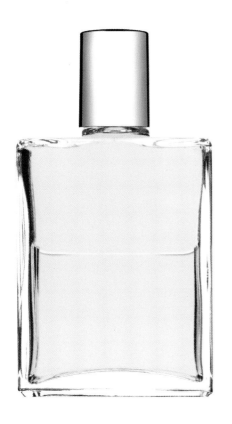

B50 Pale Blue/Pale Blue

Name: El Morya

Shakes Together As: Pale Blue

Tarot Card: Ace of Cups

Keynote: Thy will, not my will. Being able to get out of the way to allow the communication to come through, rather than from, the self.

Page 159, top: Morning mist hangs over the Brahmaputra River in Central Tibet, creating a very magical moment.
Page 159, bottom: The intense blue of the divine will shown in a delicate blue columbine in Ripton, Vermont.
Below: Mono Lake, east of Yosemite National Park, near the town of Lee Vining, California. A highly alkaline lake, the minerals dissolved in the water form "tufa towers," calcium-carbonate protrusions that make the landscape feel as if it belonged to another planet.

El Morya is the first bottle in what we refer to as the Master Set (see page 55).[50-a] When these bottles (B50 through B64) came into being, Vicky said that they had names in a way that differed from the naming of the previous bottles. In a sense, bottles B50 through B64 have names that predate the bottles' birth, names that are intrinsically connected to the color of each bottle. These bottles are born whole, complete with the name of the ray on which they arrive. At the time of their birth, Vicky was unaware of the work of Annie Besant, Madame Blavatsky, or the early Theosophists. Vicky learned from Mike of the Theosophists' understanding of the rays and the Master Beings that come in on those rays.[50-b]

B50 is the only bottle in the Master sequence that relates to the suit of Cups in the tarot (see "The Tarot Card," page 51).[50-c] The suit of Cups is associated with the element of water. All the other Masters are associated with the suit of Swords. It is appropriate that B50 is the Ace of Cups because our understanding of the blue energy is that it relates to the qualities of faith and trust, which are attributes of the water element. The pale blue is an intensification of faith and trust, which brings us to "Thy will, not my will," the message of B50, and the name El Morya.

The history of El Morya[50-d] tells us that he incarnated as a prince in the Indian province of Rajastan, became enlightened, and was known as a spiri-

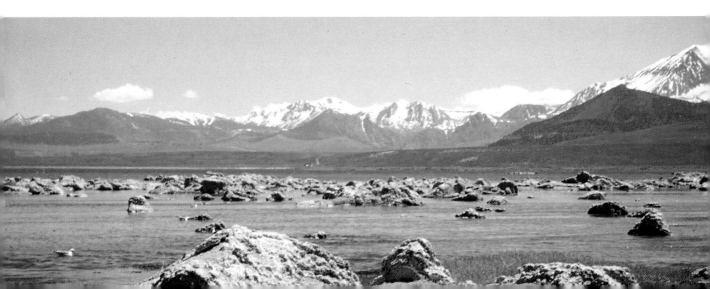

Related Bottles

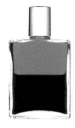

Related Colors
B1

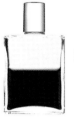

B103

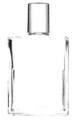

Closest Tint
B54

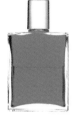

Closest Hue
B2

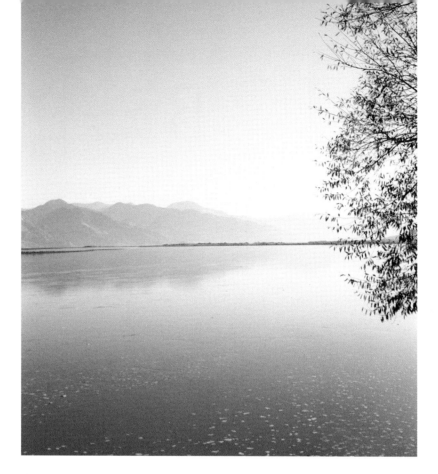

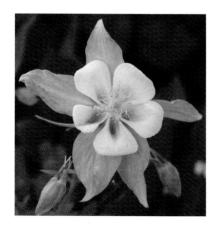

tual leader. He made a commitment to help all human beings. In both this and his other incarnation in India, El Morya's commitment to looking after people was prominent. El Morya subsequently became an Ascended Master of the White Brotherhood, a group of beings who have become enlightened on the Earth plane and have made a commitment to help all human beings evolve in consciousness.[50-e] The El Morya bottle therefore suggests that we have inner tranquility and a clear mind, that we are selfless and put the concerns of others before our own.

B50 suggests our need to find a balance between loving too much and too little. El Morya can help us with depression due to feelings of being unwanted or unloved or to difficulty expressing our feelings. B50 can guide us to our own qualities of caring and compassion.

During one incarnation, El Morya connected with a wife from a previous life experience who was known as Miriam.[50-f] Miriam became the archetypal big sister for the Judaic people. El Morya and Lady Miriam are like twin souls working together, with one or the other being more obviously helpful and effective at varied times. Therefore, within B50 is also the energy of the Divine Mother in the form of the Lady Miriam.

As discussed in "The Language of Color" (page 13) concerning the implications of hues and tints, everything that applies to B2, Blue/Blue, also applies to B50, Pale Blue/Pale Blue. In the tint the issues are more intense, or more light has been shone onto them.

An interesting fact to note from a numerological point of view is that the B50 is the amplification of B5 (5x10), the bottle that called to Vicky the most.

Apply B50 around the throat and neck.

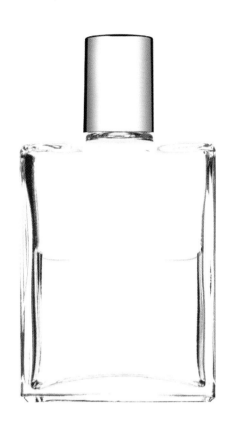

B51 Pale Yellow/ Pale Yellow

Name: Kuthumi

Shakes Together As: Pale Yellow

Tarot Card: King of Swords

Keynote: Two-way communication from that which is above us to that which is beneath us. A communication with the devic realms.

B51, Pale Yellow/Pale Yellow, is about a two-way energy connection. As humans, we are receptive to communication with angels and can communicate what the angels say to the devic world. We are the connection between these two manifestations of existence.

Kuthumi was an Indian shah (1628–1658) who also had incarnations as Pythagoras (circa 575–circa 495 BC) and Saint Francis of Assisi (circa 1182–circa 1226).[51-a] Like El Morya (see B50), Kuthumi was a member of the White Brotherhood (see note 50-e).

The name Kuthumi is pronounced somewhat like "come to me," a concept that is carried through in the energy of this bottle. Saint Francis carried this "come to me" energy, transmitting it to birds, animals, and children. The images of Saint Francis usually portray him surrounded by these beings. This same energy is reflected in the two-way energy flow from the angelic realm to humans and from humans to the devas, making B51 helpful with our perception of and

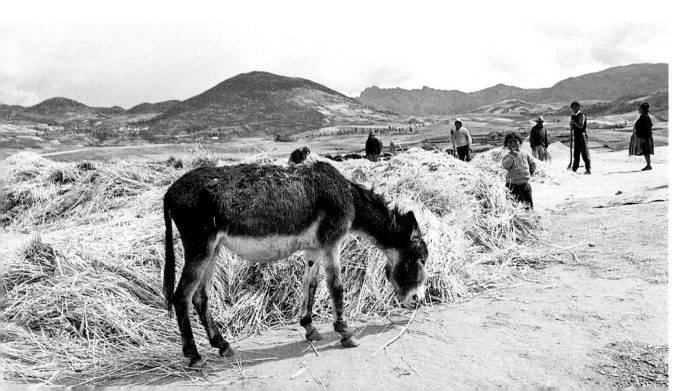

Related Bottles

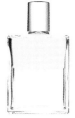

Related Color
B70

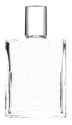

Closest Hue
B42

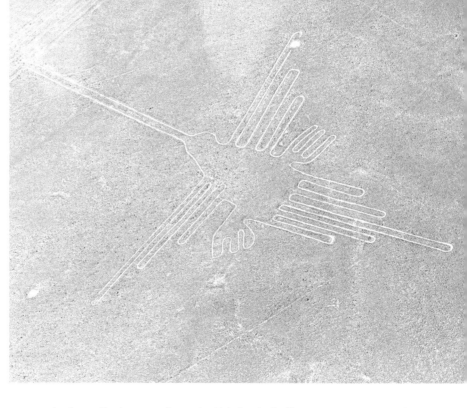

communication with devas and angels. This bottle facilitates an awareness of the entire mineral and plant realms and the beings that occupy these realms.

B51 may appeal to those of us seeking knowledge, who have mental flexibility, discrimination, clarity, and open-mindedness. It may represent those of us who fight for the rights of and seek justice for others. Yet to achieve this, we need to let go of anxiety, fear, and intolerance and avoid disputes that arise from our fears.

As discussed in "The Language of Color" (page 13) concerning hues and tints, everything that applies to B42, Yellow/Yellow, also applies to B51, Pale Yellow/Pale Yellow, in a more intense form.

In B50, the higher will (blue) is illuminated. In B51, yellow, the little or individual will of the solar plexus is illuminated. Therefore, B51 should be applied around the solar plexus.

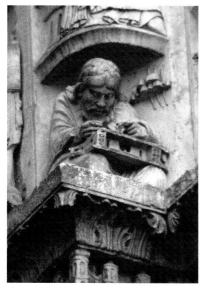

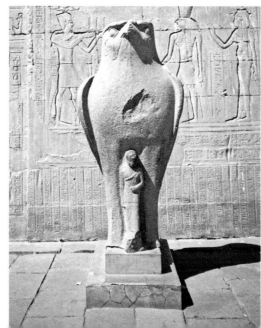

Above: Carving of Pythagoras, Greek philosopher, mathematician, and teacher of clear intellectual thought. Chartres Cathedral, France.
Left: A donkey, beloved by Saint Francis, gently grazing in Peru.
Right: Horus as the Falcon God at the Temple of Horus in Edfu.
Top right: Hummingbird at the Nazca Lines in the Nazca Desert, Peru.

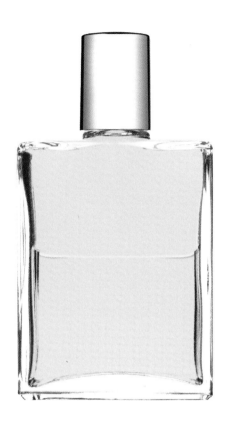

B52 Pale Pink/ Pale Pink

Name: Lady Nada
Shakes Together As: Pale Pink
Tarot Card: Queen of Swords
Keynote: The communication for self-acceptance in a profound and deep way.

Lady Nada is the consort of Christ. *Nada* is a Sanskrit word meaning "sound." Translated from the Pali/Sanskrit/Aramaic root, it means "the holy sound," the sound of silence, of soundless sound.[52-a] It is related to the holy om and thus connected with the sixth chakra. B52 also relates to the third eye and to music; it can intensify our experience and understanding of music.

There is a connection between color and the meaning of the name Lady Nada. To get in touch with *nad*, "the inner sound," and to achieve clarity, we need to have detachment at the sense doors. Each of the senses has within it a gift that forms part of our inner essence. There is a link between the organs of the body and the senses; each of the organs can be brought to more optimal functioning through the development of detachment at the sense doors. The less we identify with what our senses experience, the more likely it is that we can go beyond the senses and perfect what lies as a gift at each of the sense doors. The body thereby can come to a state of being more conscious, more whole, and more able to grow spiritually through love. In personifying B52, we would be perceptive and intuitive, able to give love to others as well as to ourselves.

Lady Nada brings us the intensification of the red qualities in the palest of pinks. These qualities include detachment, self-acceptance, and the possibility of awakening to unconditional love. Though difficult to attain, unconditional love

Right: Red fort near the Taj Mahal gardens. Originally built from mud and brick as a military fortress on the banks of the River Yamuna, in Agra, India, in 1565 A.D. when Agra was the capital. It is now a space in which to hear the voice of the silence.
Below: Rose, a symbol of love, in Ripton, Vermont.

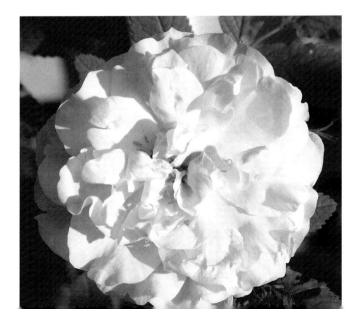

162

Related Bottles

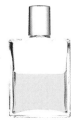

Related Colors
B11

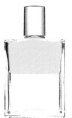

B71

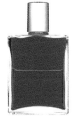

Closest Hues
B6

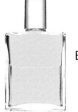

B81

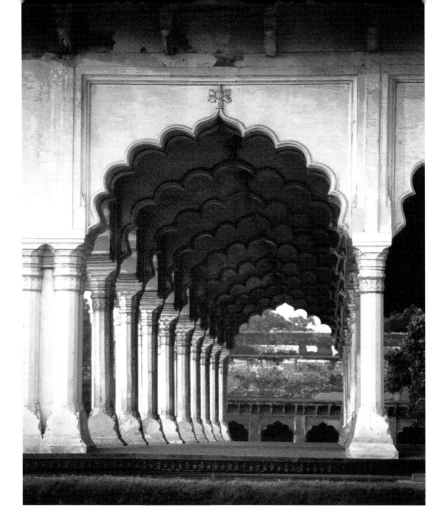

is probably the most potent of forces, and the fabric that lies behind the whole of existence.

Red is the color attributed to aversion. In Buddhist teaching aversion is a poison: that which says no, pushes away, and denies. The poison can be transformed into detachment or nonattachment, not holding on to things and having the freedom to discern when to let things go. Red represents the possibility of being in a position to watch what is happening within us, rather than identifying with it. As this transition or transformation to dis-identification takes place, a great possibility exists for us to be more aware of the inner sound, the sound that lies behind or within the body at a deep level.

When B52 points to our challenges, it suggests spiteful, critical, suspicious, or jealous tendencies. We may be susceptible to emotional blackmail, or because we are holding on to intense anger and resentment, we may be empty of love. We may not have developed the ability to detach. Consequently we may be reactive rather than actively responding anew.

In past-life therapy, B52 may help us establish contact with Essene incarnations (see also B11 and B71).

As discussed in "The Language of Color" (page 13) concerning hues and tints, everything that applies to B6, Red/Red, also applies to B52, Pale Pink/Pale Pink, in a more intense form.

Apply B52 around the body in the abdominal area. In the case of mental stress, apply one drop to the top of the head, to the temples, and to the back of the neck; rub in gently.

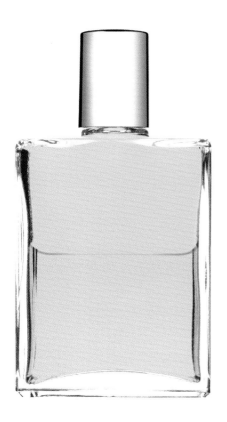

B53 Pale Green/ Pale Green

Name: **Hilarion**

Shakes Together As: **Pale Green**

Tarot Card: **Knight of Swords**

Keynote: **The Way, the Truth, and the Life. A balance within the heart where the heart has been through a process of purification.**

Hilarion, Pale Green/Pale Green, represents the intense seeker of the truth. When the seeking of truth (green) is intensified (pale green), it becomes the Way, the Truth, and the Life. Master Hilarion is said to have inspired the classic theosophical work *Light on the Path*. From this work we learn that "The great and difficult victory, the conquering of the desires of the individual soul, is a work of ages. . . . When you have found the beginning of the way the star of your soul will show its light."[53-a] Hilarion, who was a scientist in Etruscan times, developed a method to transmute energy, which could benefit all human beings. Through this he came to enlightenment.[53-b]

The sequence of time can be symbolized by the cycle of green growth in nature; thus, green is often associated with Saturn, the timekeeper. Saturn is also often associated with lead. Many theosophical masters were occupied with the alchemical task of turning lead into gold or, said another way, turning green to gold. In shining light on green (pale green), we shine light on lead, the Saturnian energy, making it lighter and more golden. The transmutation of energy is about learning the lessons of Saturn, those to do with time and a deep understanding of time and space. Hilarion came to transcendence in relation to energy by going deeply into that study and process.

When we think of vast rolling green fields, we begin to understand why people who work with body therapies, such as Rolfing, Trager, the Alexander technique, Feldenkrais, or any of the other techniques that increase the sense

Page 165, top: Carving from Saint Bartholomew's Church courtyard in New York City. Our soul star shines as we find our way.

Page 165, bottom: Green aurora in Fairbanks, Alaska, shedding light on our path.

Below: Grasshopper on the wall of a Napoleonic cottage at Ozolles in southern Burgundy, France. Like the quick movements of the grasshopper, Hilarion inspires a quickness of mind for scientific discoveries.

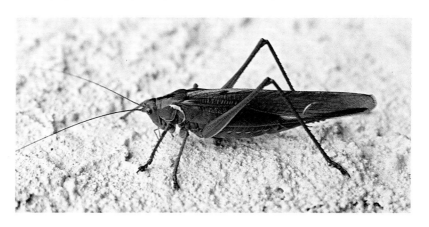

Related Bottles

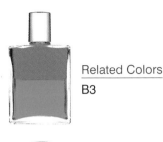

Related Colors
B3

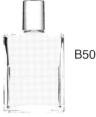

B50

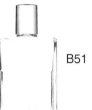

B51

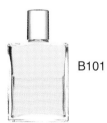

B101

Closest Tint
B94

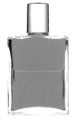

Closest Hue
B10

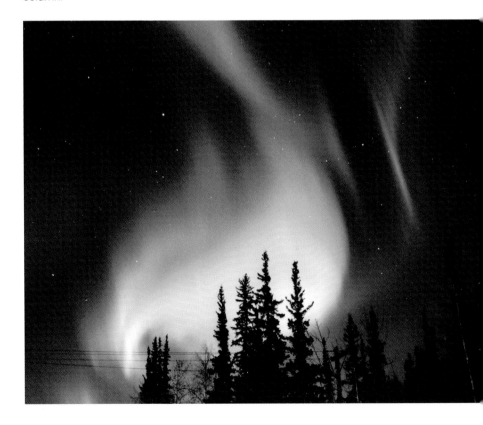

O SEND OVT THY LIGHT AND THY TRVTH THAT THEY MAY LEAD ME & BRING ME VNTO THY HOLY HILL AND TO THY DWELLING

of spaciousness within the body, often choose B53. B53 highlights our need to release feelings of frustration, confusion, or pain from separation or deceit. B53 may help us establish contact with Lemurian incarnations.

In consultation, B53 can represent those of us who like arguing and conflict or who are impetuous, in a continual state of anticipation, which prevents us from being focused in the present. This condition highlights the potential to make space for ourselves and to find our right place. If we are truthful, we are able to let go, to leave the past behind, and to move forward, discovering what lies ahead: the Way, the Truth, and the Life.

As discussed in "The Language of Color" (page 13) concerning hues and tints, everything that applies to B10, Green/Green, also applies to B53, Pale Green/Pale Green, in a more intense form.

B53 should be applied around the heart area, including the back and spinal column.

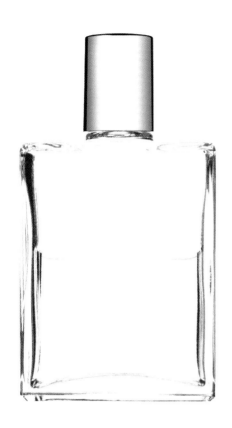

B54 Clear/Clear

Name: **Serapis Bey**

Shakes Together As: **Clear**

Tarot Card: **Page of Swords**

Keynote: **The understanding of suffering. The power of the light and purification.**

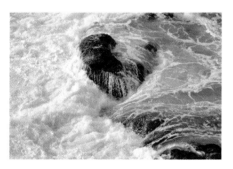

Serapis Bey was born into the family of one of the beys who ruled the Otto-Turkish Empire (1290–1603). He was a young priest/king. He reached enlightenment through developing an understanding of suffering and of the alleviation of suffering, both concepts that are inherent in the clear color. Thus, B54 suggests that we are growing through understanding of suffering.

Serapis was the inspiration for many messages of the Sufi poets,[54-a] especially the idea that devotion, above all else, can burn away the dross of our being. If more material things are burned away, it is possible to come to a new perspective of understanding. This is a pure and penetrative practice. B54 therefore also represents our awareness of revelations that come from above.

In consultation, B54 can mark us as having suffered and possibly being in great pain. It could symbolize that we are domineering and "white with rage." It may help us cease hiding who we are and look at and show our true colors.

On many occasions, Vicky said that B54 and the Quintessence Serapis Bey were the most powerful within the entire Aura-Soma range. Serapis Bey can help us find those colors that relate most closely to our soul ray. It may be helpful when other combinations are not working as intended, stimulating the Aura-Soma interactive process. Both B54 and the Quintessence Serapis Bey need to

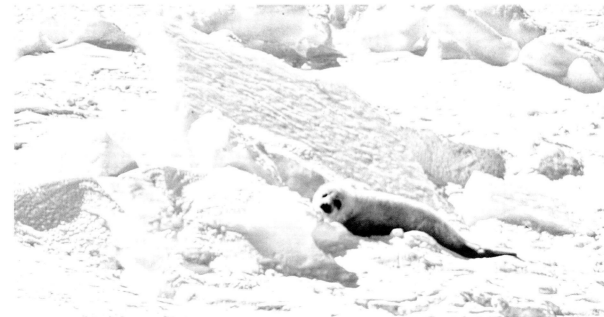

Related Bottles

All colors come
from light, and
thus all the bottles
are related to B54.

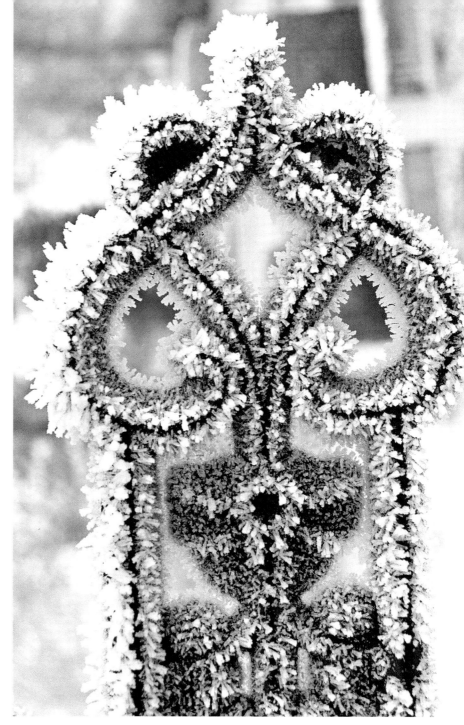

Right: Iron grave marker in Sweden.
Page 166, top: Storm surge at Castlepoint off the
end of Lighthouse Rock on the North Island of
New Zealand, an extraordinary place where the
power of nature is often demonstrated.
Page 166, bottom: Baby white seal in the Magdalen
Islands, reminding us of the purity and innocence
of a newborn.

be used with caution, supported by the use of them in combination with pink,
perhaps a pink Pomander or a pink Quintessence. Clear, if used alone, may
bring difficult issues glaringly to light. By using pink when working with B54, we
have caring, support, and the possibility of self-acceptance as we face whatever
issues and challenges may arise in the process of developing ourselves. The
pink helps with our assimilation of the light of Serapis Bey.

B54 may be applied everywhere on the body.

167

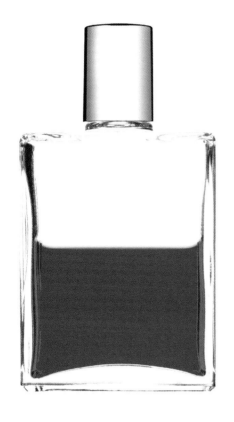

B55 Clear/Red

Name: **The Christ**

Shakes Together As: **Pink**

Tarot Card: **Ten of Swords**

Keynote: **The energy to work with and for the light.**

In B55, the Christ, clear is in the upper fraction, representing light. The red in the lower fraction represents the earth. Together, the colors represent light coming to the earth plane, just as the Divine incarnated on the earth as Christ. The Christ brings the message of forgiveness to the earth.

When the Aura-Soma bottles are placed sequentially on the Tree of Life, B55 is in the sphere of Malkuth, the Kingdom. Malkuth represents the earth. In B55, the pure light (clear) coming to earth (red) is a symbolic representation of how the Divine comes into every aspect of materiality. The bottle's placement on the Tree of Life emphasizes this meaning of divine light entering the physical world. The Christ is the reconciling force, reconciling the polarities within ourselves, particularly that between the light, which is above us, drawing us away from the earth, and the earth itself, which continually binds us toward the material.[55-a]

Shaking clear and red together forms pink, like that of Lady Nada, B52, Pale Pink/Pale Pink, but created here by two distinct colors. Red expresses love and a connection with the earth star. Perhaps this love is an answer as to why we choose to come to earth as human beings. Experiencing life on earth as a human seems to be a tremendous and unusual opportunity within the whole of

Page 169, top: Mara Rianta dancers in Masai village in Kenya, Africa. A nomadic tribe, the men herd animals while the women use native grasses to produce goods to support the family. Working together, their way of life is sustained.

Page 169, bottom: Women in Peru working with wool and caring for their children.

Below: Train in France.

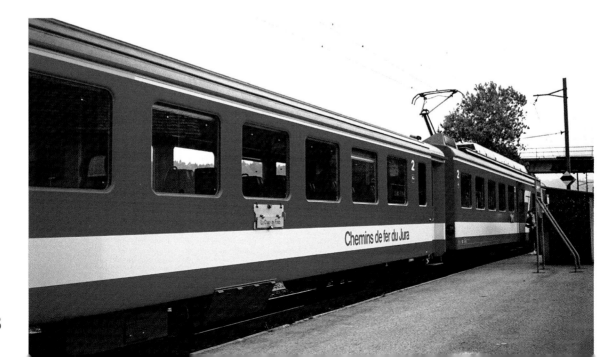

Related Bottles

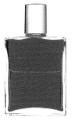

Related Colors
B6

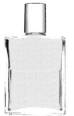

B81

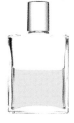

Closest Tint
B11

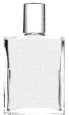

Shakes To
B52

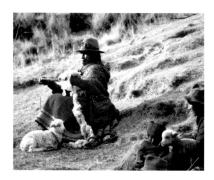

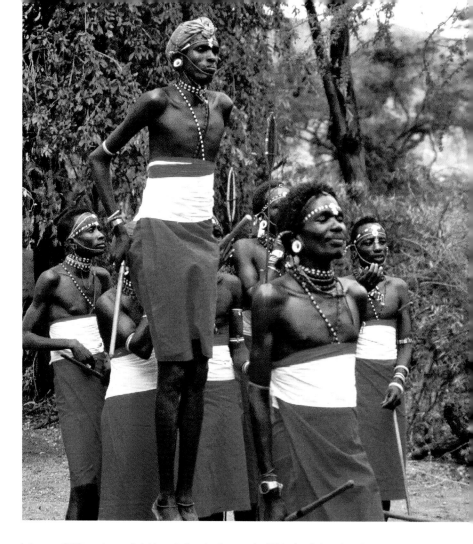

existence. B55 portrays light in relation to the earth. With the light of understanding we may reconcile what binds us to the earth and why we return to this planet. We may come through suffering to find new energy. B55 can bring our energy into the light, helping us accept who we are, all with a sense of watchful detachment. Therefore, B55 may support the process of coping with abuse. B55 could be of assistance if we wish to awaken the kundalini force.

At the same time, within this color combination is the opposite challenge of not getting caught up in our desire to return to the light. The Ahrimanic and Luciferic forces described by Steiner[55-b] are opposing inclinations. B55 could help us reconcile these inclinations to find the correct balance between being bound to the material and wanting to return to the light. In a way B55 gives us a sense of whether we are able to take on spiritual responsibility. We may need to recognize feelings of anger and resentment and let go of these feelings through emotional release, which could include crying. The insight in the clear can support us in refraining from seeking revenge.

Apply B55 around the body over the lower abdomen. Because B55 may be energizing, resulting in difficulty sleeping, it should not be used too late in the evening.

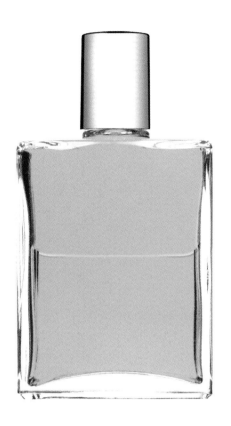

B56 Pale Violet/ Pale Violet

Name: Saint Germain

Shakes Together As: Pale Violet

Tarot Card: Nine of Swords

Keynote: Overcoming the desire to be invisible. To act as a catalyst in the world.

Saint Germain is a Master Being of many incarnations. In the late 1600s, as Prince Rakoczy of the royal house of Hungary, he supported a movement to bring about equality, fraternity, and freedom in his country, and through his works for a higher cause, he gained enlightenment and the freedom of nirvana.[56-a] He also played an energetic role in the American Revolution and as the Comte de Saint Germain during the time of the French Revolution (1789–1799), he was in a position to stimulate the French revolutionaries with the same ideals he had supported in Russia. In commemoration of Saint Germain's presence, streets in Paris and throughout France are named after him. Saint Germain is perhaps best known for his incarnations as Francis Bacon and William Shakespeare. For an understanding of the consort of Saint Germain, please see the information on Lady Portia, B59.

B56 suggests that we have entered the process of letting go of the past to become more able to be in touch with our true spirituality. We may be loving and

Page 171, top: Lavender aurora in Fairbanks, Alaska, with conductor—orchestrating and inspiring from behind the scenes a universal movement for equality and freedom.
Page 171, bottom: Amethyst crystal from Brazil.
Below: Charoite, whose chemical formula is $K(Na,Ca)_{11}(Ba, Sr)Si_{18}O_{46}(OH, F)\text{-}nH_2O$, is a rare and unusual mineral from the Chara River in Eastern Siberia. It is formed from high temperature alteration of limestone by alkaline magma intrusion.

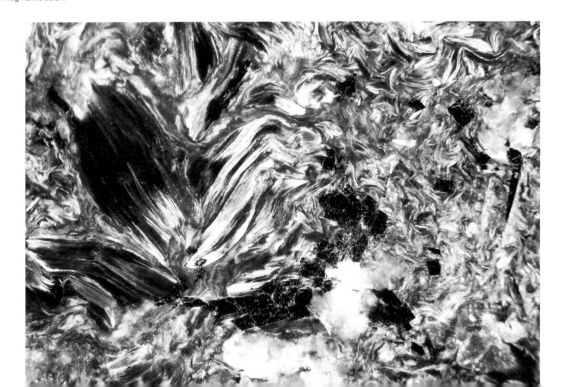

Related Bottles

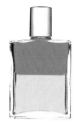

Related Color
B20

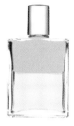

Closest Tints
B44

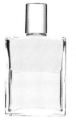

B57

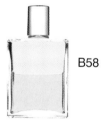

B58

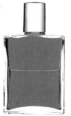

B66

Closest Hue
B16

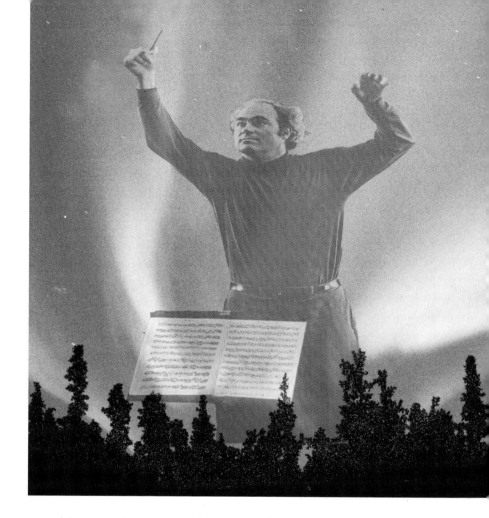

peaceful; we may be sensitive thinkers, inspirational teachers, or healers. B56 helps us synthesize our inner male and female aspects. It may help us integrate a religious experience into our ordinary life. Astrologers associate the planet Jupiter with a benevolent, expansive nature and a positive philosophical mind. B56 suggests similar qualities. Saint Germain's ability to be in many places at one time, his expansion beyond physical form, mirrors the expansive qualities of Jupiter.

B56 can point out our need to release ourselves from negative thoughts. We need to consider why we do not accept ourselves and decide where to make changes.

As discussed in "The Language of Color" (page 13) concerning hues and tints, everything that applies to B16, Violet/Violet, also applies to B56, Pale Violet/Pale Violet, in a more intense form.

Apply B56 around the hairline.

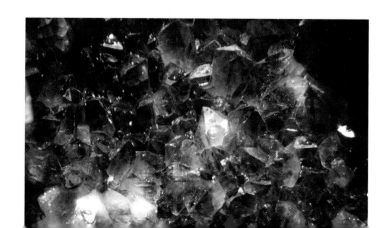

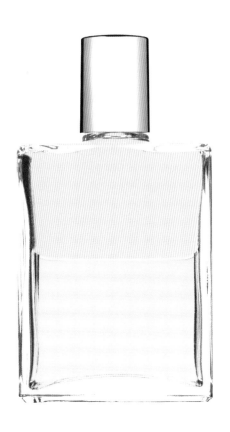

B57 Pale Pink/Pale Blue

Name: Pallas Athena and Aeolus
Shakes Together As: Pale Violet/Lilac
Tarot Card: Eight of Swords
Keynote: Creativity and right livelihood. Attention to detail.

In ancient Greece, Aeolus was known as the god of the winds, and Pallas Athena, the daughter of Zeus, was known as the goddess of wisdom. The name Pallas Athena means "spear shaker," and Athena is known for bringing spears of light to shake up and transform ignorance to insight. B56 has a connection to these divine beings both through color (the pink of the feminine and blue of the masculine) and through meaning.

In ancient Egypt, Aeolus and Athena were known as a couple, Pharaoh Akhenaton (ruled circa 1350–circa 1334 BC) and his wife Nefertiti. Akhenaton, known as a heretic pharaoh, encouraged the worship of the single sun god, Aten. The name Nefertiti means "the beautiful/perfect woman has come." In both eras these beings were concerned with dream life and the love of aesthetics and beauty. While dreams are not necessarily aesthetic, beauty can emerge in dream life even if we do not feel particularly beautiful ourselves. This bottle may help us consciously recall our dreams. It can symbolize that we accept ourselves, that we are aware of our limitations and our potential to overcome

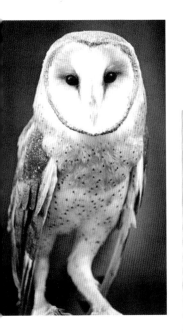

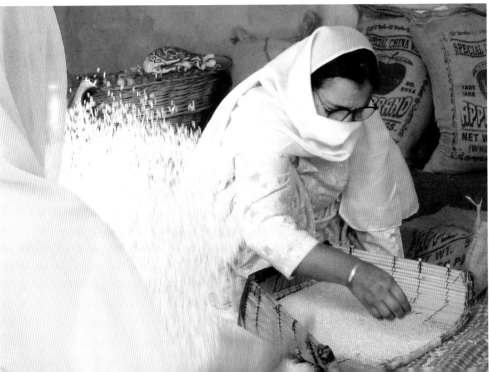

Related Bottles

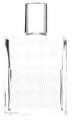

Reverse
B58

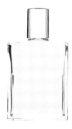

Closest Tints
B50

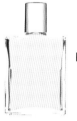

B52

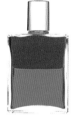

Closest Hue
B29

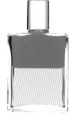

Reverse Hue
B20

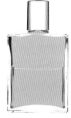

Shakes To
B56

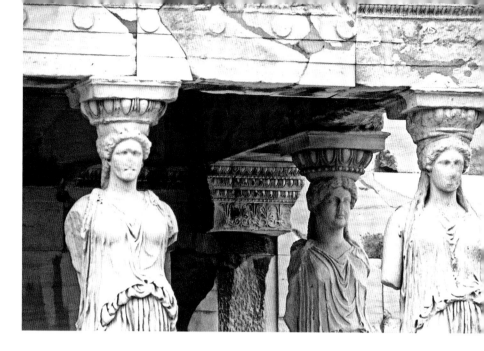

obstacles, and that we are wholesome in our understanding of the laws of the material side of life. B57 may also help us relate to incarnational experiences in ancient Egypt and ancient Greece.

According to myth, Athena was born spontaneously from the head of Zeus, thus avoiding childhood. B57 thus has a connection with childhood issues, as is also indicated by its color correspondence with B20, Blue/Pink, the Star Child. We may be having difficulties with childhood issues or relating to our avoidance of these issues. We may need to consider the male-female balance within: how one side of the body might manipulate the other. The pink and blue in B57 suggests a need to accept ourselves as we are, to let go of a sense of rejection, to let go of anger or hurts from childhood. Those of us who are drawn to B57 may be unnecessarily preoccupied with issues of survival or be narrow-minded with fanatical beliefs.

Athena is also known as the patron of the skilled crafts of ancient Greece, such as ship and chariot building, and also of traditionally female domestic activities like spinning and weaving. She is also credited with the invention of the potter's wheel, the vase, and the flute. "A major temple, the Parthenon in Athens, became hers as a result of her gift of the olive tree to the Greek people."[57-a] B57 shows us that we have an opportunity to find the balance of a skill or occupation that satisfies our survival needs and also honors what we love to do. This would allow us an inner sense of beauty, and our life might feel asthetically pleasing.

B57, Pale Pink/Pale Blue, is an upside-down and more intense version of B20, Blue/Pink, the Star Child bottle. Therefore, the concerns inherent in B20 will be more intense and perhaps considered from a different perspective in B57.

Apply B57 around the body in the lower abdominal area, around the throat, and along the hairline.

Above: Karyatids on the porch of the Erechtheion temple devoted to the worship of Athena, which is next to the Parthenon at the Acropolis in Athens, Greece.

Page 172, left: Barn owl at Blue Hills Trailside Museum in Milton, Massachusetts. The owl emanates tremendous power and makes quite a fierce display even though it weighs only one and a half pounds. The owl is a symbol of Athena's wisdom.

Page 172, right: Kashmiri women cleaning rice in preparation for a wedding ceremony. The rice becomes filled with the women's song.

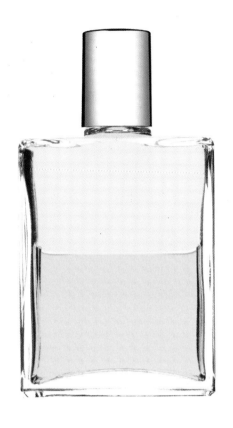

B58 Pale Blue/ Pale Pink

Name: Orion and Angelica

Shakes Together As: Pale Violet/Lilac

Tarot Card: Seven of Swords

Keynote: To help all of the subtle bodies to be in the right place at the right time. A balance within the subtle fields.

Right: Angelica herb growing tall in the garden at Dev Aura in England. Angelica cleanses impurities from the earth as it reaches toward the sky.

Below: Crow Point in Manchester-by-the-Sea, Massachusetts.

Orion, the Hunter, is a constellation named for a hero in Greek mythology.[58-a] This constellation also represents the Egyptian god Osiris, the god of death and resurrection. Interestingly, there is a theory "that would see the pyramids of the west bank's 'land of the dead' as direct reflections on the ground of the stars of the constellation Orion (Osiris), with the main Giza pyramids corresponding to the imperfectly aligned stars of Orion's belt and the Nile itself reflecting the celestial Milky Way."[58-b] The belt of Orion is said to be where the White Brotherhood (see note 50-e) is located, as suggested by the geometry and orientation of the Great Pyramid and its placement and relationship to Earth's measurements and to other significant landscape features.

Angelica is the common name of the herb *Angelica archangelica*. This herb may grow up to eight feet in height and is known for its ability to ward off the plague and all diseases of despondency and faintheartedness. Angelica is a symbol of inspiration and gladness. "It belongs to the Sun and its fiery essence directs a current of vital energy into your soul."[58-c]

In Aura-Soma, Orion and Angelica are considered angels, and they are among the biggest angels that we work with. They continually circle the Earth, drawing the curtain to bring each night and opening the curtain to bring each day. This rhythm makes B58 helpful when we travel, particularly when we are dealing with jet lag. Angelica, as an angel, has a fiery quality. We who are drawn

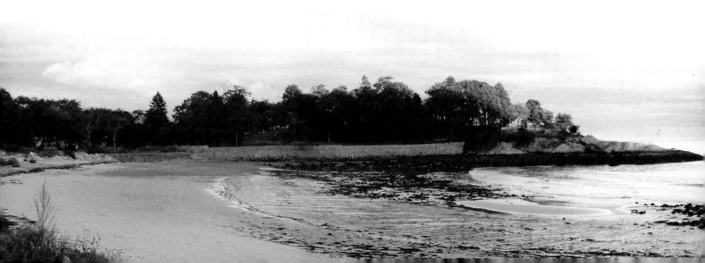

Related Bottles

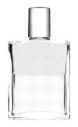

Reverse
B57

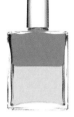

Closest Hues
B20

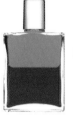

B30

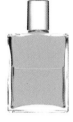

Shakes To
B56

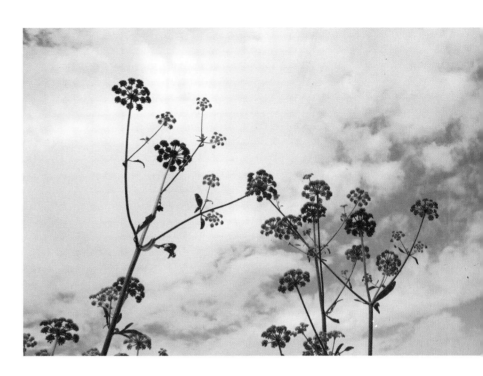

to B58 may be sensitive and balanced; we may be catalysts who can nurture peace and whose faith can build bridges between mind and matter.

We may also need to learn to accept ourselves, to let go of certain thought patterns that might limit us or hold us back. We may have family issues, including a need to heal a parental situation, a rivalry among children, or a desire not to be part of the family. When we feel that the love of our father and mother was lacking in childhood, the angels bring this love to us. Their gift of love can help support us in releasing antiquated, conditioned patterns from childhood.

Apply B58 around the body in the abdominal area, around the throat, and along the hairline.

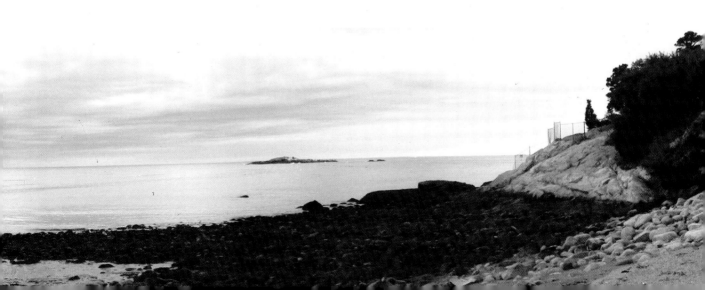

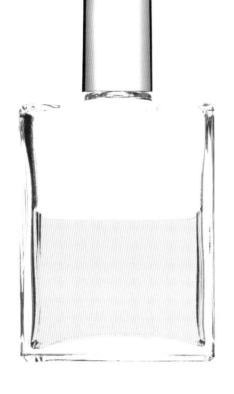

B59 Pale Yellow/ Pale Pink

Name: Lady Portia

Shakes Together As: Pale Coral

Tarot Card: Six of Swords

Keynote: Letting go of the judgment of self helps with discrimination and balance.

Lady Portia is the consort of Saint Germain (see B56). Saint Germain as William Shakespeare wrote a beautiful soliloquy for Lady Portia, sometimes called "The Quality of Mercy," in *The Merchant of Venice*, act 4, scene 1. As expressed in the soliloquy, Lady Portia tries to bring grace and mercy to all difficulties. Her message is "Judge not, lest you be judged." She is a balanced and harmonious person who accepts herself without fear of judgment. B59 suggests that our knowledge has come because we have found love. Knowledge and joy are expressed graciously in self-acceptance. Since we realize the importance of interdependence (coral), we offer caring and warmth for the benefit of everyone.

The choice of B59, Lady Portia, may imply that we are judging ourselves harshly. Perhaps we all judge ourselves, even when it is not necessary. The problem can be exacerbated because the energy of judgment can overflow, so that in time we become judgmental about everybody else. The more we are able to accept and care for ourselves within our inner experience (pink), the more we may be able to let go of judgment (yellow) in our mental and con-

The quality of mercy is not strain'd
It droppeth as the gentle rain from heaven
Upon the place beneath. It is twice blest:
It blesseth him that gives and him that takes.[59-a]

Right: Rose in Ripton, Vermont.
Page 177: Zebra swallowtail butterfly in Westford, Massachusetts.

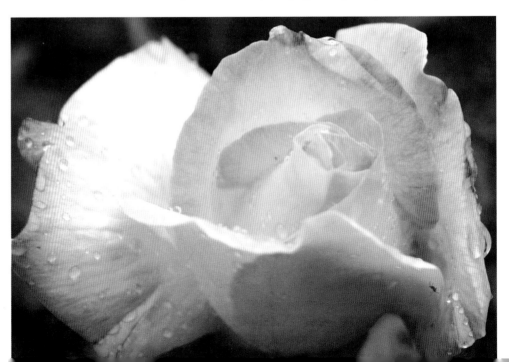

Related Bottles

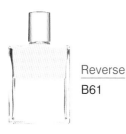

Reverse
B61

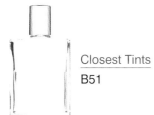

Closest Tints
B51

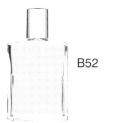

B52

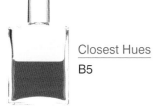

Closest Hues
B5

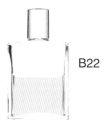

B22

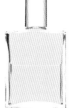

Shakes To
B87

scious mind. Therefore, B59 may be helpful for us if we have been dealing with interdependency and codependency issues, or a lack of discrimination about our boundaries. Other out-of-balance conditions include overly fearful thinking about survival issues. B59 reminds us that in judging we may miss much; it is preferable to discern all the possibilities within a situation. This could lead to great happiness.

B59, Pale Yellow/Pale Pink, is a more intense version of B5, Yellow/Red, and also of B22, Yellow/Pink, the Rebirth bottle. All that applies to those two bottles applies to B59 in a more intense form.

Apply B59 around the body in the abdominal area.

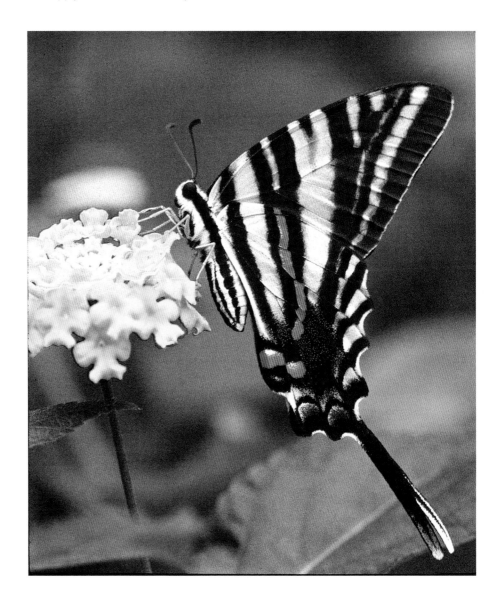

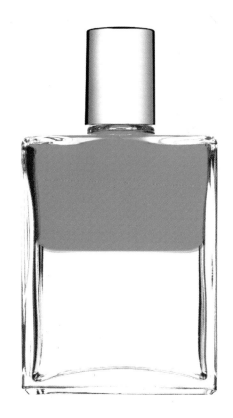

B60 Blue/Clear

Name: Lao Tsu and Kwan Yin
Shakes Together As: Pale Blue
Tarot Card: Five of Swords
Keynote: Finding the clarity within to be able to communicate from the light.

Lao Tsu was a mystic of the sixth-century BC; his name is sometimes thought to be a pseudonym for old wisdom. In the time of Confucius, Lao Tsu wrote the classic Taoist text *The Way of Life*.[60-a] He lived his life with "self-effacement and anonymity."[60-b] Kwan Yin is the Buddhist goddess of mercy and compassion. "Her force is compared to Mother Mary in the West, Green Tara in the Tibetan culture, the Virgin of Guadeloupe in Mexico, and many other ancient goddesses, the matriarchy of old."[60-c] Both Lao Tsu and Kwan Yin are considered to be Master Beings. Lao Tsu is the predominant energy in B60; within the Quintessence Kwan Yin predominates. The Quintessence Kwan Yin appears as a coral color, which is opposite to blue on the color wheel.

Lao Tsu was a master alchemist of the East. The Jade Emperor, ruler of heaven in Chinese mythology, commissioned him to make pearls of longevity; he wished to have these pearls available to give as a blessing to people who had lived a life of merit.

The clear lower fraction in this bottle relates to these pearls. The pearl of great price is born from the oyster bed of suffering, for a grain of sand within the oyster ultimately produces a beautiful pearl, shining with all the rainbow colors. The blue in the upper fraction represents peace. Peace in the conscious mind may alleviate suffering. The oyster may suffer from the pain and irritation of a gritty grain of sand. The pearl may be we who can clearly express our feelings. We have come to peace with our suffering. The light within allows us to see things as they are. B60 also carries the compassion we need when we are holding on to unexpressed sadness and other emotions. To find joy and happiness, we need to be honest with ourselves. A peaceful mind allows a release through tears and an opportunity to communicate what we have seen.

The Jade Emperor requested that Kwan Yin, the consort of Lao Tsu and a celestial bodhisattva, rule the earth with her compassion. The name Kwan Yin translates as "She Who Hearkens to the Cries of the World." Kwan Yin has been looking after many of the affairs on the earth since that time. The pledge she made, which can be repeated as an affirmation, is as follows:

"Never will I seek nor receive private, individual salvation; never will I enter

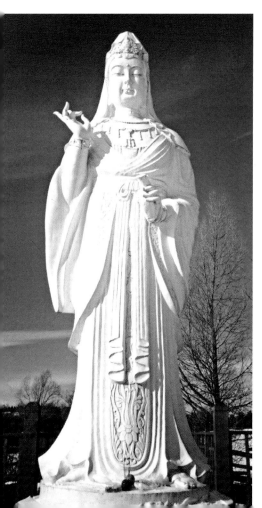

Related Bottles

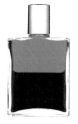

Related Colors
B1

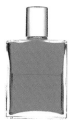

B2

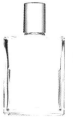

B54

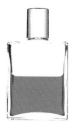

Reverse
B12

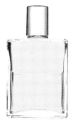

Shakes To
B50

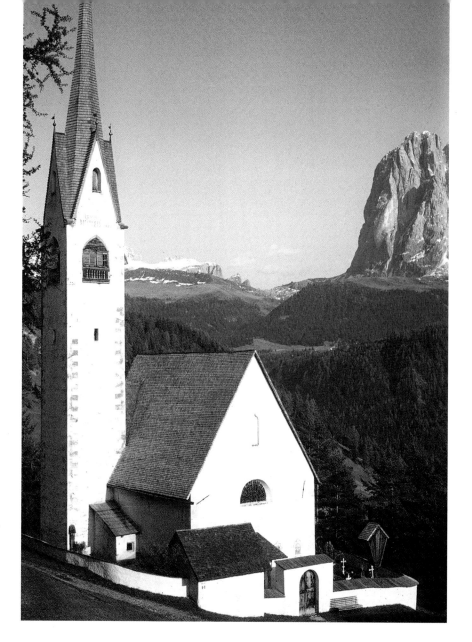

Above: Church in St. Ulrich, Italy. A border area, there is a pilgrimage route from here to the peaceful mountain.

Left: Kwan Yin statue overlooking a reflecting pond at the Taoist Tai Chi Center International Retreat in Orangeville, Ontario. Kwan Yin is a gentle protectress and a beacon of compassion.

Note: The image on page 6 is also a visual expression of this bottle.

into final peace alone; but forever and everywhere will I live and strive for the redemption of every creature throughout the world from the bonds of conditioned existence."

Kwan Yin is a member of the White Brotherhood (see note 50-e) in her own right as well as through her partnership with Lao Tsu.

B60 can act as an "in between" combination and precursor for other Equilibrium bottles in a way that is similar to B11's capacity to clear the way for other substances to be effective.

Apply B60 around the throat and neck.

B61 Pale Pink/ Pale Yellow

Name: **Sanat Kumara and Lady Venus Kumara**

Shakes Together As: **Pale Coral**

Tarot Card: **Four of Swords**

Keynote: **The deepest level of reconciliation of the role models within the self. The universal sense of the Mother/Father God.**

Sanat Kumara and Lady Venus Kumara[61-a] represent the archetypal Mother and Father, the role models for the male/female energies within the self. Often when we pick B61 we have had our role model taken away for one reason of another. Perhaps we were adopted or lost our parents at an early age; perhaps we were not able, for some reason, to relate to our parents. We may have feelings of abandonment or fears and anxieties about being alone. Having yearned and reached up from deep inside, we may have made contact with the Kumaras. B61 may represent any or all of these situations, particularly when the bottle appears in the first or second position during a consultation. The issues related to parental separation need to be taken into consideration in the understanding of this color combination.

Lady Venus Kumara is a powerful mother principle, watching over all children to make sure that their circumstances are not too difficult. Particularly when there is famine and distress, Lady Venus Kumara tries to help. Thus, this bottle

Page 181, top: Gladiolus, symbolic of strength of character, in Ripton, Vermont.
Page 181, bottom: Stonehenge, England.
Below: Mount Arenal volcano in Costa Rica.

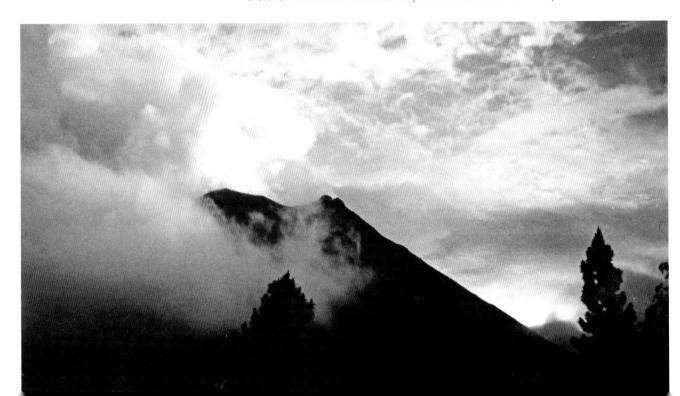

Related Bottles

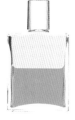

Related Colors
B76

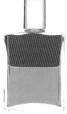

B95

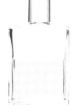

Reverse
B59

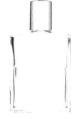

Closest Tint
B51

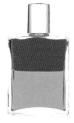

Closest Hue
B40

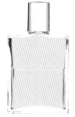

Shakes To
B87

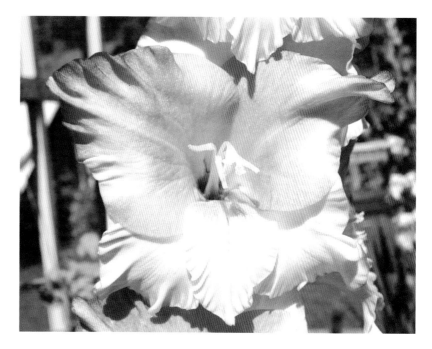

can suggest that we express deep nurturing and warmth, bringing joy. We may realize our interdependence upon all things and all people.

Pale pink and pale yellow shake together to form pale coral. Therefore, the energetic picture of B61 may contain the possibility of difficulties associated with abusive situations (see B5), possibly caused by the absence of supportive role models. The phrase "As above, so below" is associated with B61. The coral suggests the possibility of reaching a new level of consciousness, and this combination may help us establish contact with the mystical traditions in ancient Egypt and ancient Greece (2000 BC to 30 BC) and times long before. B61 has qualities similar to the feminine loving nature and the possessive hedonistic nature ascribed by astrologers to Venus.

Apply B61 around the body in the abdominal area.

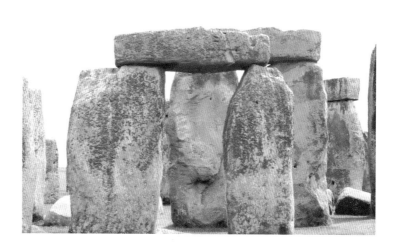

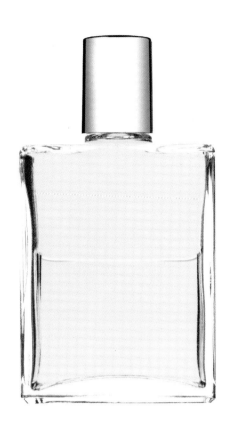

B62 Pale Turquoise/ Pale Turquoise

Name: **Maha Chohan**

Shakes Together As: **Pale Turquoise**

Tarot Card: **Three of Swords**

Keynote: **Light on the path of individuation. The clarity of the communication of the heart.**

Maha in Sanskrit means "greater," and *chohan* is Tibetan for "teacher."[62-a] Thus, the name of B62 means "the greater teacher," "the teacher's teacher," or "the inner teacher." B62 has the qualities of unexpected insight, sudden awakening, and the revelation of previously unseen dimensions that astrologers ascribe to Uranus.

Maha Chohan, a member of the White Brotherhood (see note 50-e), was the lord of civilization in Lemuria but never incarnated in physical form. Lemuria, like Atlantis all but lost to history, was an ancient civilization that, among other aspects, was focused on creativity through color and sound. Maha Chohan's

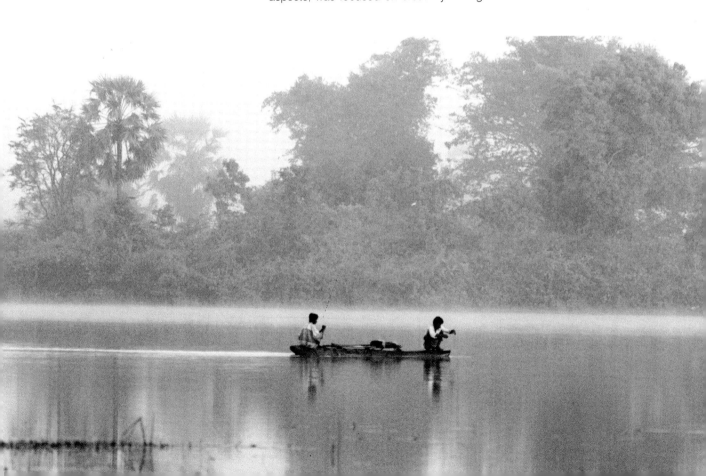

Related Bottles

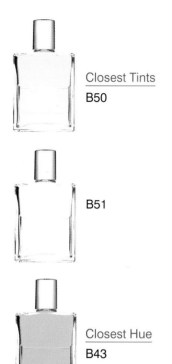

Closest Tints
B50

B51

Closest Hue
B43

Left: Fishing on a lake in Sri Lanka.
Above: Glacier Bay in Alaska. In the foreground is the bay; one of the bay's many tidewater glaciers is in the background.
Below: Green sea turtle in Barbados. Sea turtles have an amazing ability to navigate great distances across the ocean.

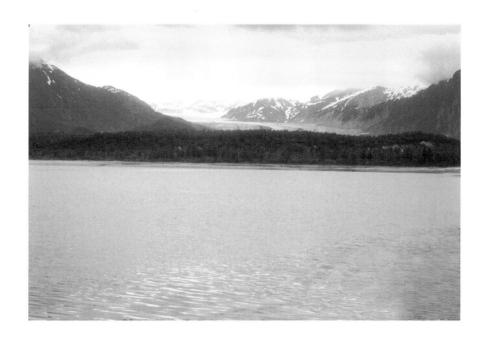

role is as the Father Creator figure, confirmed by the pale turquoise color of B62, representing intense creativity. This creativity arises from the sea of pure universal consciousness.

B62 can indicate that we have an outstanding creative ability and that we listen and understand others' problems and needs. We who are called to B62 may be humble; we may be involved in mass media or computer technology, often as a means to communicate our own creative efforts. In consultation, B62 can point toward those of us who are oversensitive or easily shocked. We may be suffering from holding on to confusion, past heartbreaks, and old fears.

All the points made for B43, Turquoise/Turquoise, are relevant for B62, Pale Turquoise/Pale Turquoise, in a more intense form.

Apply B62 around the body in the chest area and around the throat and neck.

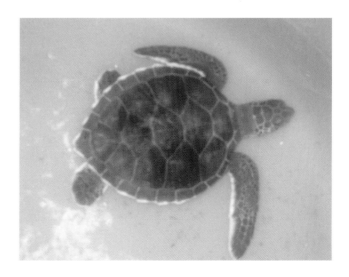

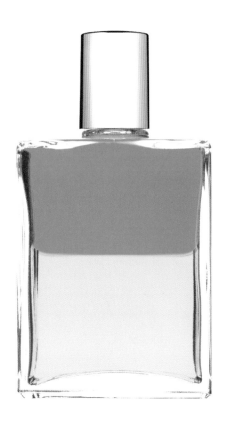

B63 Emerald Green/ Pale Green

Name: Djwal Khul and Hilarion

Shakes Together As: **Green**

Tarot Card: Two of Swords

Keynote: A truth when we give ourselves the space to be able to see ourselves as we are.

B63 is the first bottle in the Master sequence to contain two Masters: Djwal Khul and Hilarion.[63-a] These Masters of the green ray (see note 50-b) appear together perhaps because we, as humanity, are at the point of journeying between the solar plexus and the heart. We need the two Masters to work together, to consciously cooperate, to help us make this transition, to bring a new beginning with balance and harmony.

In a sense their appearance together confirms the importance of this transition. Through the understanding and use of color we are given an opening to work with the fourth dimension. As the earth evolves in her process, so humanity and the creatures upon the earth continue in their evolutionary process. Vicky Wall said, "The reason that two Masters appear in this combination has to do with humanity's journey at this point in time between the solar plexus and the emerald of the heart."

Right: Ferns and bloodroot in Sturbridge, Massachusetts. Bloodroot is used by weavers for a red dye.
Below: Field in Austria near where *The Sound of Music* was filmed.
Note: The image on page 293 is also a visual expression of this bottle.

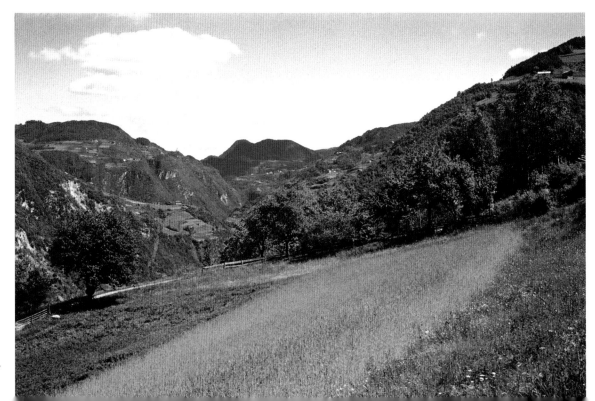

Related Bottles

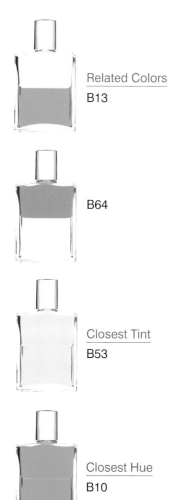

Related Colors
B13

B64

Closest Tint
B53

Closest Hue
B10

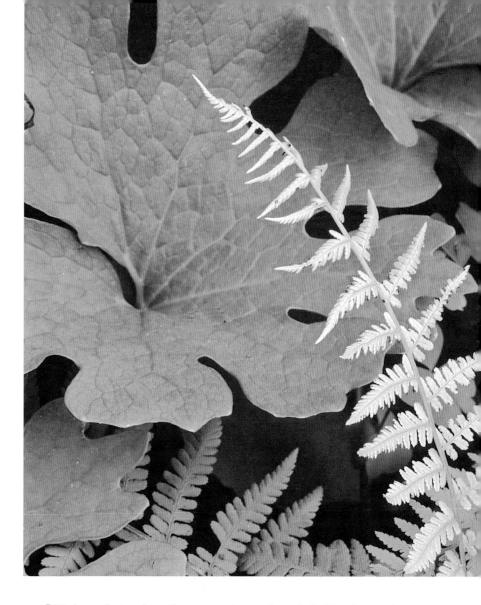

B63 shows that we have the courage to speak our truth. We who are drawn to B63, having great perseverance and determination, know where we are going and how to get there. The green suggests that we have a capacity to integrate feelings and perceive others' emotions. B63 may help us establish contact with issues of persecution (for example, from the time of the Inquisition) and can help release the resultant trauma. B63 may also suggest that we are incredibly confused, lacking joy and peace. When decisions need to be made, we may need space and time to feel out what is required. B63 can counteract a tendency to dwell on the negative side of issues, instead of looking for the positive.

This is the only bottle in the Master Set without a direct correspondence to a Quintessence; both Djwal Khul and Hilarion have their own.

Apply the contents of this bottle around the chest area.

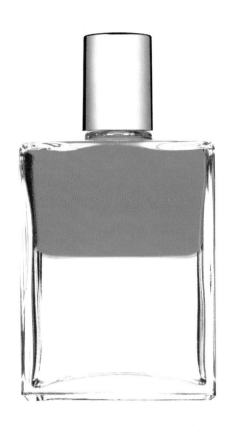

B64 Emerald Green/Clear

Name: Djwal Khul

Shakes Together As: Pale Green

Tarot Card: Ace of Swords

Keynote: The seeker's Master. Seeking of itself. The truth of the search.

Djwal Khul is the inspiration or Master closely connected with Alice Bailey. She wrote many books that she attributed to Djwal Khul's guidance. Djwal Khul is known as the Tibetan or the Seeker's Master; according to Alice Bailey, he is still living in the Himalayas. In Emerald Green/Clear we have seeking of truth for the sake of truth itself. In that sense, B64 indicates that we have the clarity of mind to seek the true self within, and to release what has been lying upon our heart. B64 is useful for people searching for hidden patterns in life, such as in astrology and in probing to understand color.

There are times when we may come to the truth directly. After, we may try to rationalize what that truth is. In so doing, we lose some of the essence of the truth. Truth, rather than coming from our thinking or our feeling, is spontaneous and comes from a deep place of innocence within us. When we try and interfere with that truth, it may become something that conveys less than the original powerful simplicity.

Right: Water cascading on Isla del Sol at Lake Titicaca in Bolivia.

Below: Sheep nestled under ferns on the Isle of Mull in Scotland.

Note: The image on the dedication page at the beginning of this book, of light pouring to earth, is also a visual expression of this bottle.

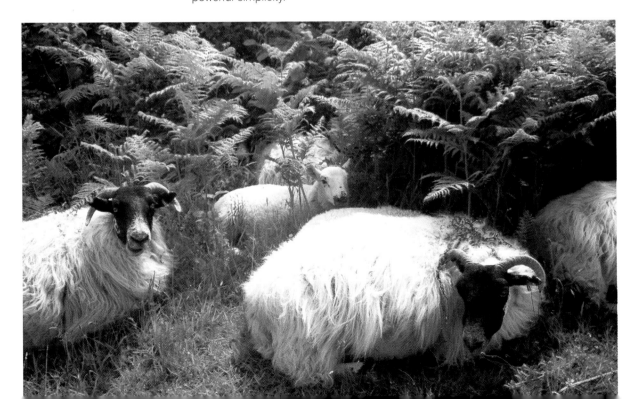

Related Bottles

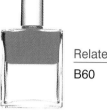

Related Colors
B60

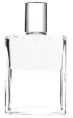

B70

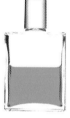

Reverse
B13

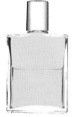

Closest Tint
B53

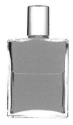

Closest Hue
B10

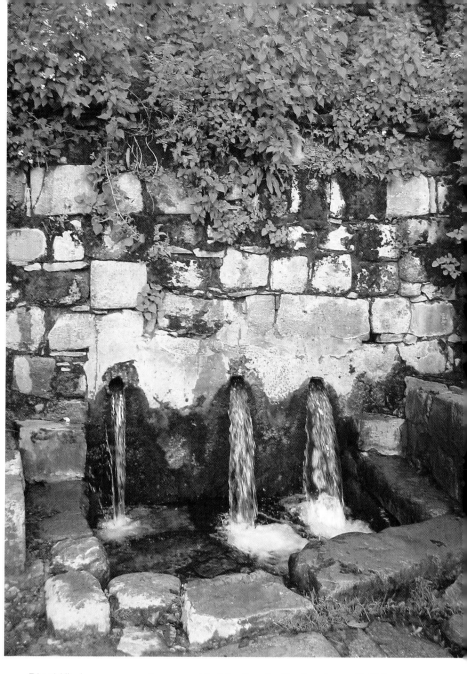

Djwal Khul appears as the emerald of the heart with clear beneath. When something touches our heart, we could say that it is the truth. Truth is linked to water. When we are touched, the truth, or water, sometimes overflows to the outside in the form of the well of tears (clear) being shed. We could say that water is truth, truth is consciousness, and the consciousness of truth is bliss. In this way, B64 suggests letting go of past anxieties and that which has not been peaceful. It may show that we need to release confusion around emotional situations and to see clearly why we have suffered, to face emotional disappointments and fears. Confusion released allows the beginning of greater clarity concerning our mission and purpose, helping create a clear channel between thought and action.

Apply B64 around the chest area.

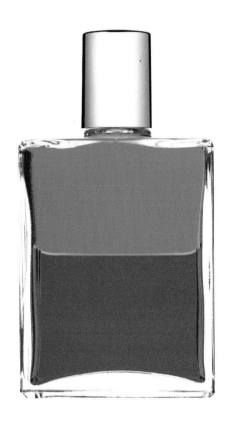

B65 Violet/Red

Name: Head in Heaven and Feet on Earth

Shakes Together As: Magenta

Tarot Card: King of Pentacles

Keynote: A deep sense of balance. The energy to perform our service.

B65 is sometimes called the "I Am Come to Earth" bottle. Violet and red are the two extremes of the visible color spectrum. In the red/infrared end of the spectrum are the slowest wavelengths of light. The violet/ultraviolet wavelengths are the fastest; paradoxically, violet is the most calming color within the visible spectrum.

B65 is similar to B30, Bringing Heaven to Earth, but with a little red mixed with the blue in the upper fraction to form violet; not surprisingly, B65 has qualities similar to those of B30. In B65 the colors are correctly positioned according to the alignment of the chakras to which they relate in the human body: the crown (violet) is above the feet (red). Violet/Red is not about bringing energy to earth; the red in both fractions shows that energy is already available.

The name of this bottle is part of Vicky's saying "Head in heaven, feet on earth"; the saying usually concludes with "center flowing free." The center or

Right: Woman shopping, using the flat bottom boats that are the primary means of travel among the floating islands and waterways of the Dal Lake region in the Kashmiri Valley.

Below: The Red Hat Society is a group of women who are symbolically expressing their joy of life and independent spirit in their bright attire. Rutland, Vermont.

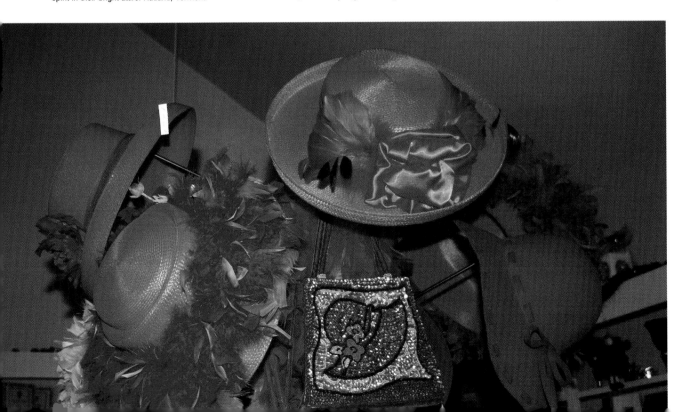

Related Bottles

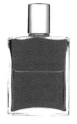

Related Colors
B6

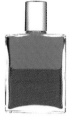

B30

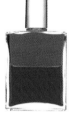

Reverse
B19

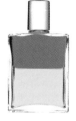

Closest Tints
B36

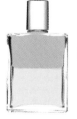

B66

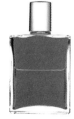

Shakes To
B67

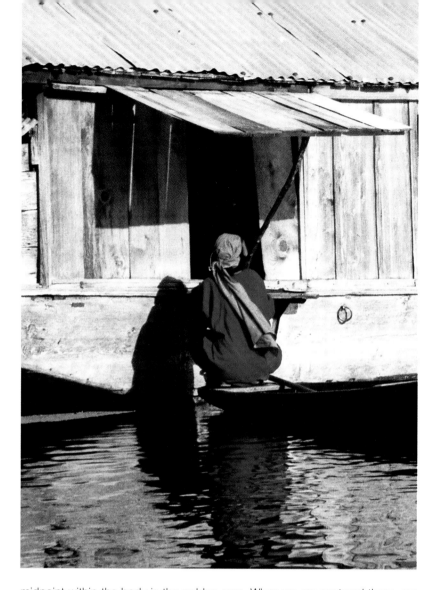

midpoint within the body is the golden area. When we are centered there, our mind is not too involved in thinking, and we are balanced, with our feet stable upon the earth and our center of gravity appropriately low. This groundedness belongs to those of us who contemplate before putting our energy into action. We are drawn to this bottle if we are intuitive and spiritual and have the ability to help guide others to their own spirituality. The violet in the upper fraction suggests B65 relates to transforming ourselves physically, emotionally, and spiritually.

B65 suggests that we might be putting energy toward people or situations that drain energy from us, and where we could be lost or abused. This bottle can be useful in guiding frequent sexual fantasies into a direction where the passion within (denoted by B6, the Lovers, hidden in B65) can be expressed constructively.

B65 may point out that we feel threatened by authority figures and may have hidden anger, which can quickly erupt. For real progress, we need to release resentment; then we have the potential for watchfulness and awakening.

Apply this bottle around the lower abdominal area and along the hairline.

189

B66 Pale Violet/ Pale Pink

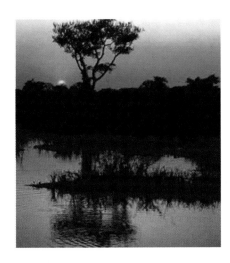

Name: The Actress/The Victoria Bottle
Shakes Together As: Pale Violet
Tarot Card: Queen of Pentacles
Keynote: To detach from our conditioning to be able to see the actors upon the stage of the self.

Page 191: Sunset on Sanibel Island, Florida.
Below, right: A performance of Cinderella.
Below, left: African sunset.

The Pale Violet/Pale Pink bottle is predominantly called the Actress, although originally it was called the Victoria bottle. The names are interlinked. Vicky and Mike would occasionally do consultations for an actress by the name of Victoria, who at the time was in a popular television series in the United Kingdom. On one occasion she explained to Vicky that although she was attracted to the Violet/Pink combination, B36, she did not think it was light enough. It was then, at Vicky's request, that Mike made B66 for Victoria. Contrary to what one might have guessed, the name had no intentional associations with Queen Victoria.

The actress who initiated the birth of this bottle wished to be loving, caring, and of service. B66 reflects this potential to express unconditional love and compassion. There is a balance between the physical (pink) and the spiritual (pale violet). At the same time, the actress had some intense survival issues, with much of her life reflecting dramatic and intense situations. Many people, whether professional actors/actresses or not, have lives full of drama. This has to do with the roles we play in life, when we are not simply being ourselves. At times, the

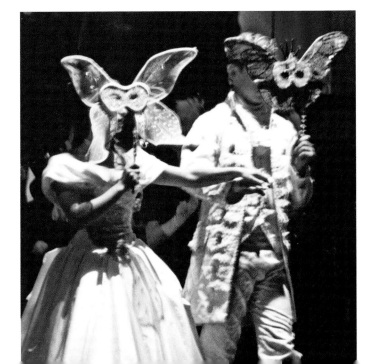

190

Related Bottles

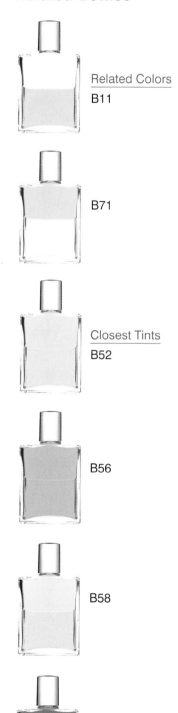

Related Colors
B11

B71

Closest Tints
B52

B56

B58

Closest Hue
B36

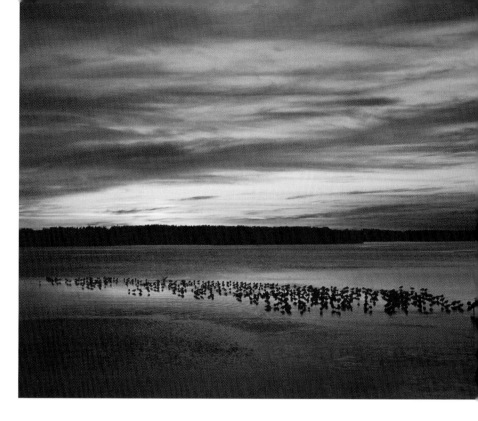

experience of playing a role obscures our real self so much that it is difficult to recognize our true self. As Shakespeare said, "All the world's a stage, and all the men and women merely players: they have their exits and their entrances; and one man in his time plays many parts."[66-a]

B66 may point toward extreme difficulties we had with our parents during childhood. We may let others down by ignoring our duties and may find it difficult to commit to a relationship. Consequently, we may be frustrated by superficiality in contact with others, even with those for whom we care.

B66 may help us recognize the actress/actor on the stage of the self or show us that we are not able to discriminate between when we are and are not acting. Detachment offered by the red, intensified to pale pink, helps us see the parts we play in life and within each day. This may teach us to expect from others only if we are prepared for the consequences. Pink energy supports the self-acceptance we require to assess our roles with compassion. This combination of colors can help bridge the gap of credibility between what is on the inside and what is on the outside of ourselves. Transformation in the mind is supported by love, and a peacefulness comes through the love, warmth, and caring that lies within.

Apply this bottle around the abdominal area and along the hairline.

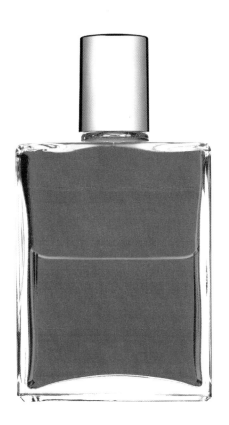

B67 Magenta/Magenta

Name: Love from Above

Shakes Together As: Magenta

Tarot Card: Knight of Pentacles

Keynote: Love in the little things. Where we recognize God is in the little things.

"Love in the little things" is the idea of putting love and care into the inanimate objects with which we come in contact each day. It is like investing in a bank account. If we invest a little bit in an account, it gradually grows; eventually it becomes a bigger account with more interest. Magenta/Magenta is about taking care with, putting caring and attention into, all the things we tend to do unconsciously or that we think do not affect the quality of our lives. When we pay attention to the little things, like polishing the doorknobs and washing the windows, we are practicing putting the energy of love into those things. As a result, when we want or need to do things that we have previously considered more worthy of our attention or more honorable, we will have a bigger and more refined resource of loving and caring energy available for those tasks.

In one way, the concepts of "love in the little things" and "love from above" might seem like opposite ends of a spectrum of love. In fact, love in the little things leads to divine love; because there is no expectation involved in the former, the possibility of divine love ensues.

Right: Window washers on sky scraper in Dubrovnik, Croatia.
Below: Bouquet.

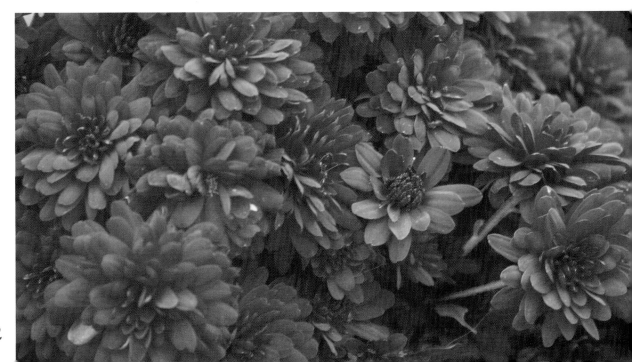

Related Bottles

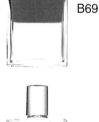

Related Colors
B2

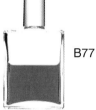

B6

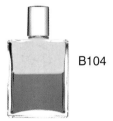

B69

B77

B104

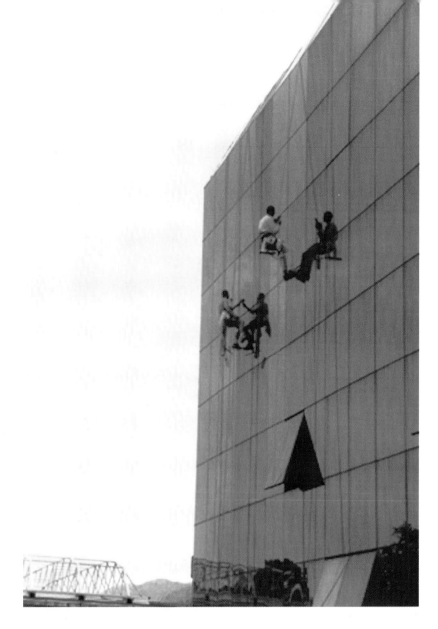

Grace is another quality found in magenta. Grace cannot be manufactured; it comes directly from that which is above us.

B67 could appeal to those of us who are loyal and reliable and who will go beyond the call of duty. We may be creative, compassionate, and selfless and have much love to give to others, to animals, and to the planet. When selected in the second position, B67 suggests that we overwork and find it difficult to have time to our selves, and that we need much caring. Looking to receive from others the quality of love similar to that which we readily give can leave us subject to many disappointments. B67 lets us learn to give without the need to receive.

B67 may help the chakras function better. It may be useful in rebirthing and other therapies, when growth has already occurred and something new is about to begin, or a new chapter in life is opening.

Apply B67 everywhere on the body. It is excellent as a body oil.

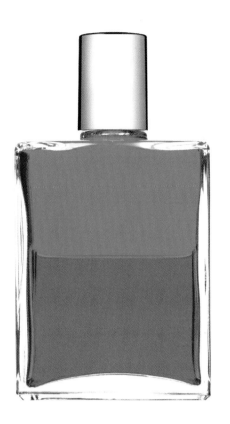

B68 Blue/Violet

Name: **Gabriel**

Shakes Together As: **Royal Blue**

Tarot Card: **Page of Pentacles**

Keynote: **The angel of peace and fulfillment. A connection with the ability to discern.**

Page 195, top: Tower Bridge in London, England.
Page 195, bottom: Abalone shell on Sanibel Island, Florida.
Below: Roof of nunnery ruins on Iona, Scotland.

B68 refers to the angel Gabriel; B95 refers to the archangel Gabriel.[68-a] Blue/Violet is an upside-down version of B37, Violet/Blue, the Guardian Angel Comes to Earth. In B68, communication is in the upper fraction (blue), and spirituality (violet) within. The angel Gabriel communicates about spirituality coming to the world. The Blue/Violet combination almost suggests a masculine angelic aspect, while the Archangel Gabriel combination, Magenta/Gold, offers a more unified male/female energy. As blue is contained in the turquoise, B68 has the qualities of B49, Turquoise/Violet, the New Messenger, linking the message and the messenger with Gabriel's role of bringing the message to the earth.

B68 can help us learn to see relationships as opportunities for our own growth. It implies that we communicate spirituality and intuitively offer healing, whether as social workers, speech therapists, spiritual teachers, or other such practitioners. We are idealists and bring ideas to the fore. The red in the base fraction suggests that B68 is attractive to those of us who embody a quality of peace, with the energy to get things done. We may appear to be brave while harboring deep resentment and frustration. If B68 appears in the third position,

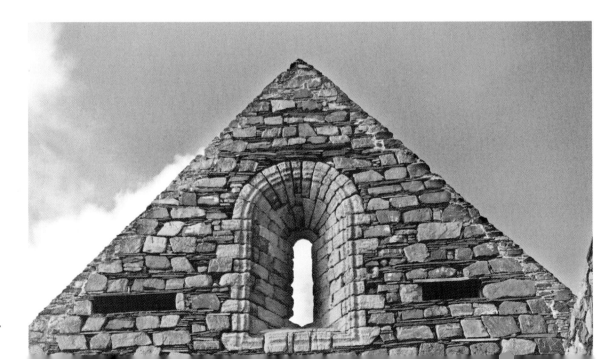

Related Bottles

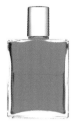

Related Colors
B2

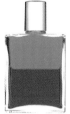

B30

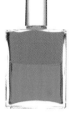

Reverse
B37

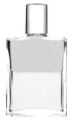

Reverse Tint
B44

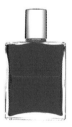

Shakes To
B96

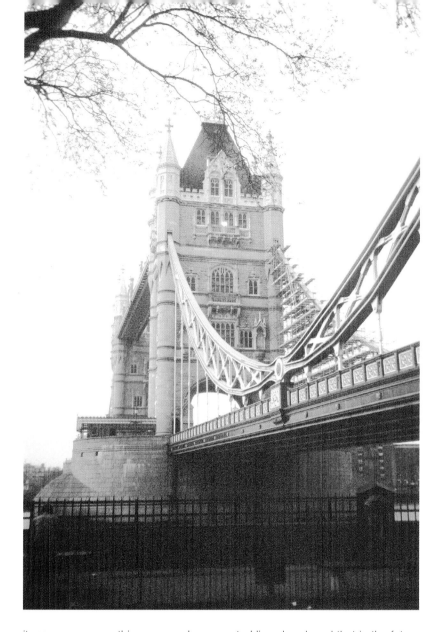

it may mean something new and unexpected lies ahead, and that in the future we will see things more clearly. We may need this increase in discernment if we speak (blue) without thinking or if we have difficulties with a father figure or idealize this role too much.

Apply B68 around the throat and neck and along the hairline.

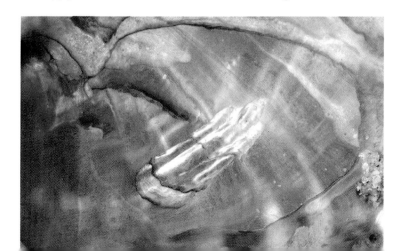

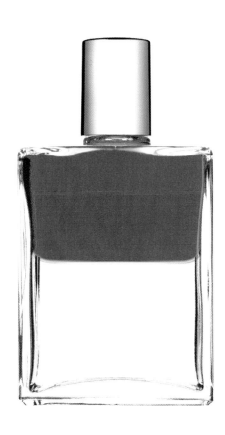

B69 Magenta/Clear

Name: **The Sounding Bell**

Shakes Together As: **Pale Magenta**

Tarot Card: **Ten of Pentacles**

Keynote: Purification as a consequence of love from above. The purification derived from putting love in the little things. Being in the moment.

In the East and West, a sounding bell is often used to call people to worship. Magenta/Clear is, in one sense, a call to reconnect with our spirituality, with what might be the true essence of spirit.

B69, Sounding Bell, is like a crystal bowl. We work with the crystal bowl to produce a sound. The sound resonates with us, resonating with how we put care and attention into making the sound with the crystal bowl. That sound in turn produces a resonance in another person. With conscious intention and love in attention to detail, we can easily increase that resonance. This is the energy of Sounding Bell. Our conscious caring and attention produces a resonance within ourselves and others.

With clear in its lower fraction, B69 suggests suffering, the well of unshed tears. As we shed these tears, as we come to understand our suffering, our experiences are cleansed and purified. The magenta in the upper fraction suggests love and caring. Together, the two colors offer the possibility of integrating

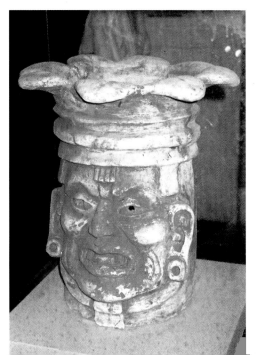

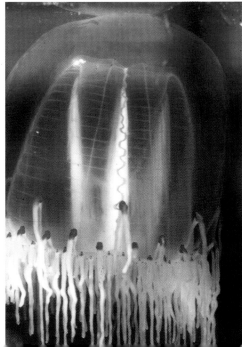

Related Bottles

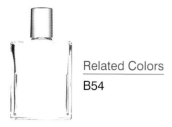

Related Colors
B54

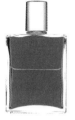

B67

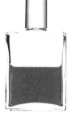

Reverse
B77

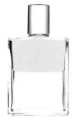

Closest Tint
B71

our suffering and caring. Being aware that love from above is always available in each moment may help us deal with the well of unshed tears. Sometimes, we do not recognize or remember this. Sounding Bell can call us back and remind us that love is there for us when we need it, even when we may not recognize that ourselves.

Those of us who are charismatic, whose light rings from within, echoing love and compassion, are likely to be called to B69. We put the love that comes through us to everything great or small and find joy within our family situation.

B69 could help us focus on that which is in front of us: by knowing we have the support of love from above, we are able to move beyond ideals to practicalities. This is necessary when we are not resonating with love and are holding back tears. We may be bored with life and, as a result, take unnecessary risks, such as emotional or financial risks. We may feel empty, not recognizing how we are suffering. Humanity's potential includes expressing the love of the magenta energy, which could help relieve our suffering.

Apply B69 everywhere on the body. It is an excellent body oil.

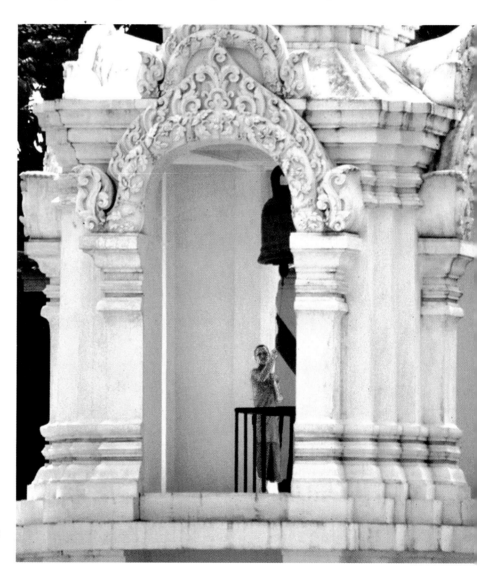

Right: Monk ringing bell to summon the others, Thailand.
Page 196, left: Corn God at the Community Museum on the Puuc route in Mexico.
Page 196, right: Jelly fish.

197

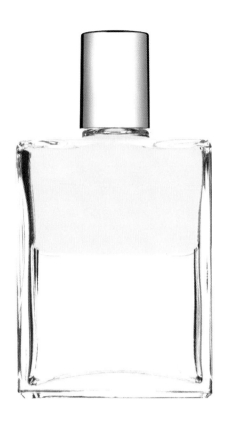

B70 Yellow/Clear

Name: Vision of Splendor

Shakes Together As: Pale Yellow

Tarot Card: Nine of Pentacles

Keynote: The clarity to see the bigger picture more openly. To gain knowledge in relation to the vibration of light.

A "vision of splendor" is when we see something wonderful, whether a field covered in hay or the golden light of the sun on the sea. B70 helps us let go of suffering (clear) within and find the joy (yellow) that is available to us in each moment, and, furthermore, to celebrate the moment in spite of suffering, to be open to the sight of beauty.

B70 offers us the opportunity to make friends with our confusion (see the description of yellow, page 18). If we do so, we may be able to glimpse a vision of something far greater than we could ever have imagined. We could say that part of the reason we suffer is that we are confused. When we let go of confusion, we can come to clarity. That, too, could be a vision of splendor. Our knowledge may be illuminated, and we may gain greater confidence in that knowledge.

Page 199, top: To infinity and beyond; clear sky, no fog, double yellow lines in Vermont.
Below: Sunny side up.

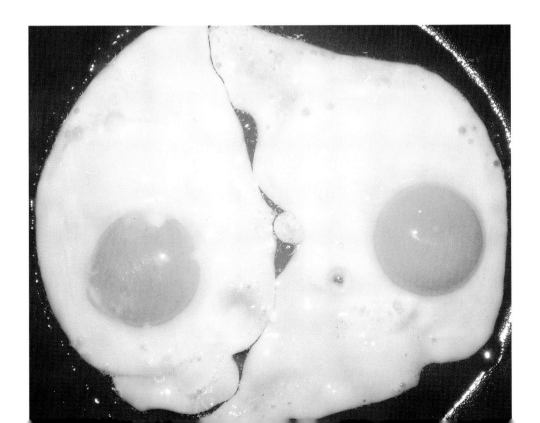

Related Bottles

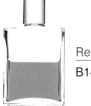

Related Colors
B14

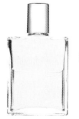

B42

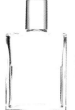

Shakes To
B51

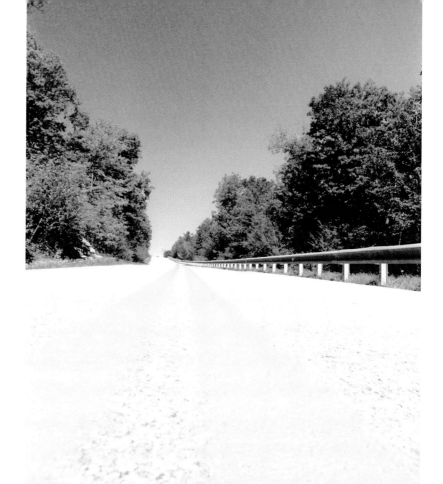

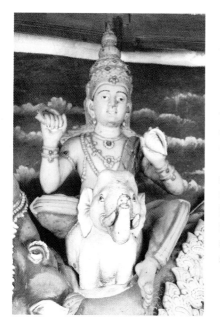

Yellow/Clear is also about shining the light in the astral fog. This describes a particular experience that occurs upon entering the astral plane. We enter the astral plane through conscious dreaming, in meditation, or sometimes spontaneously. Whichever way we enter the astral plane, we experience a yellow fogging, a yellow mist. There is more illusion on the astral plane than there is here.[70-a] Shining a light on the fog helps clarify our experience to overcome the inherent confusion; the ability to discover clarity of mind in reflection can eliminate confusion. B70 may help us integrate phenomena we find difficult to understand.

Fears and anxieties can keep us from enjoying all that life and living can offer. We may not allow others to experience the gifts that they have been given. Our fears make us suffer the most. B70 clears the way to joy through insight into the nature of suffering. It can clear the way to joy derived from the unusual; in this way, B70 sometimes can facilitate "automatic writing" (creating an empty space where we are receptive to words coming through us without our consciousness intervening).

Apply B70 around the body in the solar plexus area.

Above: Buddha on elephant. The elephant-headed god Ganesh is widely revered as a remover of obstacles, and hence as a bringer of success, among both Hindus and Buddhists. The Buddha was conceived when his mother, Maya, dreamed of his descent from heaven into her womb in the form of a white elephant. The white elephant is a symbol of strength of mind and the calm and tranquility possessed by those on the path to enlightenment.

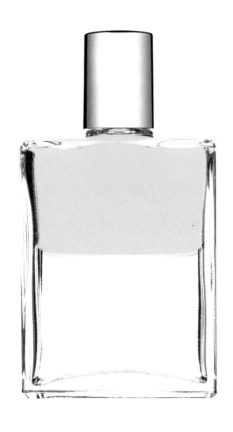

B71 Pink/Clear

Name: The Essene Bottle 2/The Jewel in the Lotus
Shakes Together As: Pale Pink
Tarot Card: Eight of Pentacles
Keynote: Taking responsibility for our thoughts and feelings opens the door to the power of love.

Right: An Aura-Soma teacher training class was held in this pink and white tent, which was a former tuberculosis clinic near Lincoln, England. The image represents the cleansing power of love.
Below: Lotus temple. The Bahai House of Worship in New Delhi, India.

Similar in coloring to the bottle, the thousand-petaled lotus has cream petals with pink tips. Although it appears to grow from a pond's surface, in reality the lotus grows in the mud. Metaphorically, we could say that the mud is within ourselves, and yet because of the mud, we are able to grow into a beautiful flower.

The lotus blossom continues the flower theme established in B11, Essene Bottle 1, the Chain of Flowers. Like B11, B71 may help us connect with Essene incarnations.

The Jewel in the Lotus is part of the blossoming process, helping us come to terms with the muddy waters within us. That muddy water has the potential to become clearer as pink energy is brought into the situation. The self-acceptance, warmth, caring, and kindness of pink offered to the muddy waters within us bring the possibility of clarity. When we achieve it, that clarity is like a beautiful shining jewel in a lotus blossom.

The jewel in the lotus is even more precious than the lotus blossom itself. It is difficult, yet possible, to attain. Initially we must cultivate acceptance, letting the mud settle so that the water may become clearer. As the lotus begins to

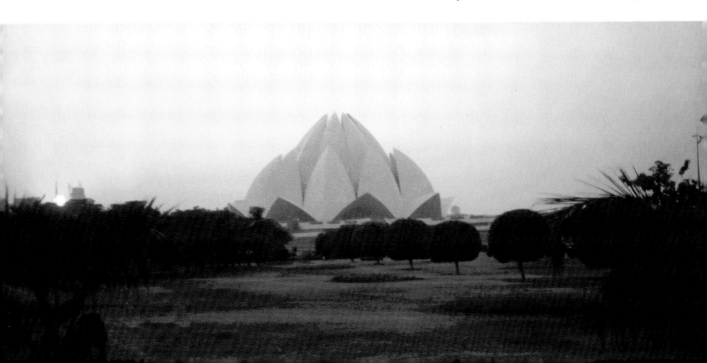

Related Bottles

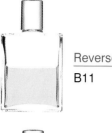

Reverse
B11

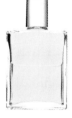

Closest Tint
B52

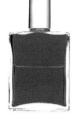

Closest Hues
B6

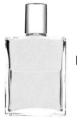

B81

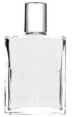

Shakes To
B52

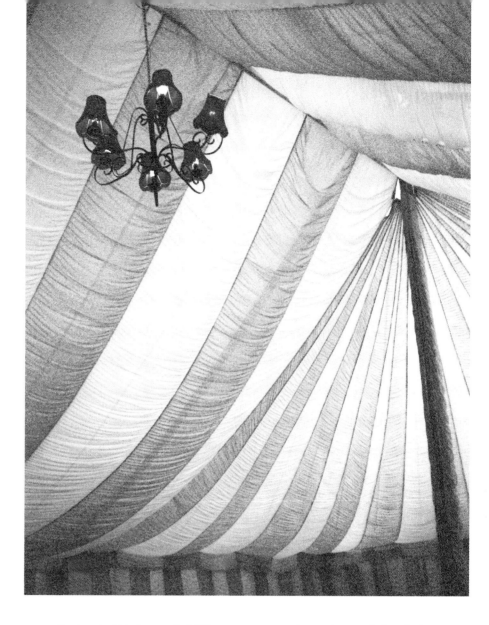

open, the jewel within is revealed. When we can accept ourselves and allow that which suffers within us to be, what we have searched for is revealed.

B71 indicates the qualities of love and warmth given to ourselves and to others, the clear insight to understand this, and the experience of true self-acceptance. Thus, B71 points to our ability to observe with compassion.

B71 may be useful when we are holding back sorrow, not tending to our own needs, or not recognizing that anger and resentment cause suffering. We may feel unrecognized. We have denied the love that we know we have and so denied that which lies deep within. It is possible that the limitless power of love can lift our consciousness.

In chakra symbolism, the lotus is at the crown of the head. B71 may be helpful in craniosacral therapy to release the cranial plates.

Apply B71 around the body in the lower abdominal area. Additionally, a drop may be applied to the top of the head.

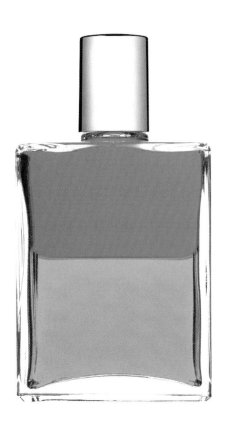

B72 Blue/Orange

Name: **The Clown/Pagliacci**
Shakes Together As: **Emerald Green**
Tarot Card: **Seven of Pentacles**
Keynote: **Joyful insights to be communicated from within.**

Among clowns, the Pagliacci tradition holds that no matter what the performer feels on the inside, he or she must perform as the clown on the outside.[72-a] This is the skill of holding an inner space so that despite whatever is going on within ourselves, we can present a different aspect to the world. B72 is about those inner and outer dynamics. In a positive aspect, it suggests that we are able to offer insight and understanding based on our own experience, communicating the essence of bliss to everyone.

We may hold an inner intention to be good, true, and of value in the world, yet to express that aspiration or ideal in the world may be a very different matter. B72 may help us bridge the gap between what is on the inside and what is on the outside. In Blue/Orange we see shock (orange) on the inside and peace (blue) on the outside. To find peace, we need to overcome dependency and codependency patterns and to release fear from the past. B72 can indicate and help with our difficulty in communicating following a deep shock. Being able to laugh at ourselves or at the circumstances that our lives present is a great gift. B72 also advises us to persevere, as the efforts of our own labor will eventually

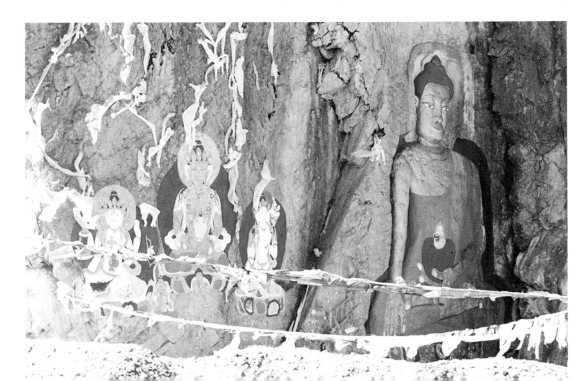

Related Bottles

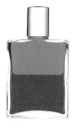

Related Color
B30

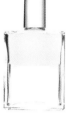

Closest Tint
B94

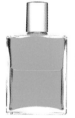

Shakes To
B10

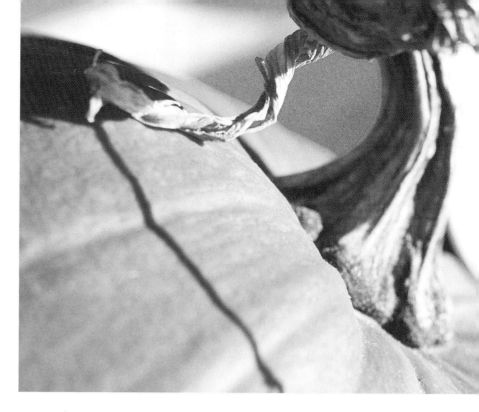

come to fruition. B72 helps create harmony (blue) with our instincts (orange), as blue and orange are complementary opposites.

Blue/Orange is said to change our cellular structure and thus possibly may be helpful for conditions involving hereditary diseases and genetically acquired illnesses. A therapist who was also a teacher and dancer near Copenhagen worked with the sound of the Equilibrium bottles, playing music with the bottles by placing tuning forks on their tops. She felt that B72 had a direct effect on DNA. Following discussions with researchers at the University in Copenhagen who were studying the effects of sound and color, she received encouragement from a professor of genetics to pursue research into the effects that this bottle could have on DNA.

B72 may be applied around the entire trunk of the body.

Top: Pumpkins in New Haven, Vermont.
Left: Medicine Buddha rock painting overlooking the Drepung Monastery where the Dalai Lama was trained in Lhasa, Tibet.
Right: Percula clown fish. Clown fish and anemone have a mutually helpful and protective relationship.

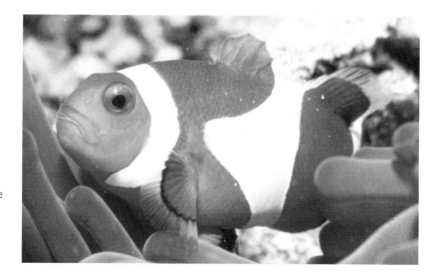

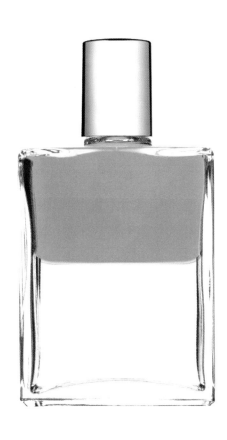

B73 Gold/Clear

Name: Chang Tsu

Shakes Together As: Pale Gold

Tarot Card: Six of Pentacles

Keynote: The connection with our incarnational star brings clarity of purpose and the understanding of the gifts within our being.

Chang Tsu was an ancient sage (399–295 BC). One story tells of how he dreamed he was a butterfly. Later, when walking by the canal with a disciple, he related his dream, saying that now he did not know whether he was a man who dreamed he was a butterfly or a butterfly who was dreaming he was a man.

Gold/Clear has to do with understanding our identification with the psyche. As we begin to allow our golden energy to become more conscious, we move our attention into the area of the true aura. Then the hologram at our center has the possibility of unfolding. As we bring the light of understanding to the experience of not being too identified with who we are, we have the opportunity for more freedom, for dis-identification. If we are aware of our wisdom and have the inner clarity to put it to good use, we may be called by B73. B73 helps us assimilate information, impressions, and food and integrate our experiences. This opens us to an inner lightening and clearing, a purification.

Chang Tsu was a master of wisdom (gold). The many examples of his work reflect the clarity of his wisdom. To gain wisdom in the conscious mind (gold

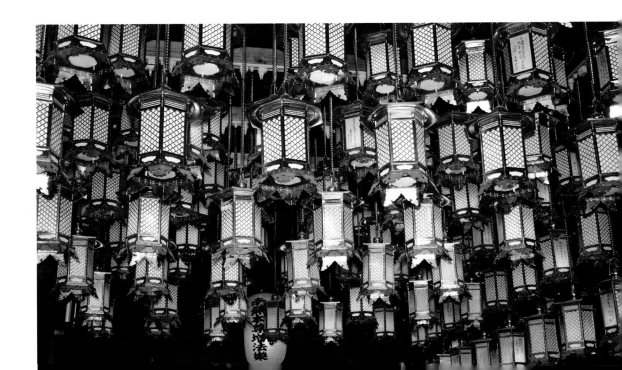

Related Bottles

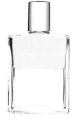

Related Color
B70

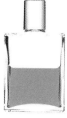

Reverse
B14

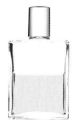

Closest Tint
B59

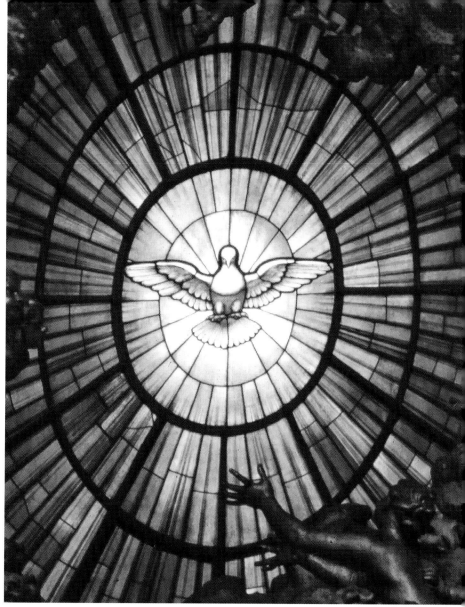

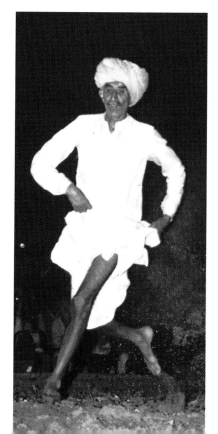

in the upper fraction) for ourselves, we need to let go of some of our suffering (clear in the base fraction). We may have a tendency toward egotism, aggrandizement, and self-glorification. B73 can appeal us if we have become materialistic and have forgotten the treasures buried within, perhaps even becoming jealous or envious of others.

Apply B73 around the body over the belly.

Above: Dome of Saint Peter's Basilica, Vatican, Rome. Gianlorenzo Bernini (1598–1680) created the *Dove of the Holy Spirit* stained glass window above the Throne of Saint Peter ca. 1660. Large stained glass windows were symbolic of divine grace. Through the understanding of suffering we become filled with light. The scorpion transforms to become a phoenix, which in turn becomes the dove, the Holy Spirit.
Left: Fire walker in Pushkar, India. Many cultures use fire walking as a means of cleansing and purifying the body. To fire walk one must transform fear into positive energy. The fire walkers chant, pray, and run around the fire many times in a trancelike state before walking through the fire on burning coals. The fire walker's mind allows him to walk through the burning coals unharmed and the entire scene creates a hypnotic mood for the onlookers.
Page 204: Inside a Japanese temple along Kobo Daishi Kukai's eighty-eight temple pilgrimage route.

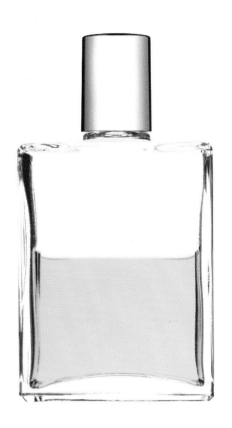

B74 Pale Yellow/ Pale Green

Name: Triumph

Shakes Together As: Pale Olive Green

Tarot Card: Five of Pentacles

Keynote: An intense test. To be able to find discernment toward a deeper balance.

B74's original name was the Aboriginal Varicose Vein bottle. A couple of people who lived in Queensland, Australia, and were of Aboriginal descent were working with the Yellow/Green bottle (B7). In the course of their work, they often found that B7 would fade in color. As it faded, they discovered, it became more effective in the treatment of varicose veins. They made a special request for a paler version of Yellow/Green, which resulted in the birth of B74. They found that this new bottle produced even better results on the veins, and so B74 became known as the Aboriginal Varicose Vein bottle.

B7, the Garden of Gethsemene, deals with the final test of faith. As a paler version of B7, B74 deals with the same, but in B74 that experience becomes more intense. We have an opportunity to respond to our emotions, doubts, and fears, even when we are afraid of having no feelings. Anxieties, deep fears, or lack of trust in our feelings can impede things from flowing as they might. Fears may not necessarily go away, but we may overcome stressors by learning to

Page 207, top: Corn in Ripton, Vermont.
Page 207, bottom: Alert and sensitive Kob along the road to Kasese in Western Uganda near the Twenzori Mountains.
Below: Reed boat water chariots in Peru

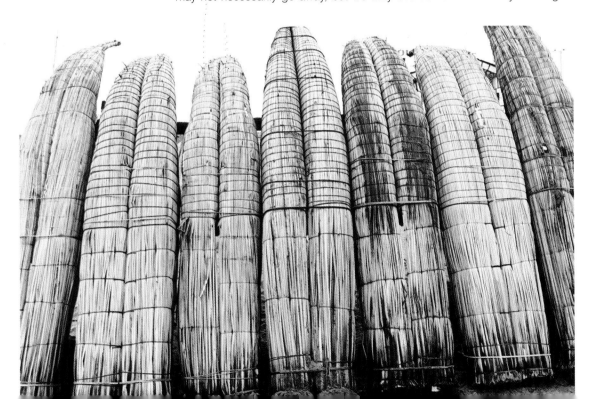

Related Bottles

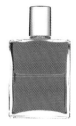

Related Color
B91

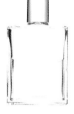

Closest Tints
B51

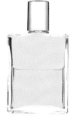

B53

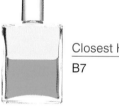

Closest Hue
B7

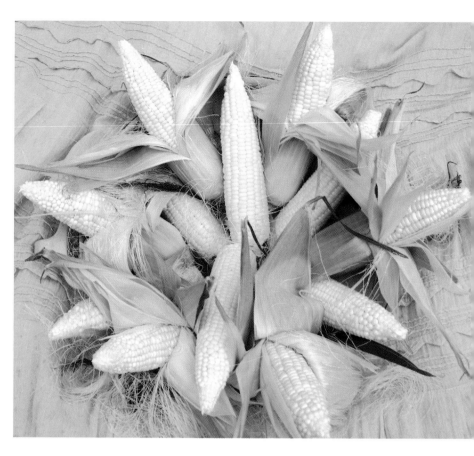

accept them for what they are and to live in that context. But spirit may triumph over matter. To have an open heart toward the issues connected with B7 is to triumph. This success brings harmony, balance, and a joy to our hearts.

B74 may appeal to us if we are true to ourselves and can express our heartfelt feelings. We have made the space for ourselves to become clear in relation to our intellect. At the beginning of a new relationship, B74 may help clarify our feelings.

Apply B74 around the body in the heart and solar plexus areas.

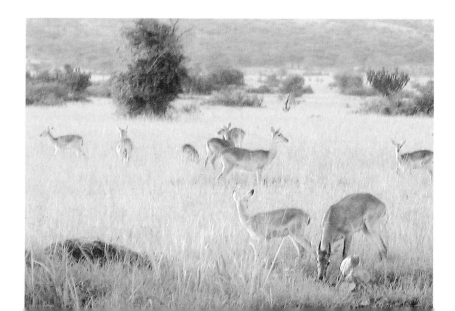

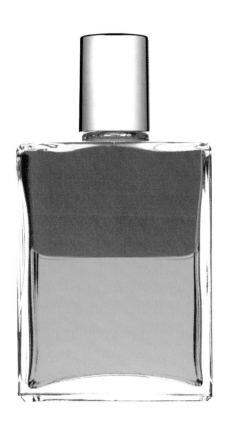

B75 Magenta/Turquoise

Name: Go with the Flow

Shakes Together As: Magenta

Tarot Card: Four of Pentacles

Keynote: A deeper understanding, particularly a reorientation in relation to the family picture.

Vicky used to call this combination the Twin Soul bottle. She felt that working with Magenta/Turquoise could help us align with or come closer to our twin soul. A twin soul may be an aspect of the self or something external. Our twin soul may help us view things from a different angle or deal with things with a new perspective.

B75 may help release built-up or blocked energy from anywhere in the system, thus facilitating the ability to "go with the flow." The colors in B75 are in a correct positional relationship: the magenta of the soul star is above the turquoise of the Ananda Khanda. The name Go with the Flow reminds us that as magenta connects with the turquoise energy, a synchronicity or flow occurs. Instead of damming the river or trying to make it run faster than it naturally will, we allow things to flow at the rate at which they are meant to flow. Love in the little things (magenta) and creativity (turquoise) come together to appropriately

Page 209, left: Water flowing. Flood sluice on a river in Elvington, near York, England.
Page 209, right: Scarf blowing, along the Rhine River.
Below: Sundial at the Ropes Garden in Salem, Massachusetts.

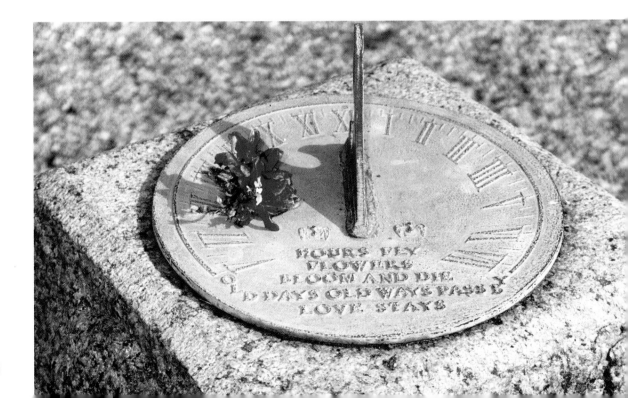

Related Bottles

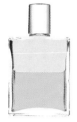

Related Color
B34

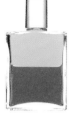

Reverse
B45

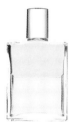

Closest Tint
B57

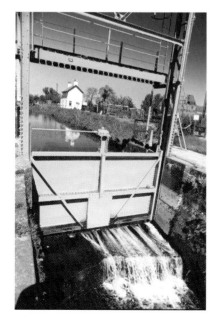

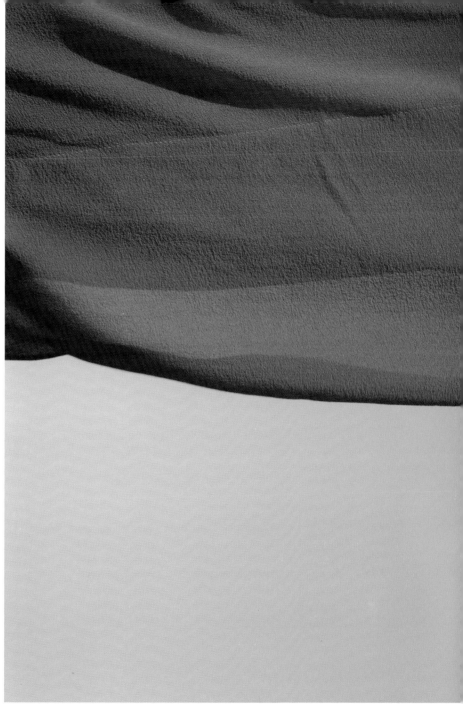

"go with the flow." These actions address our need to love, helping us to stop thinking negatively and to let go of past hurts. We can look back only from where we are. If we had arrived at a different point, the past, upon reflection, would also appear different. In the process of individuation, anger and hidden fears need to be cognized and translated, with inner discipline, to a new warm and loving flow.

Apply this combination everywhere on the body.

B76 Pink/Gold

Name: **Trust**

Shakes Together As: **Gold**

Tarot Card: **Three of Pentacles**

Keynote: **Self-acceptance leads toward the golden area within ourselves to find what we are for and the way to do what we are to do.**

Page 211, top: Houses in Burano, Italy, painted brightly so the returning fisherman might more easily find their way home.
Page 211, bottom: Daisy at Zion National Park in Utah.
Below: Resting Buddha in cave sanctuary in Sri Lanka.

If we trust in our incarnational star and the true aura, and if we find the caring and attention necessary to stay focused within the golden area, our trust in the world will increase. When we trust ourselves, we can more easily trust others. When we do not trust ourselves, we tend to trust no one.

Trust is an elusive thing, and the challenge represented by the gold in the base fraction is to face our deepest fears. The pink shows us the way to face those fears: with the energy of love. In other words, as the saying goes, love is letting go of fear. B76 encourages us to let go of confusion, fear, and anxiety and to receive care and attention. We may find it difficult to allow others to see our gifts and talents. Intense frustration can prevent us from getting in touch with our wisdom. We find it difficult to remember the past, possibly because it is too painful. But when we truly have love in our conscious mind, we can allow ourselves

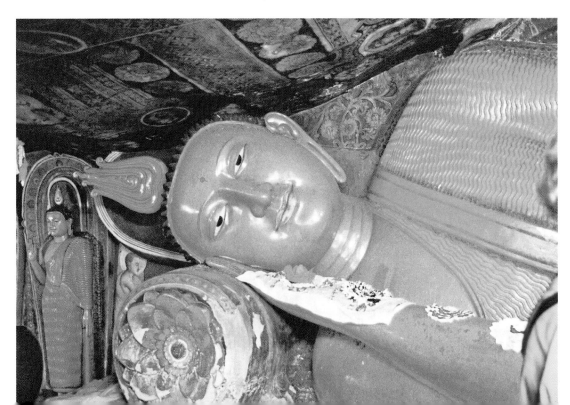

Related Bottles

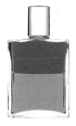

Related Color
B95

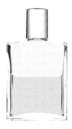

Related Reverse
B22

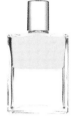

Closest Tint
B61

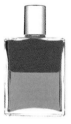

Closest Hue
B40

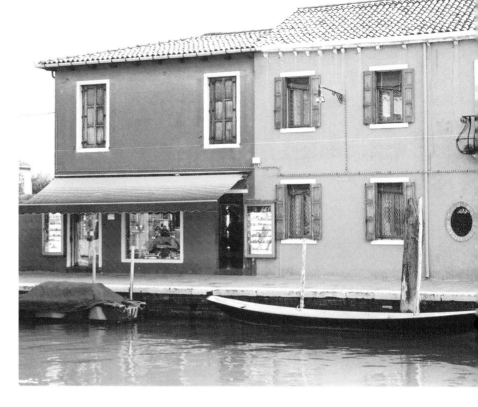

to let go of fears and progress in all these ways, expressing trust at many levels. Then we may express our wisdom through unconditional love.

Pink is concentration, focus, and love in our conscious mind. The incarnational star is in the golden area of our belly. Trusting in our belly is to trust ourselves, a firm foundation from which other things can develop. We can enter into more trusting relationships with others. As we consciously accept ourselves, we are able to refine the gold within ourselves, thus further developing trust in ourselves. The trust engendered through B76 may help us enter previous lives more easily, and it supports rebirthing.

Choosing B76 may suggest that we belong to a group concerned with the development of humanity. We are trusting and detached yet centered. Everyone enjoys being with us, and we may be very joyous. We can find our inner wisdom.

Apply B76 around the abdomen.

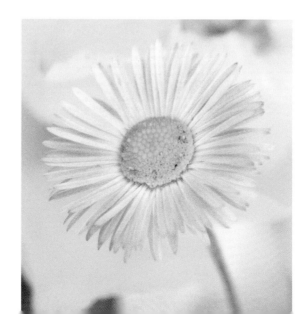

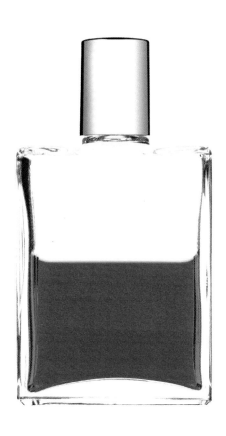

B77 Clear/ Magenta

Name: **The Cup**

Shakes Together As: **Pale Magenta**

Tarot Card: **Two of Pentacles**

Keynote: **Many things are brought together in the context of service to the light. The more open we are to receive, the more can be fed in from above.**

B77, the Cup, is the reverse presentation of B69, Magenta/Clear, Sounding Bell. A bell turned upside down looks like a cup. B77 and B69 are similar to the Essene bottles and may help us connect with Essene incarnations (see B11 and B71).

What is or is not in the cup is a theme of this bottle. If we fill our own cup, it can overflow into the world. If we do not fill our own cup, we may end up looking at the tea leaves in the bottom. But how do we fill our cup? When we remember to put love into the little things (magenta), we build up an account day by day. By putting our attention on inanimate objects, by doing things with care, we build up an energy reserve within that account. This slowly and lovingly keeps the cup full to overflowing. Without love in the little things, at some point we might dip into the cup, expecting to find something there but instead finding that nothing is left.

As full-cup people, we may have a clear mind and know the deep love we have to give to everything. We are channels for love from above to be enjoyed by ourselves and distributed to others.

However, there is a challenge to always having a full cup. If we or our cup is already full, we may have difficulty receiving anything. A little space within allows us to receive love from above, so that grace has a chance to come into our life.

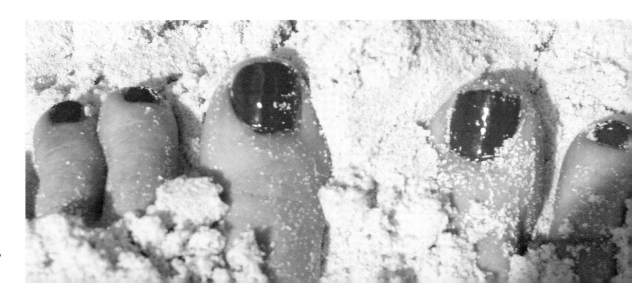

Related Bottles

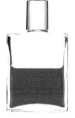

Related Colors
B55

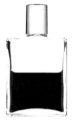

B100

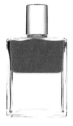

Reverse
B69

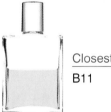

Closest Tint
B11

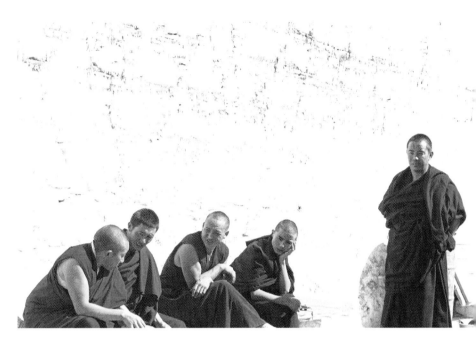

At times we may need to focus our attention in one location, instead of trying to cope with too much all at once (just as clear contains all the colors). While we may know clearly how we have suffered, we have an opportunity for grace; it is time to release this suffering in the context of love. Love and light may manifest in physical perfection: the light force becomes the life force.

Apply B77 everywhere on the body.

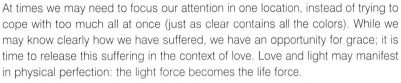

Above: Buddhist Monks at Drepung Monastery in Lhasa (meaning "Holy Place"), Tibet.
Right: Dragon fruit in Brazil.
Left: Pink toes in Barbados.

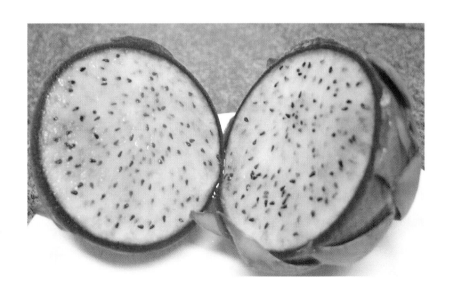

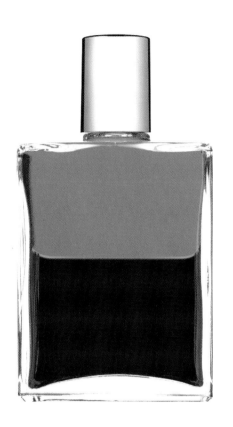

B78 Violet/Deep Magenta

Name: Crown Rescue, The Transition Bottle

Shakes Together As: Deep Magenta

Tarot Card: Ace of Pentacles

Keynote: In every ending there is a new beginning. Intense service may help us find our way to the "right" place.

Right: Male black-chinned hummingbird at Ramsey Canyon in Arizona. Hummingbirds are symbolic of devotion and eternity, of life cycles.

Below: Tea-picker in Munnar, Kerala, India.

B78 marks another shift within the Equilibrium system. This bottle was created at the time of Vicky's transition, born the day after she passed away, arriving to support both Vicky in her journey and those of us who were left behind. In one way there was a great sense of celebration at the time of her transition, and in another way, an obvious sense of loss. Celebration is always part of the experience of death, particularly when we are close to the person who has been suffering and has now moved on. There is a celebration in his or her freedom, especially in how we experience his or her movement into the realms of light and love.

B78 conveys much of that joy and sorrow. Violet energy represents the closeness of spirit. Deep magenta is the void, the emptiness, and yet it contains everything there is, a return to unity. When we look at the midline between violet and deep magenta, it is possible to see red, an indication of the energy of support for dealing with grief. This bottle can help with a rescuing of something

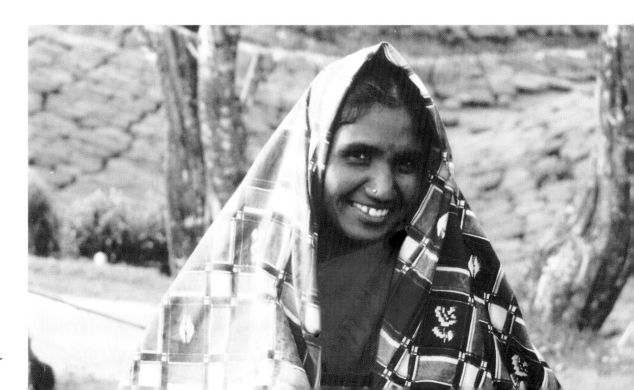

Related Bottles

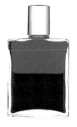

Related Colors
B0

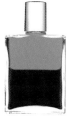

B1

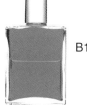

B16

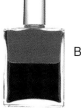

B89

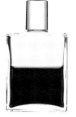

B103

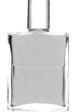

Closest Tint
B56

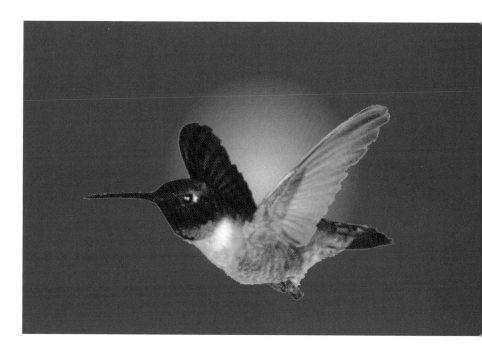

that is subtle and elusive, almost beyond our physicality, to help bring us back together in understanding.

In one sense, nothing is ever born and nothing ever dies. Violet/Deep Magenta can help us remember this, aiding our resolution of loss and grief and supporting transitions from one state to another.

The name Crown Rescue refers to the process of letting go, whether we are experiencing the ultimate transition that marks the end of the physical life and the beginning of the next phase of whatever lies beyond or letting go in the many transitional moments we experience during our life. In psychotherapy, violet and deep magenta combined help illuminate the past, thereby creating success in the present. B78 relates to the Pleiades and Ursa Major, the Great Bear.[78-a] It can be helpful for those who wish to work with devas, angels, and the unseen world.

At a more earthly level, the choice of B78 may suggest that we are peace loving, and that we put attention in the little things, not only for ourselves, but for the service we can offer to the world. We may be spiritual and true to ourselves. We may be in the middle of a psychological transformation, a spiritualization of self. B78 can also highlight the challenges of a false sense of security and inappropriate choices. To avoid an experience of loss, we could be so possessive that we hold on to grief.

Apply B78 around the hairline, throat, neck, third eye, and crown of the head.

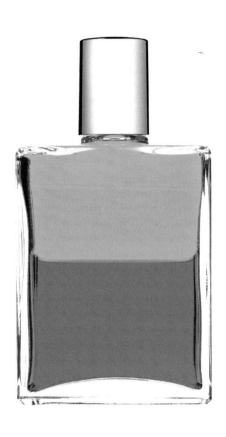

B79 Orange/Violet

Name: The Ostrich Bottle

Shakes Together As: Reddish Orange

Tarot Card: Return Journey of the Magician

Keynote: Insight and transformation. The healing of the timeline. Deep joy. Being able to hear what challenges us.

B79 marks the beginning of the return-journey sequence of the major arcana of the tarot (with the exception of B22, which is the return journey of B0). Whereas the first level, B1, showed us blue over deep magenta, a co-creator with the creator, here orange is in the conscious mind. Now the Magician has some insight (orange) into the nature of things. She/he has begun to understand the four elements and is using her/his skills in the service of others (violet).

B79 is called the Ostrich bottle. Perhaps we wish to hide our head in the sand like the ostrich. Orange in the upper fraction could represent the sand, and violet represents the head. If we put our head underneath the orange, we are in the position of the ostrich.

Yet ostriches also listen closely when their ears are in the sand. B79 suggests the offering of great insight (orange) from an active spirituality (violet). It may mark us as spiritual people who desire deep insight and to find our spiritual life, our service in the world.

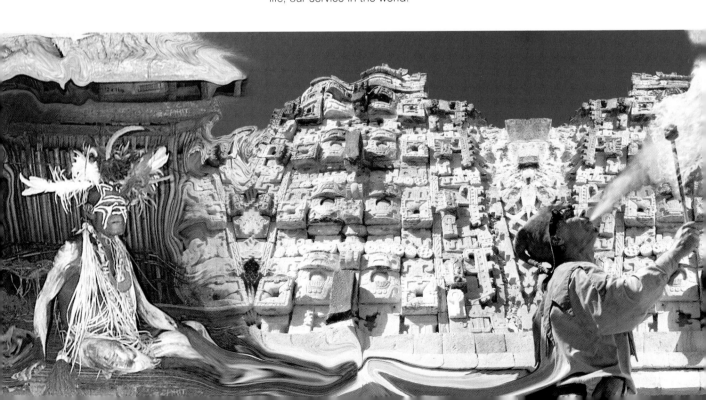

Related Bottles

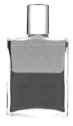

Related Color
B97

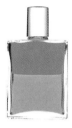

Related Reverse
B39

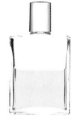

Closest Tint
B59

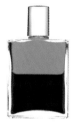

Outward Journey
B1

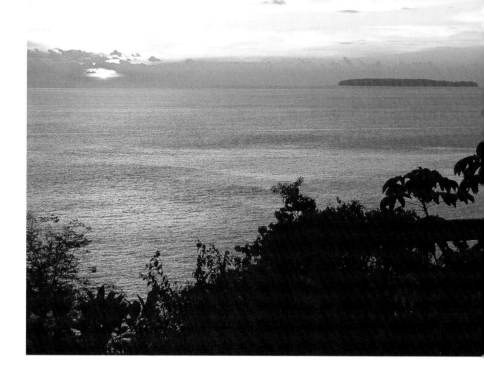

However, the effects of a shock may be preventing healing from taking place or our spirituality from emerging. Perhaps we are hesitant to see and face what lies within our depths. We may need to release inner blockages, to be able to identify with who we truly are. Like the ostrich, we may try to avoid our true spiritual self. Nevertheless, even if we try to avoid it, we cannot hide from ourselves.

The ostrich lays very large eggs; within orange lies the possibility of developing our own luminous egg, the etheric field that surrounds the physical body (see B26). Within B79 is the relationship between the spiritual nature of the violet and the luminous egg in the orange.

Because orange is also connected to shock, this bottle calls to those of us who heal others suffering from shock situations, as well as those of us who have had a shock and are developing insight and transforming. B79 may indicate that we are confronted by our own death or the death of a friend or relative; it may herald a time of intense change. It may support us in breaking free from addictions. When drawn to B79, we may be hiding from who we are, thus denying ourselves deep joy.

This color combination also may help us connect to incarnations in ancient Egypt (see B18 and B39).

Apply B79 along the hairline and around the abdominal area.

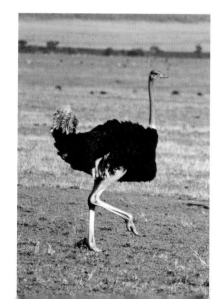

Above: Sunset at Casa Corcovado in Costa Rica.
Left: Male ostrich at Maasai Mara National Reserve in Kenya.
Page 216: Village elder on the Korosamari River in Papua New Guinea combined with scenes from Mexico.

217

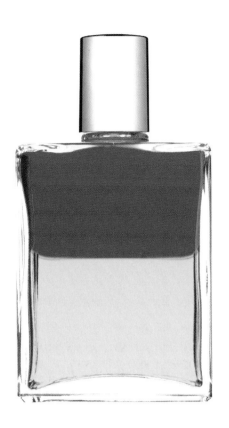

B80 Red/Pink

Name: Artemis

Shakes Together As: Red

Tarot Card: Return Journey of the High Priestess

Keynote: The energy to love and let go, to get in touch with love again. The love becomes more unconditional. The potential to awaken to the power of love.

Right: Underwater scene of coral reef at Palancar Gardens in Cozumel, Mexico.
Below: Flowers in Bondville, Vermont.

The outward journey of the tarot's High Priestess is Blue/Blue, B2. With the Red/Pink of the return journey, she is now the awakened High Priestess. The awakening has come through her full acceptance of herself (pink) within the depths of herself. The red energy in the upper fraction is the energy of awakening. B80 suggests that we have unconditional love, have experienced an awakening to be shared with others, and that we have the ability to balance our inner self with our outer self.

Red connotes issues of survival and awakening, of blood and the life force. When light is brought to red it turns pink; while both colors are symbolic of awakening, pink is more empathic (intense). Hence B80 has to do with issues of life and death, of awakening and of the power of love. Red is the energy through which we develop concentration; pink represents intense concentration. If we have the necessary concentration, we can hit the target, like Artemis the huntress, the archer.

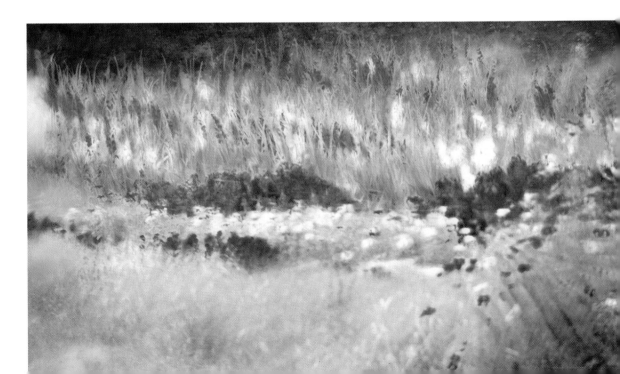

Related Bottles

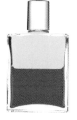

Reverse
B84

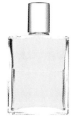

Closest Tints
B52

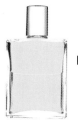

B81

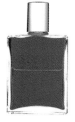

Closest Hue
B6

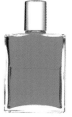

Outward Journey
B2

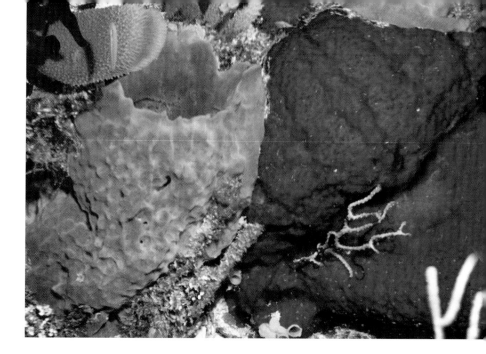

Artemis was a principal goddess in the pantheon of Greek mythology. She was the daughter of the god Zeus and the Titaness Leto and the twin sister of the god Apollo. The Romans knew her as Diana. She was known as the goddess of the moon and of wild places and wild things. Surrounded by wild creatures, Artemis is usually depicted in hunting garb, bearing horns in the shape of crescent moons. Her association with the moon balanced her twin Apollo's association with the sun. B80 can thus be seen as a Tantric bottle symbolizing a powerful coming together of the male/female energies within the self.

Artemis had a dual role as chief huntress of wild animals and divine protector of young creatures. She was also known as the goddess of childbirth and childrearing. In some worship, she was praised for bringing respite to young women who had died during childbirth, helping their soul to a swift and easy transition. She not only protected women in labor but also brought sickness and death to them. It is interesting to note this association of Artemis with childbirth in connection to the reported efficacy of B2, Blue/Blue, in times of transition, and particularly its specific benefits in the final stages of pregnancy and during labor.

As the moon receives the light of the sun, B80 suggests the qualities of receptivity and acceptance. Those of us who work in caretaking professions may, when we are depleted, work with B80 to reconnect with our resources of love and physical strength. Hidden within this bottle is B2 (Blue/Blue) and B42 (Yellow/Yellow), for it is these two primary colors—the yellow sun shining on the blue earth—that bring forth the red energy for life (see "The Language of Color," page 13). B80 can counteract a tendency to allow the material side of life to dominate. We may feel resentment because we feel that we are not loved or because we repress or reject love; Artemis may help us find a balance to release this anger and express love.

Apply B80 around the abdominal area.

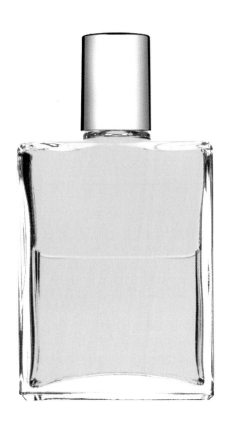

B81 Pink/Pink

Name: **Unconditional Love**

Shakes Together As: **Pink**

Tarot Card: **Return Journey of the Empress**

Keynote: **Compassion, caring, and warmth. The expression and need in relation to love.**

In Aura-Soma pink is associated with unconditional love. B81 suggests that, while able to nurture ourselves, we are sensitive and caring and need to give love to others. We might be watchful yet simultaneously able to be present to the circumstances of life.

In Aura-Soma, B81 is considered the second, or return, level of B3, the Empress, Blue/Green. B3 represents a strong connection to the earth. B81, Pink/Pink, suggests the feminine aspect of the earth, as it is the intensification of red, the color of gounding.

Pink can express itself only through green or turquoise; love must be expressed through the heart. B3, Blue/Green, the Heart Rescue, shakes

Page 221: A lovely vision in pink, Mundawa, Rajasta, India.
Below, right: The beauty of women of all ages: women returning home from church, near Mount Hagen in the Highlands of Papua New Guinea.
Below: Pink rose in Ripton, Vermont.

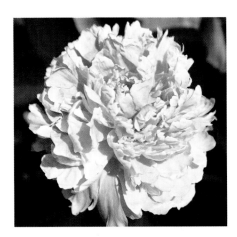

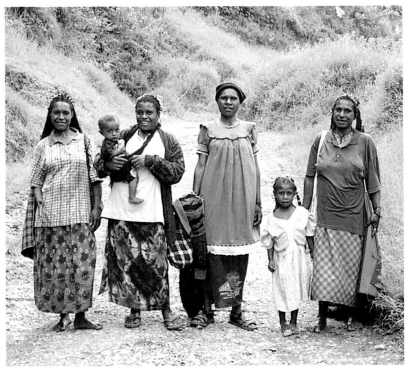

Related Bottles

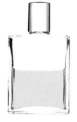

Related Colors
B11

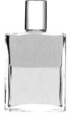

B23

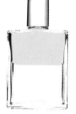

B71

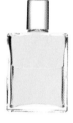

Closest Tint
B52

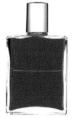

Closest Hue
B6

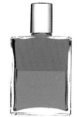

Outward Journey
B3

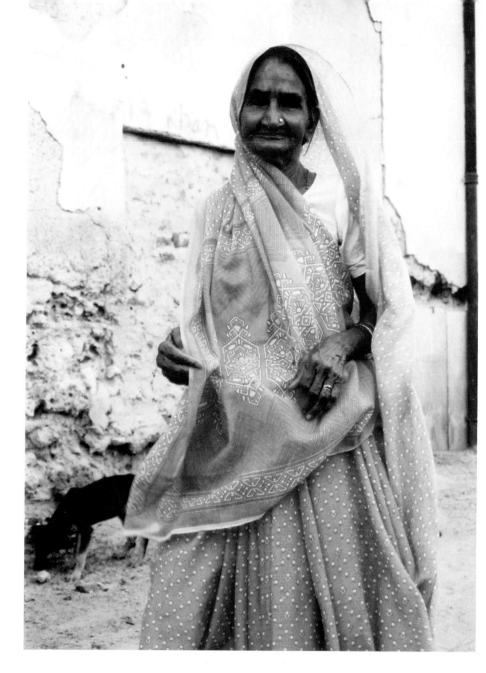

together as a turquoise. It is as if the pink is there, unconditionally encouraging the opening of Blue/Green and supporting an active expression of the heart.

Pink could be seen as the womb, fulfilled by and full of the life-force possibilities of the earth mother herself, created by love and nurtured by love. We must remember to give ourselves love. We may have had a problem during childhood, which needs to be examined now, with our mother. We may need to feel wanted or have a tendency to have too much pride. B81 supports the rebirthing process, clearing patterns connected to persecution that occurred in former lives. It may help us develop intuition.

Apply the contents of this bottle around the abdominal area.

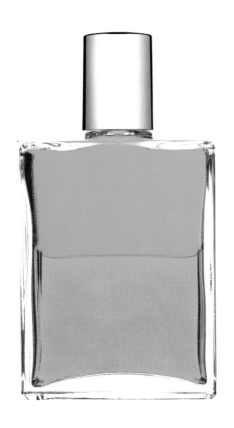

B82 Green/Orange

Name: **Calypso**

Shakes Together As: **Olive Green**

Tarot Card: **Return Journey of the Emperor**

Keynote: Insight revealed as we make space for ourselves. The revelation of the deepest joy coming from the heart.

Page 223, top: Organic carrots.
Page 223, bottom: Free to sing and work creatively in an open space, this man is preparing sago palm flesh, a mainstay of the the diet in the remote Blackwater Lakes region, near Sepik River in Papua New Guinea.
Below: Calendula, an herb used for centuries for its many medicinal properties and also for the yellow orange dye from its petals. Ripton, Vermont.

In the West Indies and Trinidad especially, green and orange seem to be part of the celebration of the calypso, of the dance and of the spirit of celebration. Green offers us the space to find a celebration within for the dance and movement of orange. B82 thus suggests that we are open-hearted, freely dance our wisdom, and joyfully share the love in our heart. We have a sense of freedom, helped by gut reactions and deep insight.

While calypso is a song of celebration, it also speaks of the pain and shock carried in the hearts of the people's slave ancestors. Slaves used song creatively to communicate with each other in a time when all other communication was restricted by authority figures. In the West Indies now, many are followers of the Rastafarian faith,[82-a] which focuses on peace, togetherness, and family. B82 may point out that we need to let go of any conflicts, shocks, and traumas from the past and to deal with underlying anxieties. If we experienced any difficulties with male authority figures, we now need to let go of them. Green/Orange may help us retrace emotions. As a result, we can gain useful insights as to why we feel the way we do.

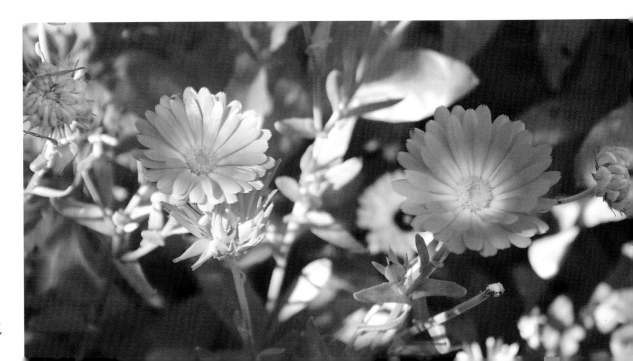

Related Bottles

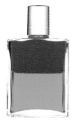

Related Colors
B27

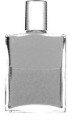

B31

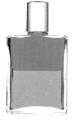

B72

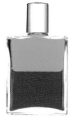

Related Reverse
B28

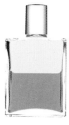

Outward Journey
B4

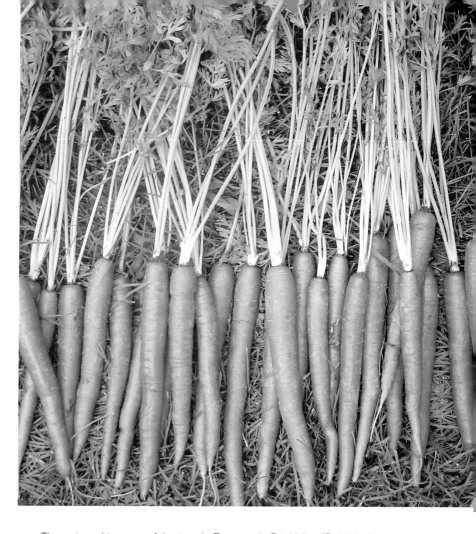

The outward journey of the tarot's Emperor is B4, Yellow/Gold. In the return journey of B82, Green/Orange, the Emperor has developed from trying to rule from his will to now ruling from his heart. The reconciliation of the three forces, the "yes," the "no," and the "I do not know," comes from our feelings rather than our thinking.

Apply B82 around the entire trunk of the body.

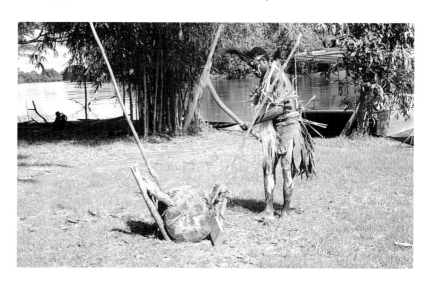

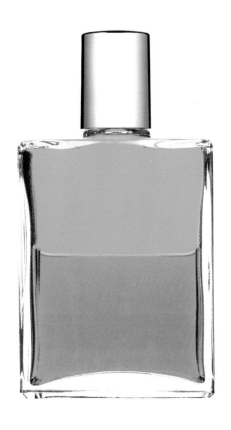

B83 Turquoise/Gold

Name: Open Sesame

Shakes Together As: Yellowish Olive Green

Tarot Card: Return Journey of the Hierophant

Keynote: The process of individuation in relation to the star of incarnation where we find the wisdom of the past expressed through the creative communication of the heart.

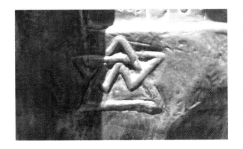

In the Arabian folktale "Ali Baba and the Forty Thieves," from the work *One Thousand and One Nights,* "open sesame" is a magical incantation that opens a door in a rock wall to reveal something previously inaccessible: an illumined cave filled with treasures of beauty and wealth.

In Turquoise/Gold, gold is hidden inside (below); it may seem to be inaccessible. Our fears and anxieties could inhibit our communication or self-expression. We may lack confidence or a feeling of self-worth. Creative communication of the heart (turquoise) from the feeling side of the being may allow an opening to the contained treasure.

B5, the Hierophant on the outward journey, offered wisdom of the past toward the future. In the return journey of B83, wisdom is offered in a creative way from the heart. The returning Hierophant opens the door for us to receive profound wisdom, which we communicate with feeling to others, perhaps preferring to share with a group rather than on a one-on-one-basis. We who are drawn to B83 may have a love of the mineral kingdom and an understanding of new

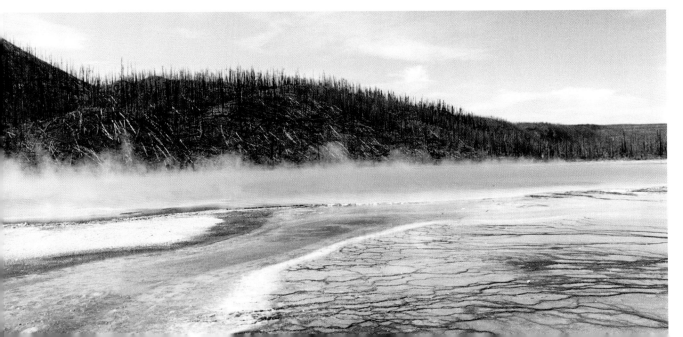

Related Bottles

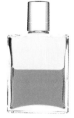

Related Color
B4

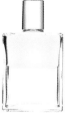

Closest Tint
B94

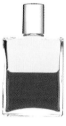

Outward Journey
B5

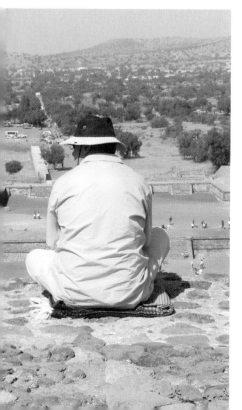

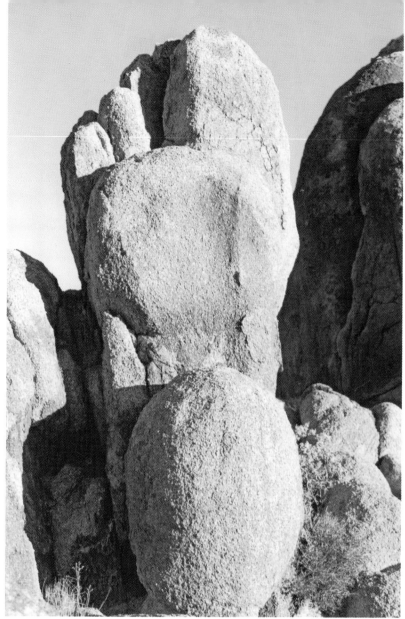

technologies, potentially opening the door to a rapport with crystals, which has been sealed off for many centuries. B83's connection to crystals can open the way to the devas that work with them. B83 may relate to incarnations in Lemuria, Atlantis, and ancient Egypt and with the Aztec, the Inca, and the mystical traditions of Europe.

Turquoise expresses the process of individuation. Here it is linked directly with gold. By getting in touch with the golden area within ourselves, the process of individuation may unfold. The name Open Sesame describes the potential of the many doors that can open as the process develops.

Apply B83 around the entire trunk of the body.

Above: Rock formation in Joshua Tree, California.
Left: Mike Booth atop a sacred site in Mexico, land of the Maya, Aztec, and Toltec.
Page 224, top: Stone carving, part of the signature on a larger statue in Audubon Park, New Orleans.
Page 224, bottom: Smoking Caldera in Yellowstone National Park, Wyoming.

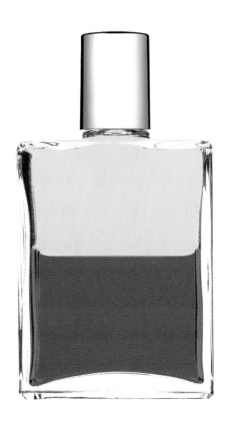

B84 Pink/Red

Name: **Candle in the Wind**

Shakes Together As: **Red**

Tarot Card: **Return Journey of the Lovers**

Keynote: **A sense of vulnerability. A strength toward a higher purpose.**

Right: The Taj Mahal, built by the Emperor Shah Jahan, in an incarnation of Master Kuthumi, as a testimony of true love to his wife.
Below: Memorial candles inside the Jokhang Temple in Lhasa, Tibet.

The song "Candle in the Wind," by Sir Elton John, in an ode to Marilyn Monroe,[84-a] is actually a statement about the feminine and how idolization of the feminine icon places that icon in a vulnerable situation. Recently, the song was rewritten and performed at the funeral of Princess Diana, another female icon of our time. The bottle Candle in the Wind is an expression of the vulnerability of the feminine, an aspect of the Pink/Red relationship.

There is a connection between the vulnerability of the feminine icon and the more complete female/male union inherent in the return journey of the tarot's Lovers. Each of us has the potential for a female/male unity within ourselves. As we move closer toward the feminine within ourselves, as we become open intuitively and more receptive, we become vulnerable. Vulnerability can be frustrating or frightening, leading to resentments in connection with the feminine. This may relate to difficulties we have with our mother model, if we feel that she did not return love in the way we gave it. Perhaps we have difficulty acknowledging the love we need or could give. Eventually we may compassionately understand the

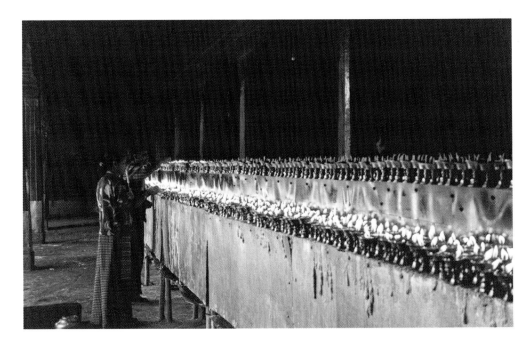

Related Bottles

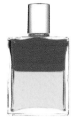

Reverse
B80

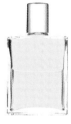

Closest Tints
B52

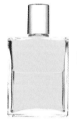

B81

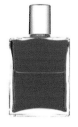

Closest Hue
B6

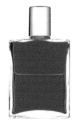

Outward Journey
B6

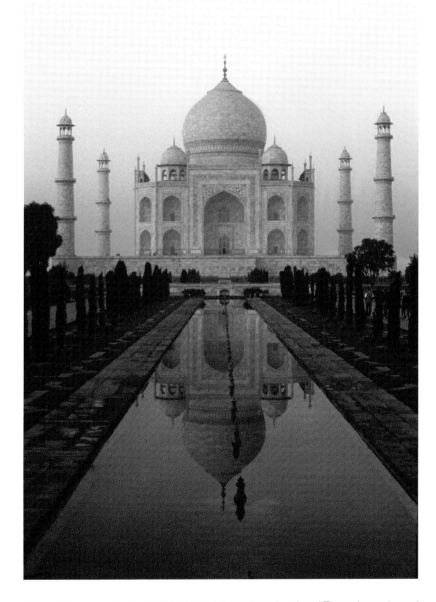

different loves and vulnerabilities that child and mother, I and Thou, the male and female within, experience. B84 may call us if we have awakened to our female intuition through self-acceptance, if we have the discipline necessary to change the patterns of the past.

Receptivity and openness imply vulnerability; being prepared to be vulnerable is the story of B84. This acceptance leads to the energy and passion we need to give unconditional love, to put caring into action. While a candle needs a certain amount of air to breathe and burn, if there is too much air, the candle will be snuffed out. The candle is a source of light, symbolic of many aspects of caring and warmth. Wind is symbolic of change. Intertwined, they describe this bottle.

Pink/Red supports Tantric work, the transformation of sexual energies into spiritual energy. This does not necessarily imply sexual practice.

Apply B6 around the abdominal area.

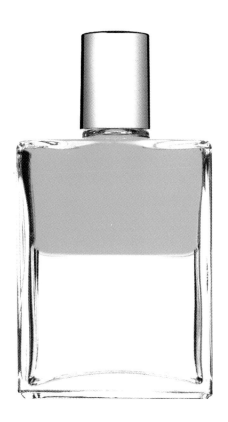

B85 Turquoise/Clear

Name: Titania, Queen of the Fairies

Shakes Together As: Pale Turquoise

Tarot Card: Return Journey of the Chariot

Keynote: Light within; the path of individuation unfolds in the conscious mind.

Titania is the queen of the fairies, as portrayed in Shakespeare's *A Midsummer Night's Dream*. All of the Little People (the fairies) have a mother or queen figure. Living in the realm halfway between tangible reality and the unseen realm, the fairies personify a living aspect of the earth. The queen of the fairies looks after these beings, who are incredibly tender and precious and yet, in another way, support nature in its coarsest aspect. Nature is an incredibly potent force. Titania has a grip on this potency, yet she also deals with the subtle ethereal realm, beyond physicality.

Right: A house for the little beings of the unseen realms, in a garden in Selkirk, Scotland.

Below: Sulphur springs at Yellowstone National Park, Wyoming.

> *First, rehearse your song by rote*
> *To each word a warbling note:*
> *Hand in hand, with fairy grace,*
> *Will we sing, and bless this place.*
> (ACT 5, SCENE 1)

The magic of Shakespeare's tale depends on the events synchronistic with Titania's awakening from sleep. In the return journey of the Chariot, the final test of faith (B7) manifests as synchronicity. The sphinx, the guardian spirit in traditional tarot imagery of the Chariot, transforms to become Pegasus, the

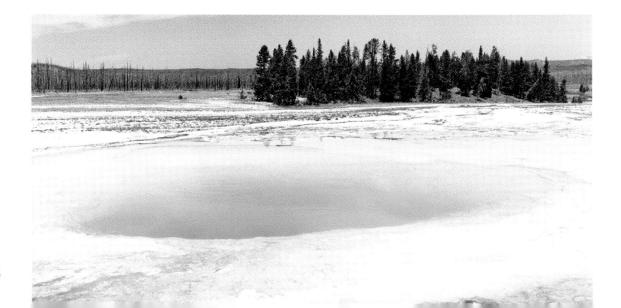

Related Bottles

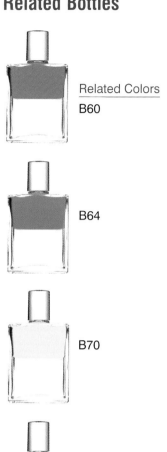

Related Colors
B60

B64

B70

Reverse
B86

Closest Tint and
Shakes to
B62

Outward Journey
B7

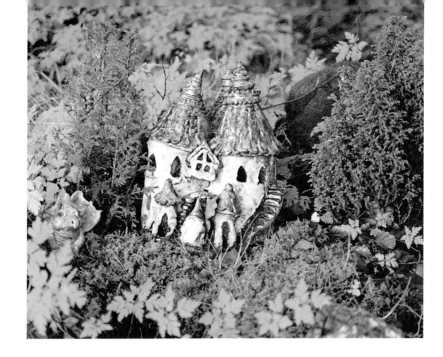

winged horse symbolizing the immortal soul and synchronicity. Pegasus was Vicky's nickname from when she drove an ambulance during World War II; she had an intuitive gift that allowed her to arrive when and where she was needed. Synchronicity is a product of the process of individuation (turquoise); coincidences happen as a result of a change in being. The test of faith that had a static quality in B7 unfolds in B85 as Pegasus takes us on a journey.

As we become more in touch with the Ananda Khanda, the turquoise energy, it becomes more full of light. The light here is in relation to the turquoise; the process of individuation produces an intensification of the creative communication of the heart, which, in turn, allows an opening to something subtler and more ephemeral. Both B85 and B86 have this quality. The creative energy expresses itself with a quality that is at once more delicate and more intense. There is the possibility of increased awareness of the unseen realms, whether of the devas, fairies, angels, or gnomes, or an awareness of the earth energies and their unfolding on the planet at this point in time. The king and queen of the fairies symbolize the profundity of the subtle realms and the possibility of being in contact with those realms through creativity. As the Ananda Khanda becomes more full of light, as clear is brought to the turquoise, all of these things become possible.

Ancient wisdom systems deal with consciousness, with subtlety, expressing an awareness of things that exist in the margin between the natural world and the unseen world. We who are drawn to B85 may be charismatic and able to communicate the light with feeling, perhaps enjoying new technology to keep in touch with others through the Internet or e-mail, moving in this borderland. We may be linear thinkers and yet find joy in creative expression, learning in the context of teaching. By enhancing creativity and the energy of the creative, Titania and King Oberon represent the possibility of connecting with the subtle realms and making them more tangible.

B85 may help us release creative blocks and allow in a new light. Yet we may have difficulty with the masculine side of ourselves, caused by holding on to hidden fears. Applying B85 around the chest area may help us when our feelings are trapped inside, and we are unable to shed tears or to express ourselves creatively.

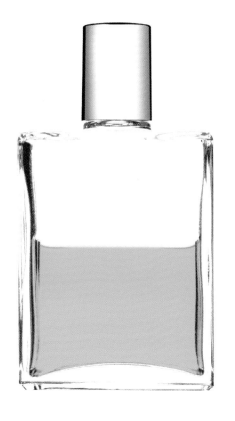

B86 Clear/Turquoise

Name: Oberon, King of the Fairies
Shakes Together As: Pale Turquoise
Tarot Card: Return Journey of Anubis or Justice
Keynote: Understanding of the light upon the path of individuation.

Oberon is the husband of Titania, queen of the fairies. In Shakespeare's tale *A Midsummer Night's Dream,* Oberon, the king of the fairies, releases Titania from the spell of misplaced love to a remembrance of her true feelings (act 4, scene 1). Both Titania (B85) and Oberon indicate an awareness of the subtle realms, especially of the devic kingdom. They support an aptitude toward that which is subtle; they encourage a sensitivity to the beings of the nature kingdom. In Titania's company, Oberon wishes:

> *Every elf and fairy sprite*
> *Hop as light as bird from brier:*
> *And this ditty, after me,*
> *Sing and dance it trippingly. . . .*
> *Now, until the break of day,*
> *Through this house each fairy stray,*
> *To the best bride-bed will we,*
> *Which by us shall blessed be.*
> (ACT 5, SCENE 2)

Page 231, top: Reeds growing in Lake Titicaca. Known as the abode of the gods and site of a creation myth, Lake Titicaca in Bolivia is the world's largest high altitude lake.
Page 231, bottom: Yellowstone Falls, Wyoming.
Below, left: Trevi fountain, with faint notes from local street musicians winding their way through the air, in Rome, Italy.
Below, right: Canal in Venice. As a powerful city-state, Venice was recognized for the keen perceptions and communications of its ambassadors and for the creative brilliance of composers such as Gabrieli and Vivaldi and artists such as Tintoretto and Carpaccio.

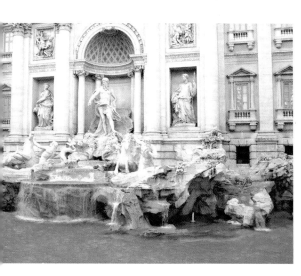

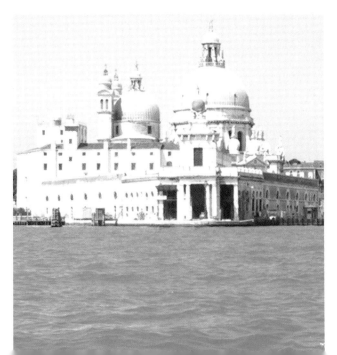

Related Bottles

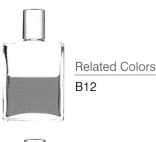

Related Colors
B12

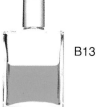

B13

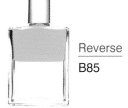

Reverse
B85

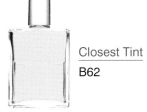

Closest Tint
B62

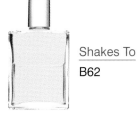

Shakes To
B62

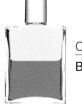

Outward Journey
B8

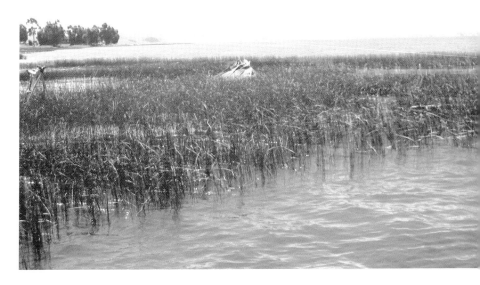

In Egyptian mythology, Anubis, the jackal-headed god, is an associate of Horus and Thoth. He guards the inner wisdom by bringing balance; he helps lead the soul through the underworld, where the purity and truthfulness of the heart may be assessed and preserved. The clear over the turquoise in B86 suggests that Anubis's insight (clear) penetrates powerfully into the creative communication of the heart (turquoise), producing an illuminated rainbow of light from the seven chakras. The insight of B86 could bring a clear mind and the ability to communicate heartfelt feelings. We may be drawn to B86 if we are able to balance our own positive and negative energies. We could have great creative depths, which we present in a light-full way. Light has penetrated each of our energy centers or chakras.

Apply B86 along the hairline and around the chest area to address difficulties in communicating feelings due to intense suffering. This may allow us to let go of hidden fears, becoming more assertive in communications.

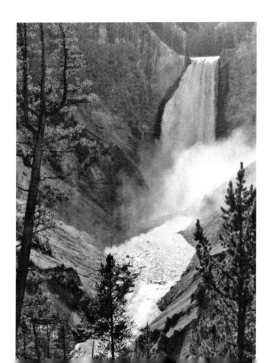

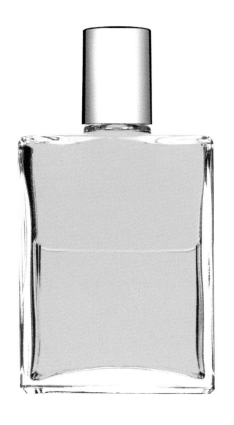

B87 Pale Coral/Pale Coral

Name: Love Wisdom

Shakes Together As: **Pale Coral**

Tarot Card: Return Journey of the Hermit

Keynote: To be able to see ourselves beyond the reflection of self. The wisdom of love.

Page 233, top: The Great Wall of China, built over 2000 years ago by Emperor Qin Shi Huangdi to keep out the huns and other nomadic tribes to the north.

Page 233, bottom: Apprentice pillar in Rosslyn Chapel, associated with the yet to be revealed mysteries of the grail quest.

Below: Sign on the exterior of one of the oldest caves in Northern India. The cave was the home of a sage and later became a sacred place of pilgrimage.

In B87 pale coral appears for the first time. At first we called this combination Unrequited Love. Unrequited love is love that is not returned in the way in which it is given or that is not returned at all. B87 expresses the situation in which, for some reason, the love we offer is unreturned in the way that we offer it. Thus B87 may be helpful when we are dealing with shock, abuse, or unrequited love in present as well as past incarnations. The choice of B87 may suggest that we have suffered some form of abuse in the present life or previously; we may have difficulties with relationships from the past.

In the return journey, the Hermit goes within himself to perceive what lies beyond his own reflection of self. As he looks past his own reflection he sees something else, something new. His eyes open to his inner contemplation, his own sensitivity. B87 is an expression of the witness: a witnessing not from a detached point of view but as an active involvement. To develop awakening and awareness of the witness requires full participation, and this coral offers us.

B87 is now called Love Wisdom. It expresses our potential to give love and wisdom to the world, to accept ourselves, and to "wake up." We may be called by B87 if we have an understanding of interdependence that has brought us deep joy. We may have a sense of emergence, of a new consciousness, often referred to as the New Man or New Christ energy, which is the emergence of the Christ energy of which Rudolf Steiner spoke. Steiner said that at the end of the twentieth century and at the beginning of the twenty-first century some

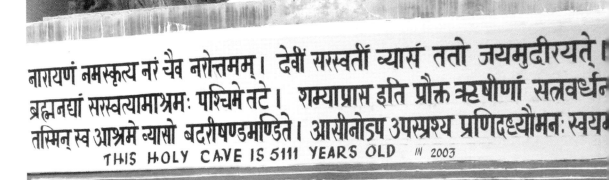

नारायणं नमस्कृत्य नरं चैव नरोत्तमम् । देवीं सरस्वतीं व्यासं ततो जयमुदीरयते ।
ब्रह्मनद्यां सरस्वत्यामाश्रमः पश्चिमे तटे । शम्याप्रास इति प्रोक्ऋ ऋषीणां सत्त्रवर्धन
तस्मिन् स्व आश्रमे व्यासो बदरीषण्डमण्डिते । आसीनोऽप उपस्पृश्य प्रणिदध्यौमनः स्वयम्

THIS HOLY CAVE IS 5111 YEARS OLD IN 2003

Related Bottles

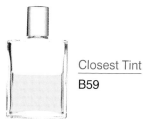

Closest Tint
B59

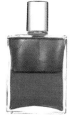

Closest Hue
B105

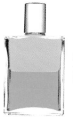

Outward Journey
B9

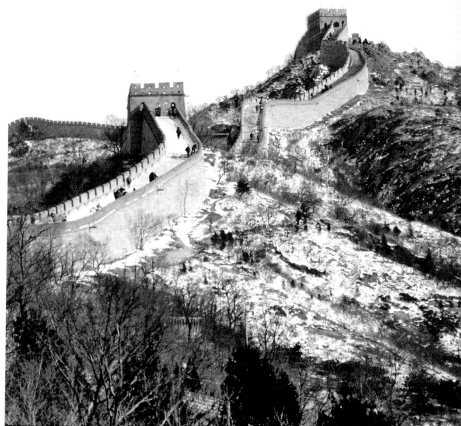

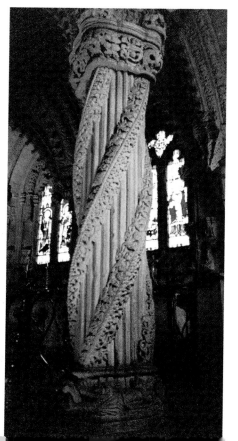

people would have a personal experience of the Christ energy. This experience would arise then to usher in a new wave of consciousness.[87-a] Synchronously, as the new wave of coral energy is birthed, so, too, will this new human being's consciousness arise.

B87 may help us establish a connection with past lives spent in the North American Indian tradition.

B26 is applied around the lower abdomen and along the left side of the body, from the left earlobe down to the left ankle. B87 is applied in the same way but along the right side.

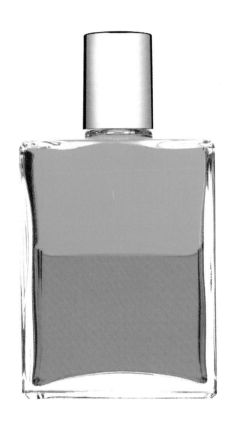

B88 Green/Blue

Name: Jade Emperor
Shakes Together As: Turquoise
Tarot Card: Return Journey of the Wheel of Fortune
Keynote: As we plant so shall we reap, but it is the way we plant that makes a difference.

B88 it is the second level or return journey of the Wheel of Fortune, B10, Green/Green. The difference between these two levels is the absence of yellow in the bottom fraction of B88. According to Chinese mythology, the Jade Emperor is the ruler of heaven (see B60). He searched for the secret of longevity and had the peace within (blue) to rule heaven with the truth (green).

Green/Blue shakes together to create turquoise, expressing creativity. Feelings of spaciousness allow us to find peace and harmony. B88 shows us the peace within ourselves and lets us communicate our feelings and our creativity. As we allow ourselves the space to be in touch with our feelings, our ability to communicate increases.

B88, Green/Blue, is an upside-down version of the Heart bottle, B3, Blue/Green. The choice of B88 may suggest that we are nature lovers, ecologists, or otherwise working for reform in the consciousness of Gaia. This bottle may also help us connect with incarnations in Atlantis, in Lemuria, and with the Knights Templar.

B88 indicates an understanding of the difference between karma and dharma. We must live through that which arises in our present life, the result of the seeds

Page 235, top: Little blue heron fishing at the J.N. "Ding" Darling National Wildlife Refuge on Sanibel Island in Florida. This solitary wading bird feeds by alternating slow stalking with wild running.
Page 235, bottom: 88 piano keys.
Below, left: A Jade Emperor, also known as the August Personage of Jade, or less formally, Grandpa Heaven, New York City.
Below, right: Frog—symbol of the spring, fertility, and renewal. Kiss a frog and reveal an emperor. Gayle Meadow Pond in Winhall, Vermont.

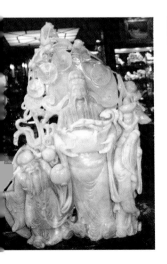

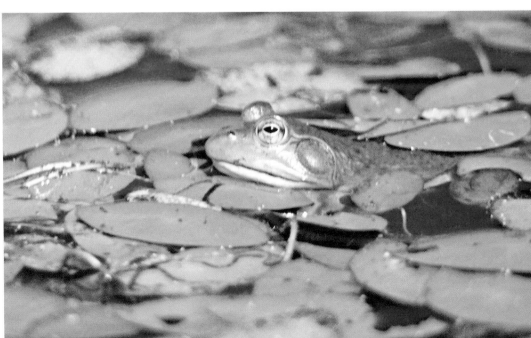

Related Bottles

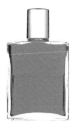

Related Colors
B2

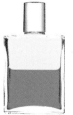

B8

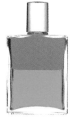

Reverse
B3

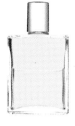

Closest Tint
B50

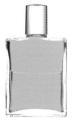

Shakes To
B43

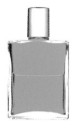

Outward Journey
B10

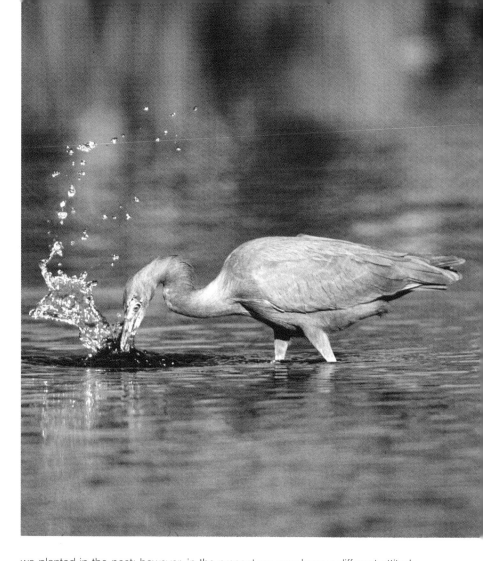

we planted in the past; however, in the present we may have a different attitude toward, or a different way of working with, our experience. While an individual seed may not be particularly long-lived, longevity can be expressed in the cycle from seed to growth to new seed. If we plant seeds of happiness in the present, we are likely to find blossoms of joy greeting us in the future. Equally, if we plant seeds of unhappiness, then it is those that are likely to sprout in our future. Perhaps the Jade Emperor is not external but an aspect that we could find within ourselves. The ruler of the heaven within ourselves comes as a consequence of understanding cause and effect. In this light, B88 could suggest that we have difficulty with our masculinity or that we fear authority. In consequence, we may experience difficulty in expressing emotions, feelings, and truth. We can find peace within the depths of ourselves as we deal with that which occurs in time and space.

Apply B88 around the chest area and over the entire throat and neck. It can be especially helpful in assisting us when we feel that we do not belong on Earth.

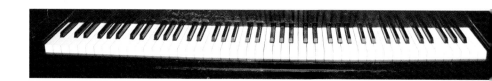

235

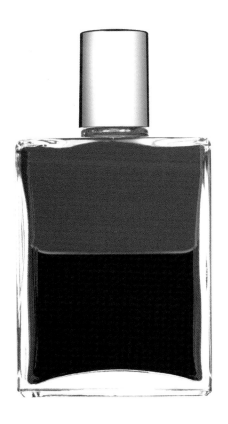

B89 Red/Deep Magenta

Name: Energy Rescue/The Time Shift

Shakes Together As: Deep Magenta

Tarot Card: Return Journey of Strength

Keynote: A time shift, a gateway to a new understanding and a new possibility toward enthusiastic well-being.

Red/Deep Magenta is the return journey of B11, Clear/Pink. B11, the outward journey of strength, is associated with the lion, the proud king of the jungle. A task associated with B11 is taming the lion, or overcoming spiritual pride. In the return journey of strength, pride is overcome; we become integrated with the lion, and we begin to realize our potential in everyday life.

The red in the upper fraction of B89 is a very strong energy when linked with the deep magenta. We may be drawn to this bottle when we are depleted or are experiencing extreme lethargy; it can help restore our energy and vitality. The name Energy Rescue originated in part because shortly after this bottle was born, several people associated with Aura-Soma suffered electrocution. Red/Deep Magenta was found to be helpful when applied in this situation, offering strength when energy had dissipated or when energy levels needed to be rescued. Contained within B89 is B6, Red/Red. B89 can therefore represent and be useful for those of us who do not utilize the energy we have and who decline the opportunities that life presents to us. We could lack attention to detail, being too busy to look at the shadow within, depleting ourselves of the energy we need to

Page 237, top: The Lion Gate, Mycenae, circa 1250 BC. The lions are the emblem of the royal dynasty of Mycenae, the house of Agamemnon, from a time when the divine right of the king to rule was conferred by the gods. According to José Argüelles, we are now in the Solar Inhalation Cycle, which will be completed in 2012 and promises a potential great transformation.

Page 237, bottom: Train station in a small village in Norway. In Norwegian, *hell* can mean "luck" or "cliff cave."

Below: Mount Arenal at night, Costa Rica.

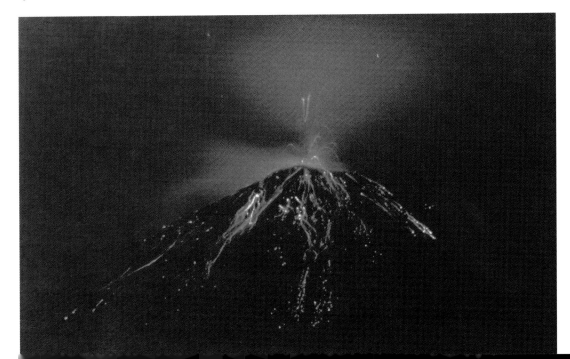

Related Bottles

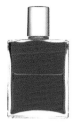

Related Colors
B6

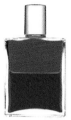

B19

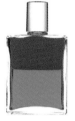

B29

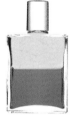

Closest Tint
B104

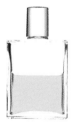

Outward Journey
B11

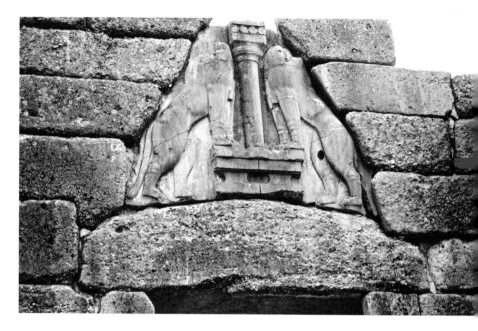

awaken transformation. The transformation can help us have the energy to bring forth our healing instincts. B89 can appeal to us if we are intuitive and spiritual, with an extraordinary relationship to and understanding of time.

This bottle was born on July 26, 1992, when the Mayan calendar marked an end of a cycle. Therefore, this bottle is also called the Time Shift bottle. The shift is to a new paradigm. For the past two thousand years the cultural paradigm has been that time is money. As intimated in the ancient Mayan codices,[89-a] we are coming to the era of a new paradigm: time is art. It is the qualities of personal touch and caring that we bring to what we do, rather than how much we produce, that characterize this new paradigm.

B89 is suitable for Tantric exercises and can help people who work with earth energies, protecting them from negative earth-energy radiation.

Apply B89 around the lower abdominal area.

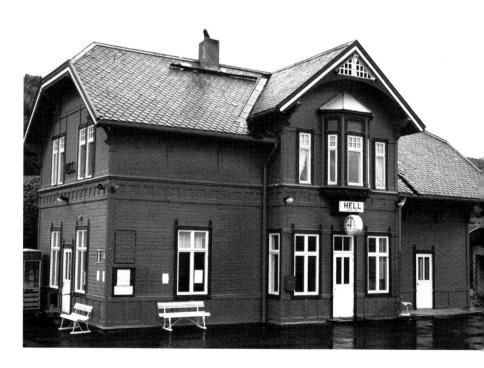

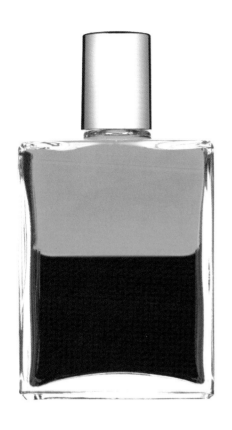

Note: The image on page 292 is also a visual expression of this bottle.

B90 Gold/Deep Magenta

Name: Wisdom Rescue
Shakes Together As: Deep Magenta
Tarot Card: Return Journey of the Hanged Man
Keynote: The initiate finds the way to be active in the world.

B90 is the return journey of the Hanged Man, B12. The gold represents awakening to the wisdom understood in the past. B12 is associated with an initiate, with someone who has completed an initiation process and reawakened the wisdom (gold) held in the past. By consciously bringing attention into our belly, the golden area of our body, we enliven the ancient wisdom that lies within us.

Initially the Hanged Man, the initiate, is upside down, symbolic of the need to look at things from a different point of view and to have action suspended until clarity ensues. In B90 the Hanged Man becomes the Redeemer. He has made sense of the initiatory experience and can apply his innate wisdom to daily life. He has done this by finding love and compassion within, and he is now able to put love into the little things. Choosing B90 suggests that we can discover immense joy and wisdom through what we have to share with others. B90 might aid those of us who have condemned ourselves so much for our little mistakes that we cannot express our strengths.

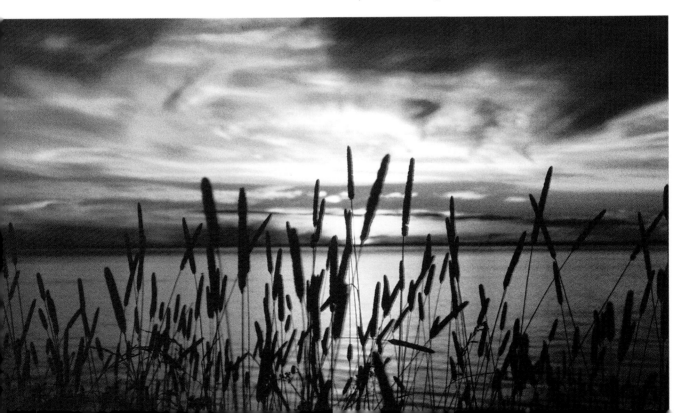

Related Bottles

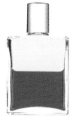

Related Colors
B5

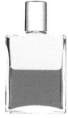

B18

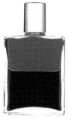

B89

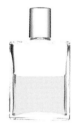

Closest Tint
B59

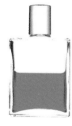

Outward Journey
B12

Above: Bengal tiger, native of India, immortalized in the poem by William Blake, which begins "Tiger, tiger, burning bright, In the forests of the night." The tiger is a symbol of strength and fearlessness.

Left: Cattails growing on the shore of Lake Champlain, Vermont.

Right: Eastern box turtle. An individual turtle may live over 100 years. Evidence of the species itself exists in the ancient fossil records.

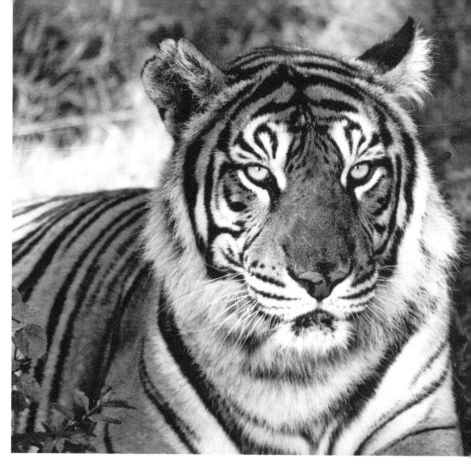

Both B89 and B90 are concerned with the potential for shifting to a new paradigm. Wisdom Rescue, in particular, is associated with the Convergence, an event that was held August 16th and 17th, 1987, to mark that shift astrologically, in a timing that coincided with a shift shown in the Mayan calendar. (The Maya have a calendar of noteworthy accuracy that has been relevant for centuries.) The deep magenta in the base of B90 suggests tapping into an eternal source to support the wisdom being offered. B90 may help us connect to incarnations with the Maya, Aztec, or Toltec.

B90 may suggest that we have confusion in our mind and experience frustration because we do not recognize the depth of our love. Applying this bottle around the abdomen can help us let go of deep fears and anxieties and recognize our innate love.

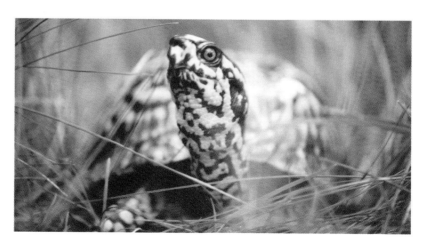

239

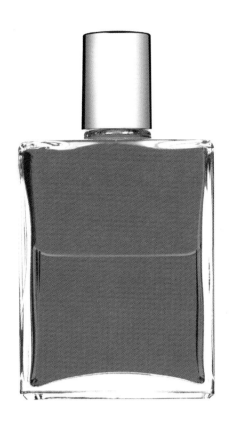

B91 Olive Green/Olive Green

Name: Feminine Leadership of the Heart

Shakes Together As: Olive Green

Tarot Card: Return Journey of Death

Keynote: The trust in the Holy Spirit. Love brings up everything unlike itself for the purpose of healing. The hope, not in the sense of anticipation, but in the sense of a positive attitude toward that which will come to be.

Page 241, top: Terracotta warriors in Xian, China, created and buried to accompany and protect the emperor in his afterlife.

Page 241, bottom: Woman capably paddling flat bottom boat while her child sleeps curled up behind her, on Dal Lake in Kashmir, India.

Below: Moss growing on house roof in Pittsfield, Vermont.

B91, Feminine Leadership, is the return journey of Death. In B13, Death, the Grim Reaper, waits for no person, but in B91, the feminine intuitive offers empathetic love to death, and death goes through a transformation.[91-a] Death's sickle brings an awakening, the light of hope and change, to each of the chakras. B91 presents another relationship with our emotions, in which our ability to witness the ups and downs of life allows us to experience a flexible and harmonious response to what we feel.

The olive green energy of feminine leadership bridges the journey between the third and fourth chakras. The only way across the solar plexus is through the feminine intuitive, the olive area (see "The Subtle Anatomy," page 23). To go beyond relationships and experiences based on fear and power (yellow), we must develop trust in our feminine intuition, the olive that blends yellow and green.

B91 is often chosen by those of us who trust our feminine intuition, who are

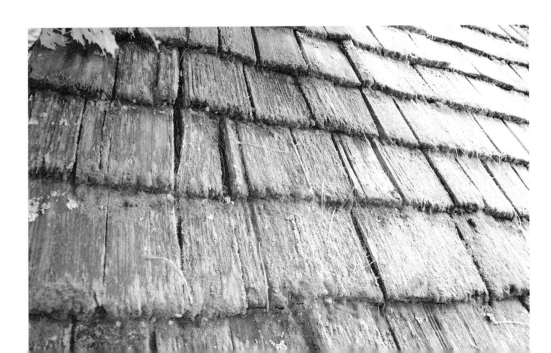

Related Bottles

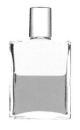

Related Colors
B7

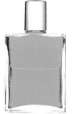

B10

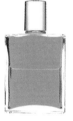

B41

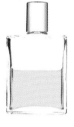

Closest Tint
B74

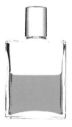

Outward Journey
B13

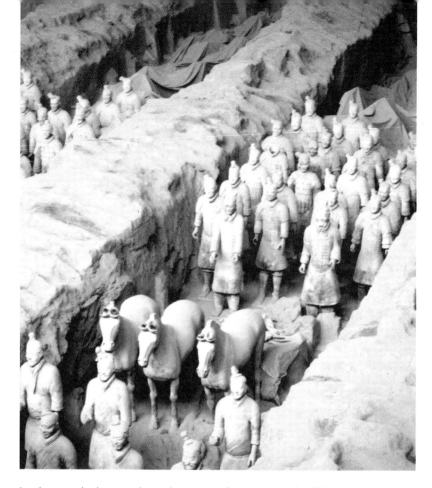

leaders, and who passionately express from our hearts. This bottle suggests that we are truthful and have integrity. We may have the ability to understand scientific and spiritual matters and to explain them to others in such a way that they may be understood. B91 could help resolve fear of feminine power, fear of the feminine side of the self, and fear of authority. We may be drawn to B91 if we are in emotionally unsuitable relationships and are repeatedly creating the same mistakes and patterns in our relationships.

B91 can help us come into the right relationship with the unknown. It can help us find clarity in cases where we believe we are aggravated by extraterrestrials.

Apply B91 around the chest and abdominal areas.

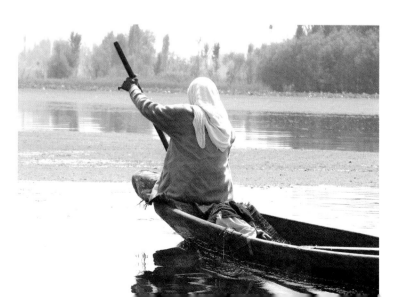

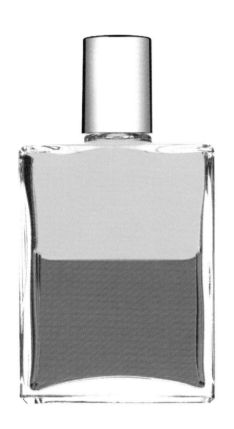

B92 Pale Coral/ Olive Green

Name: Gretel

Shakes Together As: Olive Flecked with Pale Coral

Tarot Card: Return Journey of Temperance

Keynote: Feminine leadership, independence. Cooperation, rather than competition. Peace as a priority.

While the task of Temperance, B14, is to balance the power of fire (inspiration) with the qualities of water (the emotions), B92, Gretel, has integrated this dichotomy. Gretel embodies the interdependent cooperation of the male and female personas within the self (coral), as well as the gift of intuitive feminine heartfelt leadership (olive).

B92, Gretel, and B93, Hansel, came into being at the same time; they were the only two bottles in the whole Equilibrium range to be born as a pair. In the folktale, Hansel and Gretel are lured by an old witch into her cottage. The witch plans to eat the children. She locks up Hansel to fatten him for dinner and puts Gretel to work. Eventually the witch tells Gretel to light the oven, but Gretel says she cannot. The witch has to do it. Then Gretel pushes the witch into the oven and immediately releases Hansel. Hansel and Gretel leave the witch's cottage, free to play in the woods again.

Right: Portal to another dimension, along the Puuc route in Mexico.
Below: A being of noble gentleness, this elephant with chain is in a baby nursery in Sri Lanka.

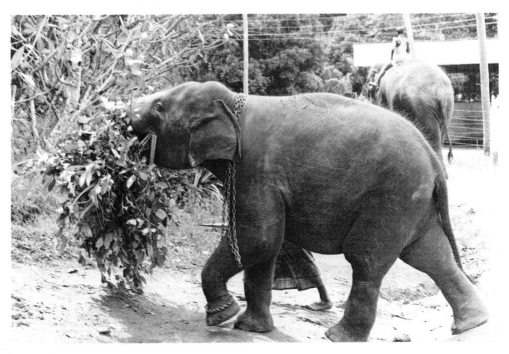

Related Bottles

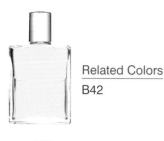

Related Colors
B42

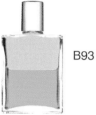

B93

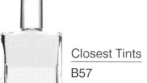

Closest Tints
B57

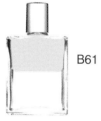

B61

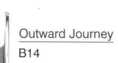

Outward Journey
B14

B92 suggests that we may be in a difficult situation because of our inner conflicts and negativity; in the tale, the negative is represented by greed, susceptibility to temptation, and the forces of malice. However, the female aspect of our inner child (Gretel) trusts in her intuition and overcomes negativities. Female leadership becomes important in the tale; the old witch represents the feminine of the past, while Gretel symbolizes the new feminine taking the initiative. In this way, B92 indicates personal change and growth toward self-reliance, finding the love and wisdom with which to quell our fears. With compassion, we can lead others to develop trust in the process of life and hope for the future. Hansel, allowing the young woman to control the situation and ultimately save him, represents the male aspect of the inner child placing his trust in the female aspect. This releases him to find true joy and happiness.

B92 and B93 support us in striving for peace in the face of what seems like irreconcilable conflict. The olive in the base fraction of B92 gives hope for the future that we may use our creativity (the turquoise in B93) constructively. Awakening energy may bring a new understanding, a new consciousness upon Earth, the New Woman/New Man of the coral.

The energy of B92 also has to do with the energy of Zeus/Jupiter; according to Western astrology, Jupiter offers grace and generosity.[92-a] B92 supports further work with the inner child. It is also helpful when we have difficulty concerning finding our right livelihood.

Apply B92 around the belly and chest areas.

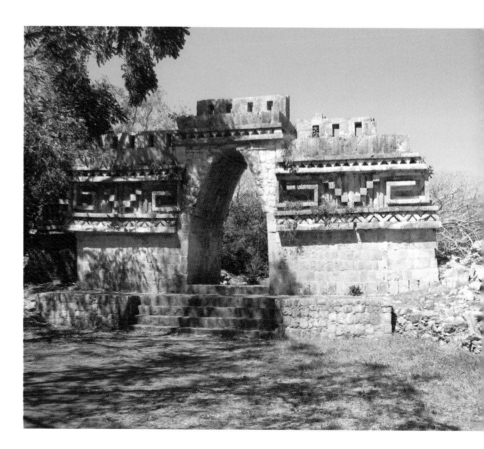

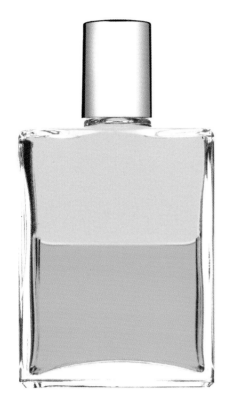

B93 Pale Coral/ Turquoise

Name: **Hansel**
Shakes Together As: **Deep Violet**
Tarot Card: **Return Journey of the Devil**
Keynote: **Facing the shadow to be able to find the truth of the heart as we see more aspects of ourselves.**

Below: Puente la Reina ("bridge of the queen") was built in the eleventh century by the Queen of Navarra at the confluence of two rivers. The bridge, at one time under the protection of the Knights Templar, is 12 feet wide allowing two horsemen to pass comfortably. It is an important stop along the Camino de Santiago, the path also known as the Milky Way.

B93, Hansel, was born as a pair with B92, Gretel; please see B92 as well.

The individuation process (turquoise) involves developing the ability to be a witness to ourselves and at the same time to be aware of the collective. In the folktale, Hansel is primarily a witness to the process of the feminine discovery of strength; it is Gretel's love for him (and ours for our inner male child) that gives her the strength to discover her leadership. The pale coral in the upper fraction makes it possible to transcend dependent and unfulfilling relationships; the coral supports more interdependent, shared awakening. B93 connotes an ability to encompass an integration of the inner and the outer witnessing and to go beyond the duality of the self, to find cooperation between the inner male and inner female. Then it is possible to see things clearly as they are now and not how we would like them to be or, in a sense, to be clairvoyant.

Hansel tells us we must allow ourselves to face, to witness, how we are

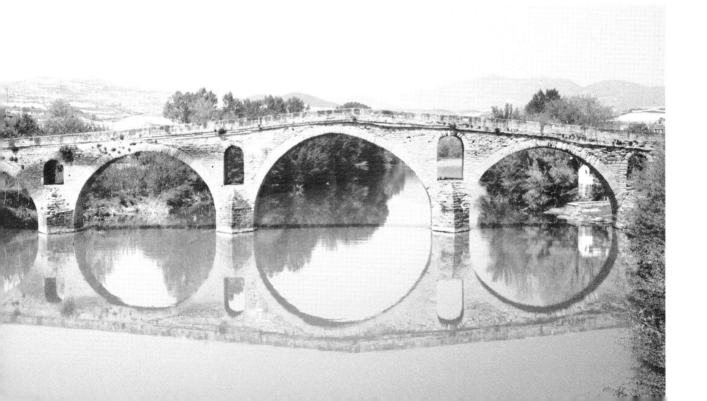

Related Bottles

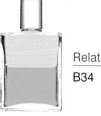

Related Colors
B34

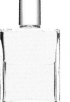

B42

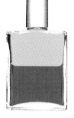

B92

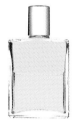

Closest Tint
B57

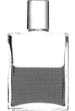

Outward Journey
B15

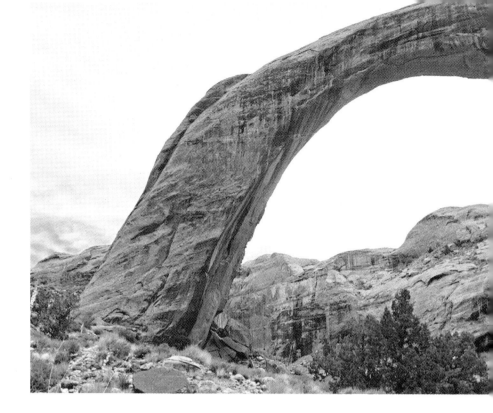

dependent upon others, and to see what is truly there, not what we imagine to be there. B93 can be of assistance in this letting go. This process of self-examination helps us find the trust to communicate our feelings (turquoise) with a few individuals as well as with many people. B93 nurtures our ability to cultivate loving attention and the wisdom with which to transform negative to positive.

Apply B93 around the entire trunk of the body.

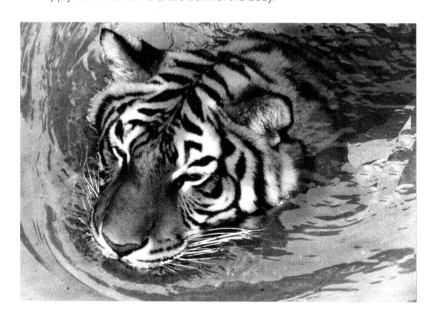

Top: Rainbow bridge, sacred to the Native Americans, is a naturally occurring sandstone arch in Arches National Park, Utah.
Bottom: Bengal tiger free to swim. As we digest and integrate our shadow, we allow our individuality to emerge. This is illustrated in the following limerick, attributed to Cosmo Monkhouse: "There was a young lady of Niger / Who smiled as she rode on a Tiger; / They came back from the ride / With the lady inside / And the smile on the face of the Tiger."

245

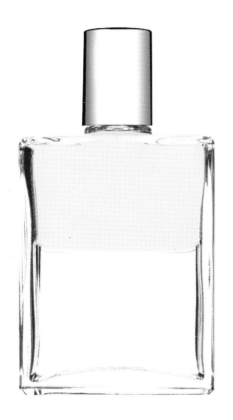

B94 Pale Blue/ Pale Yellow

Name: Archangel Michael

Shakes Together As: Pale Green

Tarot Card: Return Journey of the Tower

Keynote: An intense truth is revealed in relation to the evolution of consciousness.

The entrance of the archangels with B94 marks the beginning of a new chapter in the Equilibrium range. Archangel Michael's appearance here seems auspicious, as he watches over the evolution of the earth and of humanity at this point in time.[94-a]

In B94, Archangel Michael brings his sword of discernment and intelligence (pale yellow) to the heart center of the planet. He grounds the Michaelic energy into the heart to usher in the New Aeon. The pale blue of "Thy will, not my will" (B50) with the pale yellow of the little or individual will come together to create pale green, the color of B53, whose keynote is "The Way, the Truth, and the Life." If we hold "Thy will" in our conscious mind and move our personal ideas and opinions out of the way, something of the pale blue, of the greater will, may come through us. We may find peace as we let go of our inner confusion. Then the pale yellow, the illumination of the little will, our personal will, is in harmony with the higher will. These intentions come together in our heart (green). We may be at peace with authority, no longer fearing authority, because a "greater authority" of peace prevails.

Page 247, top: Glastonbury Tor. Both the Tor and Mont-Saint-Michel are nodal points on the Michaelic line of the earth's grid system.
Page 247, bottom: Forget-me-not, symbolic of love and loyalty, in Ripton, Vermont.
Below: Mont-Saint-Michel on the north coast of France. Archangel Michael brings an inspiration of true freedom of thought and of global consciousness.

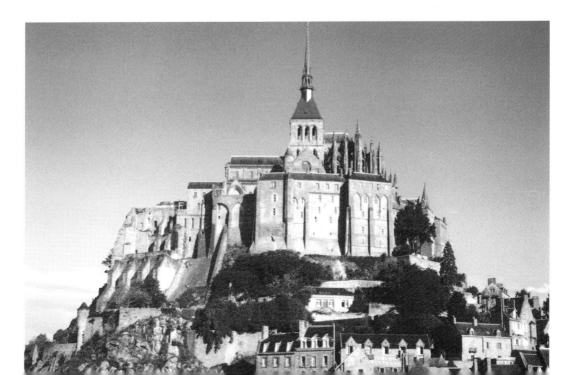

Related Bottles

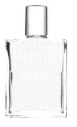

Closest Tints
B50

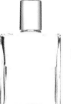

B51

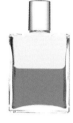

Reverse Hue
B8

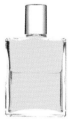

Shakes To
B53

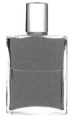

Outward Journey
B16

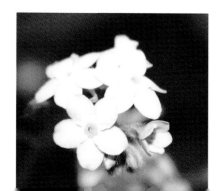

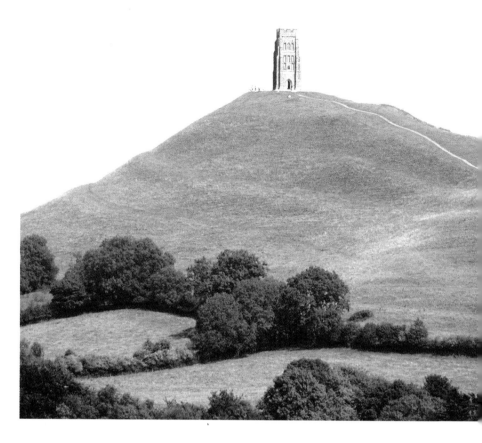

Michael is the representative of the New Christ energy in our time and the time that is to come. He ushers in awareness on a personal level of the nature of the redeeming force within us. As we each understand this, we become representatives of the Michaelic energy.

Symbolically, archangel Michael places his sword on the tower of the Glastonbury Tor (a hill in Glastonbury, England). B94 is the return journey of the Tower, B16. The Tower symbolizes metanoia, a change of mind. In B16 it is as if the tower of Babel were collapsing; all the artifacts of our mind are being challenged. The collapse of the tower provides an opening to the other world through the heart within the heart. In B94, Michael brings from spirit a new life for a new time, a new light force into the planetary grid system, helping human consciousness grow to another level of understanding. The Michaelic energy gives us a new understanding of the Christ energy. It is an awakening energy, an energy of reconciliation between two opposing forces in ourselves (see B55): that which binds us to the earth and that which is trying to pull us away from the earth. Michael brings part of the Redeemer's message.

B94 indicates a time of great change when many familiar things fall away to reveal something new. B94 represents the need to balance the emotions, to let go of jealousy, fear, and the feelings of wishing to be where someone else is or wanting what someone else has. When we do this, we can experience the joy that we have within.

B94, Pale Blue/Pale Yellow, is the reversed, more intense version of B8, Yellow/Blue. As such, the qualities of B8 are intensely present in B94, but with a different perspective.

Apply B94 around the heart and navel areas and the throat.

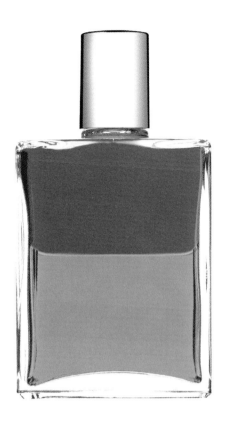

B95 Magenta/Gold

Name: Archangel Gabriel

Shakes Together As: Gold with Flecks of Magenta

Tarot Card: Return Journey of the Star

Keynote: The messenger from the stars so that we may get in touch with our true purpose.

Right: Bouquet with lotus blossoms outside of a temple in Bangkok, Thailand. Symbolic of purification of body, mind, and soul and the potential for enlightenment, linking that which is above with that which is below.
Below: Blossoming stars in the Derwent valley, Tasmania.

B95 is the second bottle in the Archangel sequence. The soul star (magenta) and the incarnational star (gold) join in the return journey of the tarot Star B17. The coming together of the two stars brings information and energy from a divine source of love from above into the golden area of the body. This magenta energy journeys through the Ananda Khanda and the emerald of the heart before touching the golden area. When magenta arrives at the incarnational star in the golden area, it activates the hologram of the true aura within our being, provided that we have given conscious attention to grounding (bringing the light of attention to the red root). The archangel Gabriel is the messenger who assists us with that possible activation of the true aura. In the return journey of the Star, the soul star and the incarnational star become illumined. The sound of inspiration, the phoenix that rises from the ashes, now rests in the heart. We can hear the still small voice within; the Holy Spirit expresses itself through the emerald of the heart.

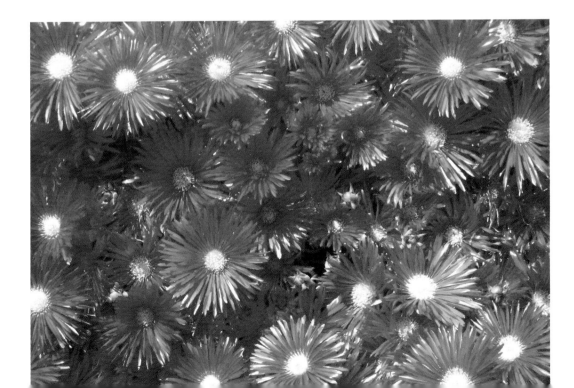

Related Bottles

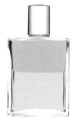

Related Colors
B23

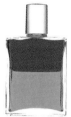

B40

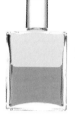

B76

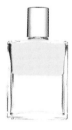

Closest Tint
B61

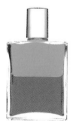

Outward Journey
B17

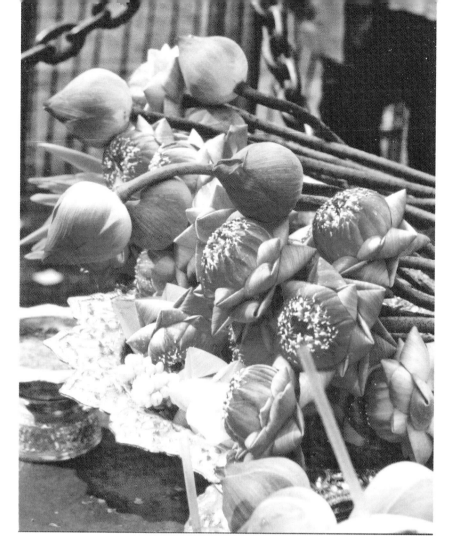

The archangel Gabriel is thought to have been the archangel watching over the evolution of humanity before the archangel Michael took over this responsibility. His time of prevalence was AD 1510–1879.[95-a] The importance of developing the link between the incarnational star and the soul star results from the growth of humanity during that epoch, and the need now is for us to actualize the potential for individuation in harmony with our divine purpose.

In some respects B95, Archangel Gabriel, is the higher aspect or principle of B68, Gabriel. B95 contains Red/Gold, B40, the I Am bottle, and thus the concerns expressed for B40 are also inherent in B95.

B95 suggests that we are receiving divine love and have the inner wisdom to understand the meaning of such love. We perform all actions with care and warmth, putting love into the little things. We may be drawn to this bottle if we suffer from deep fears or confusion and need to be true to ourselves; despite the fears, we need not to fall into old habits or patterns. The red hidden in both fractions of this bottle could indicate hidden anger and frustration, but red is also the energy that encourages awakening. We may be going through a great change in our life; the combination of magenta and gold indicates a new beginning.

Apply B95 around the body directly below the navel, and also apply one drop on the top of the head.

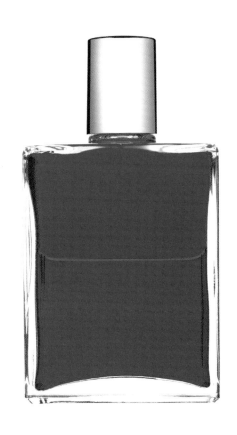

B96 Royal Blue/ Royal Blue

Name: Archangel Raphael

Shakes Together As: Royal Blue

Tarot Card: Return Journey of the Moon

Keynote: To bring the creative possibility of conception into form. Clarity in relation to the higher energetics of being.

In B96, royal blue is present in the base fraction for the first time in the Equilibrium range. The third archangel, Raphael, receives something from the reflective light of the moon, reaching for, bringing down, and integrating the feminine intuitive energy. The royal blue of the sixth chakra brings the higher intuition and higher mind functions from the higher center. Raw creativity and a creative nurturing energy are expressed through Raphael. He is the angel of healing as well as of science and knowledge.[96-a]

When communication comes to us, we have a chance to witness it before we communicate it to the world. We have an opportunity to choose to take responsibility for it. Raphael gives a profound seeing and a perception of something from another level.

Royal Blue/Royal Blue is the return journey of the tarot card the Moon, B18, Yellow/Violet. Both B18 and B96 remind us that as humans we may aspire to the highest, reaching to the mountaintops. The royal blue of the brow chakra may suggest that Archangel Raphael goes beyond the ordinary perceptions to bring down a reflection of the intuition experienced by far seeing. The royal blue also suggests clarity in seeing, hearing, and feeling, supported by detachment, and developed with the presence of red in the royal blue. Red could indicate a need for discipline and an opportunity to let go of anger, frustration, and resentment. In the Yellow/Violet of B18 we await receptively the light of wisdom. Royal Blue/ Royal Blue, B96, suggests the importance of allowing the creativity that comes to us to be expressed.

We may be drawn to B96 if we have found deep peace that we can give to others. We can stay focused, undistracted by comments and actions of others.

Apply B96 along the hairline, on the brow, and on the feet. A little B96 rubbed over the forehead may clarify the senses of seeing, hearing, trusting, smelling, and touching.

Left: Harvest moon overlooking Frenchmen Bay at Acadia National Park in Maine.

Related Bottles

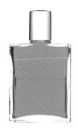

Related Colors
B2

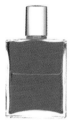

B6

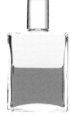

Outward Journey
B18

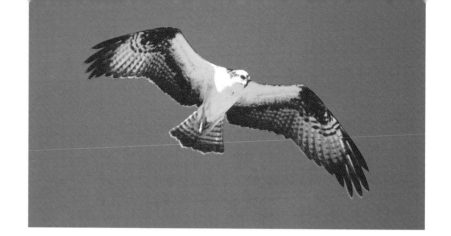

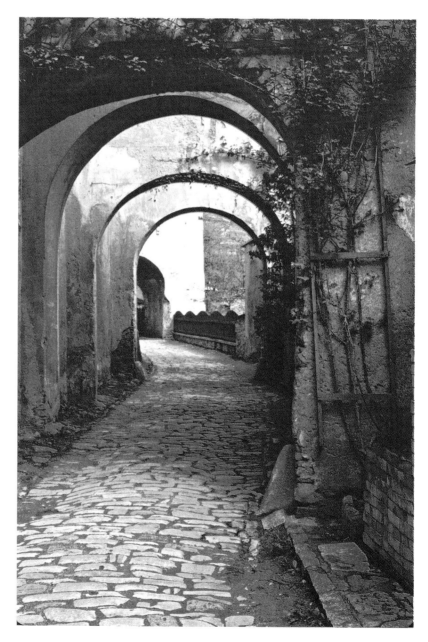

Above: Osprey in flight on Sanibel Island in Florida. An osprey's sight is more developed than that of other birds of prey. Ospreys are able to scan a broad area and judge the distance of their prey below the surface of the water. They then plunge feet first into the water.

Right: Cobblestone pathway to the castle in Durnstein, Czech Republic, where Richard the Lionhearted was imprisoned on his return from the Third Crusade. He was found and rescued when he heard the song of a troubadour and responded.

Note: The image on page 49 is also a visual expression of this bottle.

251

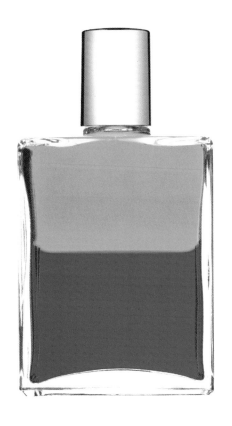

B97 Gold/Royal Blue

Name: Archangel Uriel

Shakes Together As: Emerald Green

Tarot Card: Return Journey of the Sun

Keynote: Clarity in relation to the true purpose of our self. A deeper understanding of the heart.

Page 253, left: Sundial at Chartres Cathedral in France.

Page 253, right: Sunflower, Lancaster County, Pennsylvania, Amish country. An expression of our relationship with the Divine.

Below: Golden leaves of the fall reflected in water at Connor's Pond Dam in Petersham, Massachusetts.

B97, Gold/Royal Blue, fourth in the Archangel sequence, shakes together as emerald green, the color of the heart, symbolic of the time to get in touch with our service and purpose in the world. The golden energy that surrounds the incarnational star in the belly comes into the conscious mind; the royal blue of Raphael, B96, is in the base. In B19, the outward journey of the tarot's Sun, the Sun is like the Little Prince.[97-a] It is as if our solar plexus, like the Little Prince's, is so strong and radiant that sunflowers turn toward us rather than toward the sun. The sun, whether in B19 or B97, can encompass and touch all the signs of the zodiac as a source of light shining forth solar energy. This suggests our potential to radiantly communicate our feelings for others. B97 shows us that deep peace within is beginning to be expressed. We are centered, have a heart of gold, and have great enthusiasm for life. In the return journey of B97 we connect to our values and purpose; all of what we could be is brought into us. Our

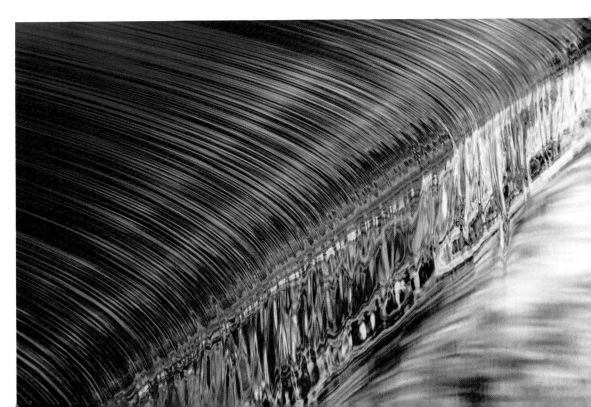

Related Bottles

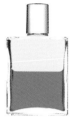

Related Colors
B8

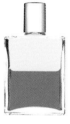

B18

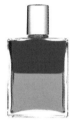

Reverse
B32

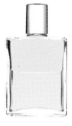

Closest Tint
B57

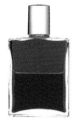

Outward Journey
B19

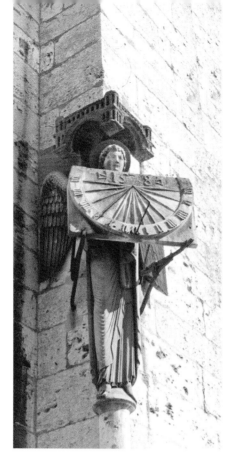

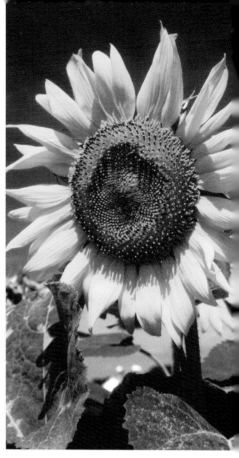

true potential is realized through experience, allowing us to express ourselves with deep inner peace.

Uriel in Hebrew means "fire of God" or "God is my light." Although Uriel is known as the archangel who rules the earth element, he also reaches to the sun and offers sunlight to the world. Uriel brought alchemy to earth and was the giver of the Kabbalah to humankind. According to legend, this archangel stands with a fiery sword at the gate of the lost Eden. Lost Eden symbolizes the condition of forgetting to love God. The fiery sword, the "fire of God," shows that negative matter, which consists of selfish and impure desires, is destroyed when we truly focus our love on God.

Uriel is also described as the archangel of salvation who visited Noah and teaches the path of the heart, the path of pure love. We need to release deep anxieties so we can connect with these inspirational qualities that are being fed in from above. B97 offers an opportunity to examine our values. It is important to remain appropriately humble.

Apply B97 along the hairline, on the brow and temples, and around the heart and solar plexus.

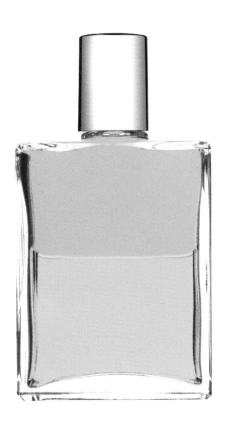

B98 Lilac/Pale Coral

Name: Archangel Sandalphon/Margaret's Bottle

Shakes Together As: Magenta

Tarot Card: Return Journey of Judgment

Keynote: A four-way energy connection: above and below, to the left and to the right. The inner child within ourselves becomes the angel that we are.

Margaret was Vicky's partner and companion for many years. She and Vicky ran a clinic together in Amersham, England. Margaret was present through the birth and early years of the development of Aura-Soma (see chapter 2). In 1992 Margaret and Mike were together in South Africa walking along a street of orange-colored dirt. On either side of this orange road were jacaranda trees with their lovely lilac blooms. As they were walking, Margaret said that one day these colors would make a very beautiful bottle. In June 1998, Lilac/Pale Coral was born, just a few months before Margaret was to make her transition. B98 is called Archangel Sandalphon; it is also called Margaret's bottle, in memory of the walk underneath the jacaranda trees and because its birth ushered in her passing in October 1998.

Page 255: Dawning of a new day: November sunrise on Black Duck Creek at Chincoteague National Wildlife Refuge in Virginia. This is a beautiful area of dunes and marsh on a barrier island, where warm weather lasts into November.

Right: Community of coral and fish at a coral reef in Palancar Gardens in Cozumel, Mexico.

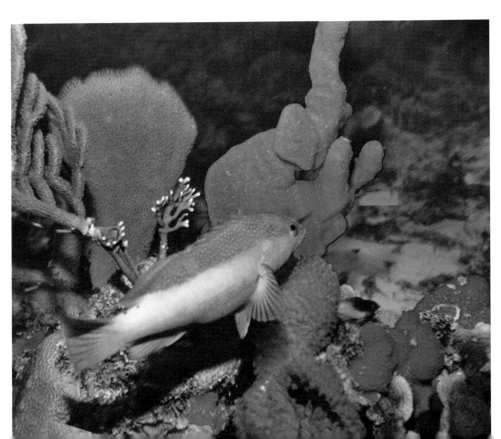

Related Bottles

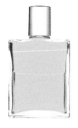

Related Color
B87

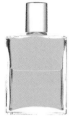

Closest Tints
B56

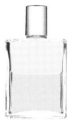

B58

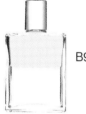

B94

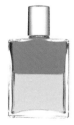

Outward Journey
B20

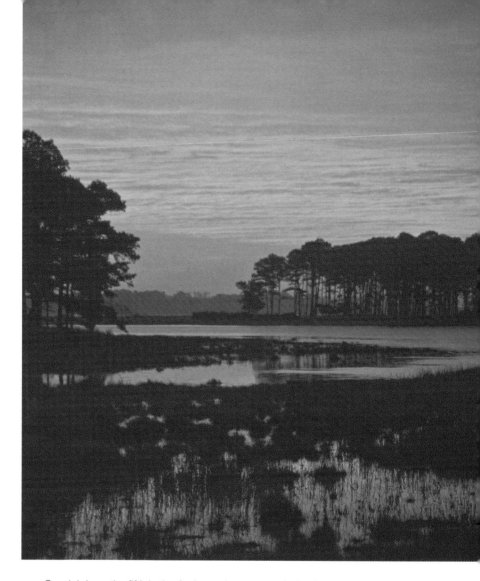

Sandalphon, the fifth in the Archangel sequence, is the Archangel associated with the sphere of Malkuth on the Tree of Life. He is concerned with the whole of existence upon earth, with the transmutation of negativity in the conscious mind (lilac), and with the New Man (see B22 and B87) within coral and across all levels of being. If we are attentive enough to consciously transmute negativity, we can reveal the New Man within. The New Man shares joy, bliss, and insight visible to others. B98 indicates that we have a capacity for unconditional love (pink in the upper and lower fraction) that is helping us through a process of change. The higher will assists in our communication with devas and angels.

B98 is also the return journey of Judgment. In the outward journey of B20, Star Child, Blue/Pink, the male (blue) and the female (pink) energies are separate, yet they can be joined when shaken and integrated to create the birth of the Star Child. In B98, the male and female energies have united (lilac), and the child and its angelic connection are strong (pale coral). B98 helps us deal with abuse suffered in the past and allows healing of unrequited love. It is easy to love ourselves when we are always a catalyst for change.

Apply B98 on the top of the crown and on the lower abdomen. B98 may support craniosacral work, helping the cerebrospinal fluid to flow more easily. For this, B98 could be applied over the whole length of the spinal column.

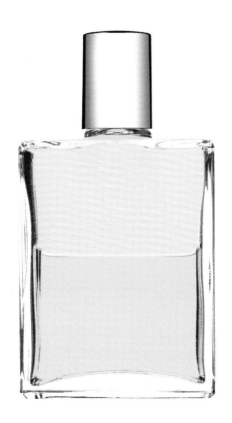

B99 Pale Olive Green/Pink

Name: Archangel Tzadkiel/Cosmic Rabbits

Shakes Together As: Pale Violet

Tarot Card: Return Journey of the World

Keynote: A new opening to the love of self is a step toward our purpose in the world.

Right: Doors and windows that let us open to possibilities and step into the world.
Below: Stepping into the waters of life, lake in Fiji.

In B99, pale olive appears for the first time. The connotation of fluidity in olive suggests greater freedom in B99 than in B21, the outward journey of the World. When pink arcs across from the incarnational star in the golden area to the emerald of the heart, it passes through the yellow energy into the olive. Pink becomes brighter when it reaches the olive, where it is on the threshold of entering the emerald of the heart and allowing the heart's energy to be expressed (see "The Subtle Anatomy," page 23).

Sixth in the Archangel sequence, Archangel Tzadkiel is concerned with humans' development toward the fourth dimension. He is an angel of mercy who prevented Abraham from sacrificing his son. Tzadkiel is also one of two standard-bearers who follow directly behind the archangel Michael as he enters battle. Archangel Tzadkiel's divine qualities are freedom, mercy, and transmutation. He is of the seventh ray and the violet flame (see note 50-b).

B99 lets light shine upon feminine intuition. Thus, it may be useful in helping us learn who we really are and get in touch with our true purpose and mission. B99 suggests that it is time to be free of fears and to accept ourselves. The

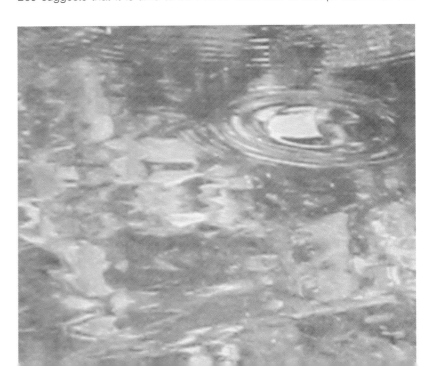

Related Bottles

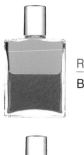

Related Color
B46

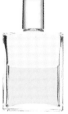

Closest Tints
B58

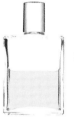

B59

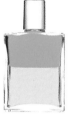

Outward Journey
B21

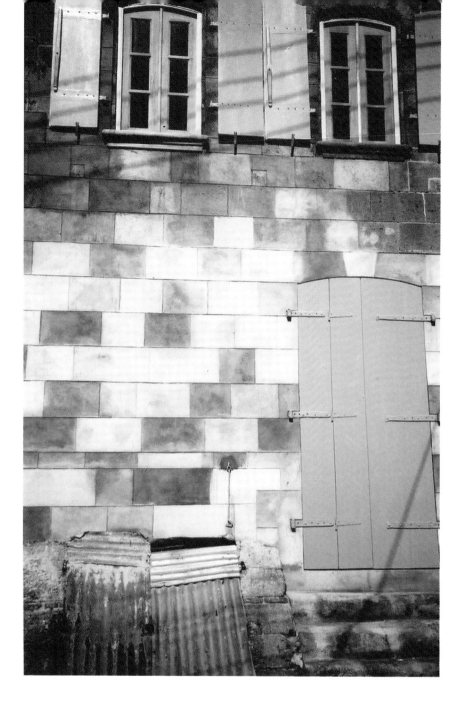

energy is there for awakening to ourselves. Frustrations and resentments can hold us back. The feminine in ourselves is supported by B99's unconditional love and unconditional self-acceptance. With these qualities we can be pioneers for freedom, secret agents for truth, with the courage to step into the world with love, to open our heart, to step into the waters of life.

Apply B99 just above the solar plexus in a band around the body, around the pelvic girdle, and over the base of the spine.

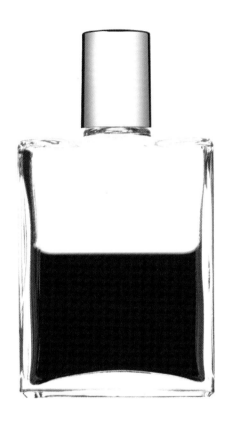

B100 Clear/Deep Magenta

Name: Archangel Metatron

Shakes Together As: Deep Magenta

Keynote: Shining the light into the shadow. A new dawn in the inner worlds.

The archangel Metatron is the same being as the prophet Enoch in the Old Testament. Enoch had clairvoyance and supernatural vision. He saw wheels upon wheels moving together through time and space. Metatron is the Time Lord. He is able to stand in the eternal and look at the whole of time. We as humans would label this as the past and the future; Metatron looks at it all at the same time from a vast perspective, beyond our comprehension. Archangel Metatron led the Hebrews through the forty years in the wilderness and wrestled with Jacob. He has been known as the link between the human and divine.

Metatron's twin brother is the archangel Sandalphon. Metatron is known as the king of angels and also the angel of the covenant. He joins together Heaven and Earth, the clearest clear and the deepest dark magenta. One of Metatron's capabilities is to help put us back in touch with a true sense of our being.

In this combination light (clear) is in the conscious mind, the upper fraction, and deep magenta is in the subconscious/unconscious mind, the lower fraction. Usually, the difficulties that arise in our lives are based not on the problems we create consciously but on that which is most difficult to face. B100 offers the possibility of shining light into that which is difficult to see, into the shadow,

Right: This medieval clock in Salisbury Cathedral in England was built in 1386 and is believed to be the oldest working clock in the world. The Salisbury Cathedral is also home to the original Magna Carta.

Below: White mountains in central Alaska on the winter solstice of 1991, at solar noon, the high point of the sun's journey across the sky. The spruce trees in the foreground are heavily bowed over by snow, but come spring will stand upright again. The monochromatic nature of the light is typical of the Arctic and subarctic in winter.

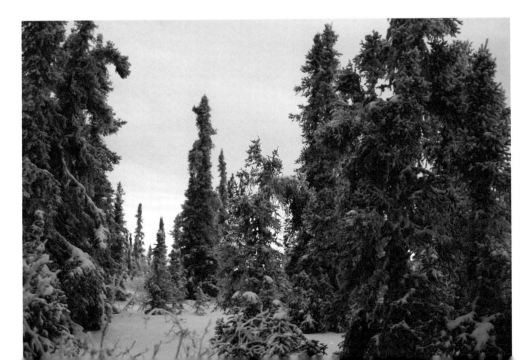

Related Bottles

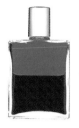

Related Colors
B0

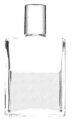

B11

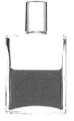

B55

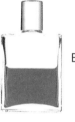

B77

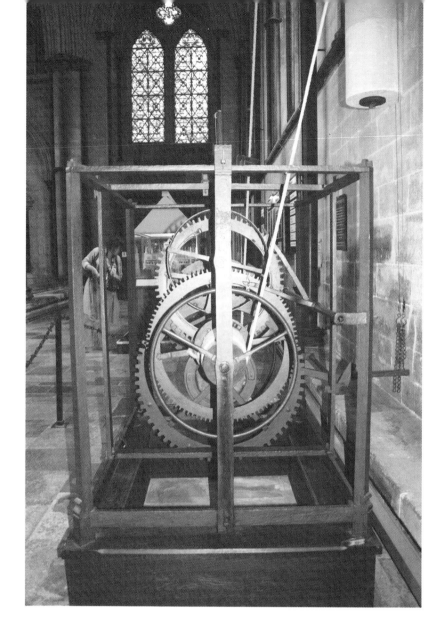

into the darkness. Metatron brings awareness to those obstacles that block our self-awareness. B100 suggests that we may put on a brave face, but we have suffered, and we are aware of the type of and reason for our suffering. Now we have an opportunity to release suffering from the deepest level. When we can see the truth of our selves, we can come to an understanding of the forces within our own unconsciousness.

All of the Rescue Set bottles that have deep magenta in the base are contained in B100, as the clear in B100's top fraction contains all the colors.

Apply B100, the seventh in the Archangel sequence, anywhere on the body, but particularly over the back of the head and neck and around the temples. It also can also be applied on the soles of the feet, as in reflexology.

The combinations B100 through B104 have the names of archangels. As yet it has not been revealed how these bottles relate to the tarot or to the Tree of Life, with the exception of B102, which appears to be linked with the Tower, B16.

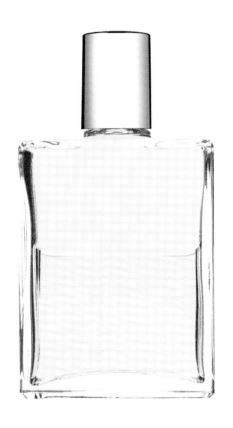

B101 Pale Blue/ Pale Olive Green

Name: Archangel Jophiel

Shakes Together As: Pale Turquoise

Keynote: The way back to the garden of the heart. The opening of a new level within our being.

The eighth in the Archangel sequence, B101, Pale Blue/Pale Olive, is the intense version of B3, Blue/Green, the Atlantean or Heart bottle. B101, like B3, is pertinent to the lost continent of Atlantis. Jophiel may help us attune to the higher will, to help us to be more aware of our peace.

Archangel Jophiel's specific role in Hebraic text was to lead Adam and Eve out of the Garden of Eden.[101-a] Perchance if Jophiel knew the way out, he would also know the way back. He has a connection to the will of God (pale blue) and the laws of existence (pale green), which together manifest through the feeling heart (pale turquoise). Within Jophiel is a connection with our stellar ancestry; this in turn links with the feeling side of our being, perhaps bringing us closer to an understanding of ourselves as beings of light.

The pale blue indicates intense communication: communication that comes through us unfiltered, unmodified by us in any way, a higher communication that

Right: A Wedding ritual: Setting out on a new life on the Sepik River in Papua New Guinea.

Below: A peaceful view from a hill at Teluk Batumonan, Komodo Island, Indonesia.

Note: The image on page 286 is also a visual expression of this bottle.

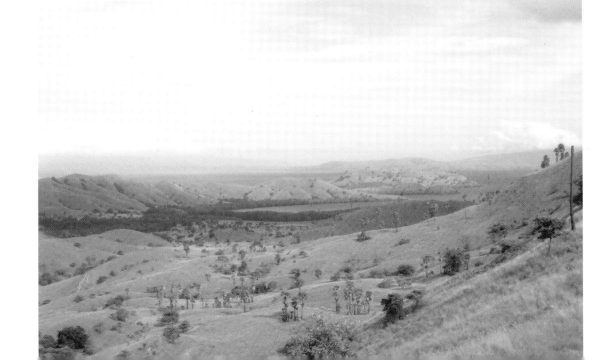

Related Bottles

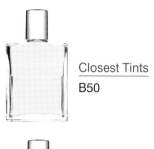

<u>Closest Tints</u>
B50

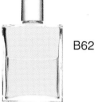

B62

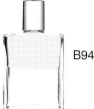
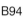

B94

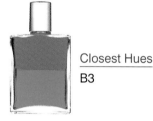

<u>Closest Hues</u>
B3

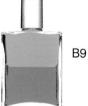

B9

is sourced from larger forces. The pale olive is created by the interface of light coming into the olive. The energy moves toward the green from the yellow.

Blue and olive are found on either side of the heart (see "The Subtle Anatomy," page 23) and in B101 are found in their intense (pale) form. Pale blue is located above turquoise, which is located on the right of the heart. This color language suggests that Jophiel can guide us back to the garden of our heart, where the original male/female relationship, the Adam and Eve within us, may find its right unity.

This bottle also reminds us to look at jealousy and envy, either coming toward us or arising within us. Sometimes it is difficult to find the space for ourselves because of intrusion. This color combination asks that we reach up inside ourselves: that we are given the space we need, according to the higher will. B101 addresses feelings of inadequacy, of not being good enough, of a lack of a sense of self-worth. B101 gives us a wonderful opportunity to deepen our feminine intuitive capabilities, helping us feel hopeful about our new growth. If necessary, Archangel Jophiel may unblock our creative expression, as it shakes together as a pale turquoise.

As with all the bottles that contain clear, B101 may be applied anywhere on the body. It is particularly helpful when rubbed over the heart region, including the sides and area of the upper thoracic spine, to form a complete band around the body. It may also be used over the upper part of the chest and around the shoulders.

See "Aura-Soma and the New Aeon," in chapter 6 for further information about B101.

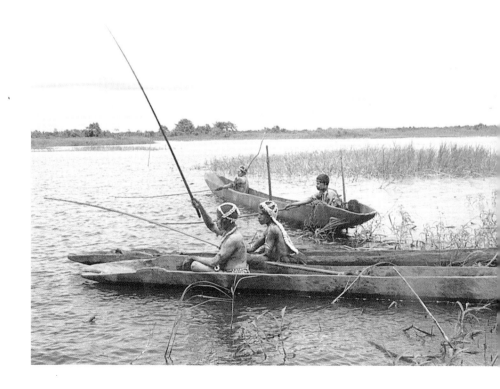

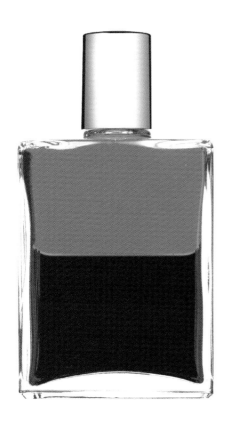

B102 Deep Olive Green/Deep Magenta

Name: Archangel Samael

Shakes Together As: Deep Magenta

Keynote: O-live, where we find a new beginning in relation to the hope within ourselves. Upon what do we build the foundations of our lives?

Samael is described as the most beautiful of the archangels, and he has been called the angel of death and the poison of god. Like Metatron, Samael is said to have twelve wings. He is linked to the planet Mars, which is often thought of as the planet of war and conflict. Traditionally, Samael's tarot attribution is the Tower,[102-a] which in Aura-Soma relates to B16, Violet/Violet, for the outward journey and B94, Pale Blue/Pale Yellow, for the return journey. In some anthroposophical studies, Samael, linked with Mars and the Tower, is thought to have ruled humanity's evolution on the earth from 1190–1510, a time characterized by the Crusades.[102-b] This epoch of Samael was prior to the era of the archangel Gabriel and the subsequent era of the archangel Michael.

Page 263: Female Ostrich with eggs at the Maasai Mara National Reserve in Kenya. The ostrich incubates shared eggs. This ostrich has eggs of more than one bird in a nest, which is just a small indentation in the open plain on the African grasslands. Those eggs not under the bird will probably not hatch as they will become overheated in the direct African sun. The mother bird, by stretching her neck, tries to protect the eggs and the young from the hot African sun and from predators. From this challenging start, new life emerges.

Right: Deep pool surrounded by greenery that hides it from the site of the Mayan sun temple in Chichén Itzá, Mexico.

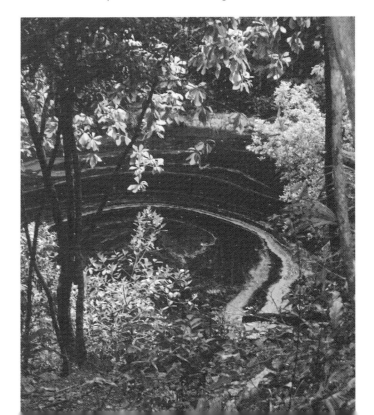

Related Bottles

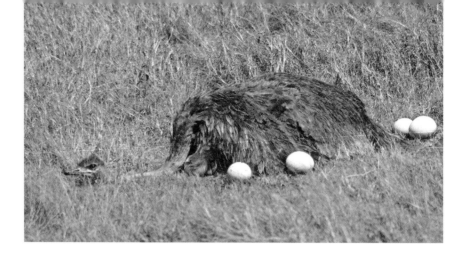

Related Colors
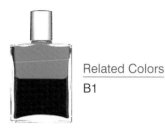
B1

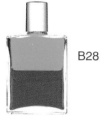
B28

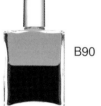
B90

Closest Tint
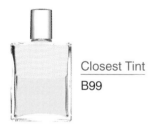
B99

Outward Journey
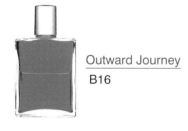
B16

Return Journey
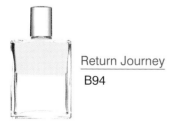
B94

B102 is the ninth bottle in the Archangel series. In B102 the first shade in an upper fraction in the entire Aura-Soma range is born: deep olive appears. Deep olive indicates the possibility of a deepening of feminine intuition. Yellow is hidden within the deep olive, suggesting that hidden fears exist in the conscious mind. When these fears are resolved, the possibility of incredible joy exists. Deep olive offers a guiding light of hope toward the future.

Olive and magenta are color opposites on the color wheel. The deep magenta in the lower fraction brings love from above, from the source. Magenta is about putting loving attention into every single thing that we do; deep magenta in the base fraction suggests giving love to all the little things in the unconscious/subconscious mind, thus enabling us to bring care into all that we do and to give love to all that lies in the shadow of our selves, to that which we may tend to deny.

Hidden within deep magenta is red, perhaps representative of frustrations; hidden within deep olive is blue, offering peace and calm. This peace in the conscious mind may help the energy of the red to be used for awakening rather than be expressed as rage. Green and red are also contained within the olive and magenta of B102 and also are opposites on the color wheel.

Samael comes to help us to see clearly where our false values lie and how we need to address them. B102 addresses fears, be they irrational or valid. Hidden fears may have suddenly come to the surface. A deepening anxiety begins to be overwhelming. With Samael the possibility of resolving these fears exists; for example, a new job may come to be. Samael has to do with loss through war, particularly when it is not possible to express love. Part of the story of Deep Olive/Deep Magenta is the falling away of one circumstance so that something new may be born. B102 is not necessarily a bottle that produces a rapid change or brings about a different situation. Samael brings the possibility of a new hope for a change of being. There are many things to be addressed concerning our decisions and the direction in which we are traveling personally as well as planetarily. The depth of the deep magenta with the olive green shade means a situation of perfect balance.

B102 may be applied over the whole area between the bottom of the sternum and the upper abdomen as well as over the lower part of the chest in a complete band around the body, including the lower thoracic spine. This bottle may bring relief when applied over the back of the head and around the crown, particularly when an emotional or pressure headache is troublesome.

See "Aura-Soma and the New Aeon," in chapter 6 for further information about B102.

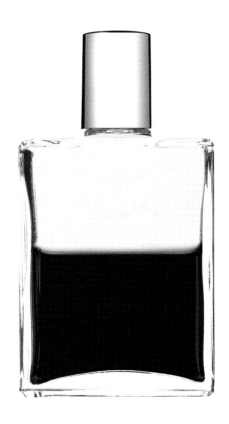

B103 Opalescent Pale Blue/ Deep Magenta

Name: Archangel Haniel

Shakes Together As: Deep Violet

Keynote: The support and the higher will. The light at the end of the tunnel begins to glimmer in the distance.

Archangel Haniel, B103, is the first Equilibrium bottle to appear opalescent, an effect caused by mica fragments floating in the oil fraction of the bottle. Mica is both insulative and protective of the energies therein. Within B103 are energies associated with the higher will. The light opalescent blue in the upper fraction is indicative of this, the greater purpose manifesting through the unfolding of the divine plan on earth.

Archangel Haniel, the tenth in the sequence, comes with a message: we are either part of the problem or part of the solution. It is our choice how, both mentally and emotionally, we align ourselves. We can choose how we will express our personal will relative to the higher will. B103 describes us as having an ability to communicate from the depths of ourselves with a quality of inner peace, with a warmth that expands to others. B103 may appeal to us if we are in harmony with our life purpose, able to put love into different areas of our life, with an ability to see beneath the surface.

Haniel gives us the opportunity to see, in the midst of difficult circumstances and conditions, the possibility of a solution, even while we may not understand the reason for, or the nature of, these difficulties. It is possible that within a bigger picture these difficulties may help us arrive at the light at the end of the tunnel. B103 may appeal to us when difficulties with parental models and with authority figures have had an impact on our inner life; we need to restore our own authority, because we have previously given it away. B103 offers a sense of protection as we express what we are for and our true purpose. We can find nurturing in the mundane activities of life and fulfillment and happiness in the ordinary, while cultivating faith in our alignment with the higher will.

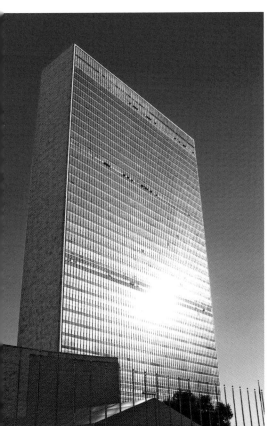

Left: United Nations building in New York City. There is an ancient prophecy in the Hopi tradition that one day the leaders of the world will gather in a Great House of Mica where through rules and regulations they will solve the world's problems without war. The many panes of glass reflect the light as does Mica.

Page 265, top: Scree in the Ogilvie Mountains of Alaska. The sense of protection of the divine will that is reflected in the mica of the upper fraction of B103 can also be seen in this image. Even in this inclement environment, one of the most challenging tundra regions, there is enough protection among the rocks for little plants to grow.

Page 265, bottom: Reflecting ball in front of the United Nations.

Related Bottles

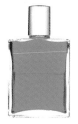

Related Colors
B2

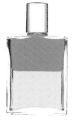

B20

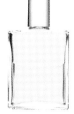

Closest Tints
B50

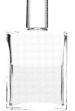

B58

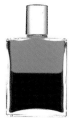

Closest Hue
B1

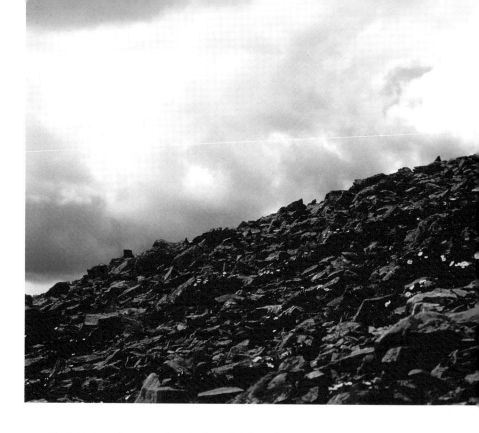

Haniel is here to support us in the unfolding of our purpose. This archangel has an immense beauty and is said to govern the planet Venus. The form in which Haniel appears protects that beauty. The archangel protects the communication that comes to us and from us as we develop our alignment with that which is above us.

Apply B103 around the throat area, including the back of the neck and underneath the hairline all the way to the atlas bone in the spinal column.

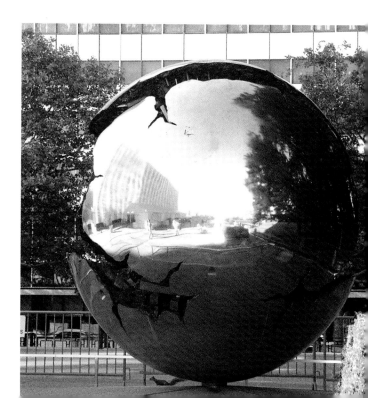

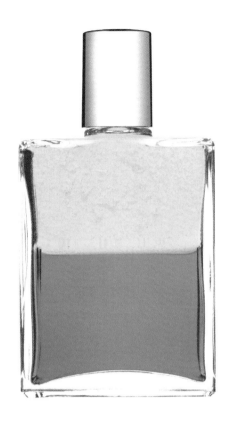

B104 Iridescent Pink/ Magenta

Name: Archangel Chamael

Shakes Together As: Rose Pink

Keynote: It is as it is. A new beginning for love. A new order of being.

Archangel Chamael brings forward the feminine aspect within ourselves and the planet. Archangel Chamael, one of the protectors of heaven, is one of seven archangels that attend the throne of God. In his role as protector he also, in times of need, protects such places as cities, nations, airports, and sacred spaces, as well as people's health and well-being.

B104 is the most recent arrival, the eleventh in the Archangel series. Iridescent Pink/Magenta helps us be more conscious of and receptive to the feminine side of our being, especially our intuition, and to accept, with trust, that everything "is as it is." As we develop an ability to witness our feelings, we can realize more consciously that we need not separate or create distance from our feelings when life is challenging. Chamael can give protection in times of critical need.

Page 267: Petals fallen to the ground in Elvington, England, are beautiful in their own disorder.
Below, left: Morning mist in a garden in Shelburne, Vermont.
Below, right: Roseate spoonbill.

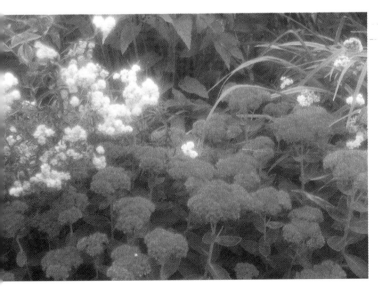

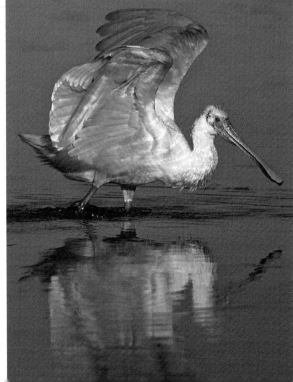

Related Bottles

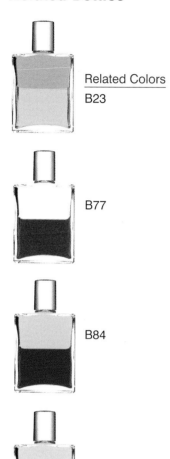

Related Colors
B23

B77

B84

Closest Tint
B52

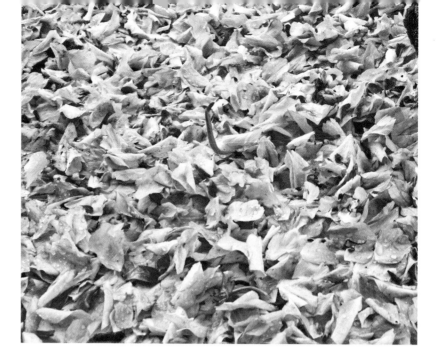

Iridescent pink is in the upper fraction of this bottle, in the conscious mind. The iridescence comes from the addition of mother-of-pearl, which relates to the tears of suffering created when we separate at any level within our self. Mild suffering that occurs when our wants and desires are not being fulfilled may be caused by our failure to accept ourselves as we are. Pink (red with the light shining through it) can indicate detachment in an intensified form. Accepting ourselves as we are and loving who we are will diminish the suffering.

A silver connection and floating silver within the iridescent pink helps the feminine intuition to be made more conscious. Silver supports the possibility of healing the feminine aspect of ourselves deep within and finding a different comprehension of deep levels of receptivity. B104 may appeal to us if we have difficulty relaxing and are troubled by inner conflicts. We may discover our love and compassion as we let go of feelings of anger and violence; we may see ourselves more clearly. If we can accept ourselves a bit more, we feel less inner conflict. The feelings of anger and violence can abate.

This process gives us space inside for love and compassion. Magenta in the lower fraction, in the unconscious mind, brings this compassion and the divine love from above. B104 helps us find within ourselves compassion and love to share. Through self-acceptance we create the possibility for peace and harmony. Instead of rejecting and pushing away parts of ourselves, we may find space in our hearts for all of us to exist. Then we have the energy to put our caring into all the little things. A sense of balance helps us love ourselves and extend love to others. Self-acceptance helps us dissolve projections onto and judgments of others. Being judgmental with ourselves will not allow the being we really are to surface. Being judgmental with others may cause rifts or separations that are difficult to resolve.

This color combination, as it contains the pink (red) of the root and the magenta of the soul star, can be applied anywhere on the body. B104 is especially appropriate across the whole of the lower abdomen and around the back, over the lower part of the spinal column.

Vicky's blessing comes with this bottle, as B104 can become B14 and then B5 (1 + 0 + 4 = 5), Yellow/Red, the bottle that called to Vicky the most (see B5 and page 282).

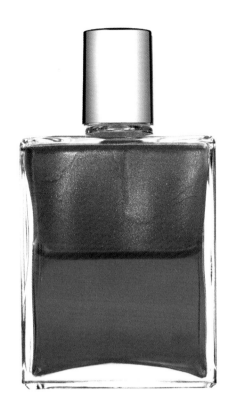

B105 Iridescent Coral/Coral

Name: Archangel Azreal

Shakes together as: Coral

Keynote: Going beyond separation, receptive to the feminine and touching unity.

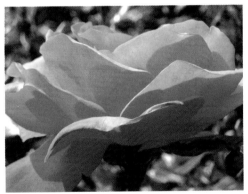

The coral hue appeared with the birth of B105 on March 8th, 2006. Archangel Azreal, also known as the unnamed archangel or the nameless one, created a ripple backward in time. It could be perceived that it was the *tint* of coral that had already been present in B87, B92, B93, and B98. The pale coral that emerged earlier expresses the more ethereal, less tangible, and more intense coral issues.

The reddish tone of the hue of coral, reinforced by the emphasis of *real* in A*zreal,* reminds us of the importance of grounding the potential of coral—cooperation, community, and universality. Coral, a tertiary color, suggests the importance of actualizing the orange potentials of creativity and of healing the timeline (see B26).

Archangel Azreal arrived when Saturn was in Leo, representing the opportunity to alchemically transform lead into gold, hinted at by the iridescence appearing golden in the upper fraction. With awareness and acceptance, an alchemical transformation to active compassion and love-wisdom can occur.

Grace comes with the birth of B105, as Venus had just entered the early degrees of Aquarius, passing the opposing Saturn and suggesting an emer-

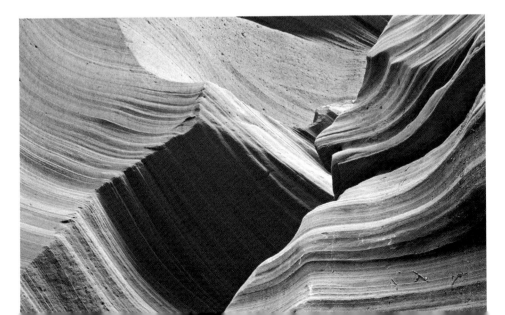

Related Bottles

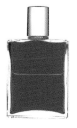

Related Colors
B6

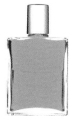

B26

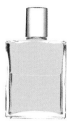

Closest Tint
B87

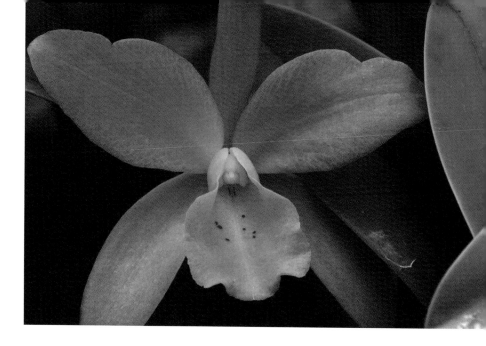

Top: The feminine energy of the orchid in Fort Myers, Florida.

Below: Autumn blueberry fields in Maine, showing the beauty of unity.

Page 268, top: A rose, receptive to the light, on the banks of the River Derwent in Tasmania.

Page 268, bottom: The power of namelessness, near Page, Arizona.

gence of the divine feminine in the Leo/Aquarian aeon, the Golden age. B105 brings the energy of the goddess, a feminine receptivity between the first and second chakras, balancing the externalization of the goddess and the revelation and appreciation of the goddess within ourselves. With B105 we may experience inner unity, an integration of the inner male and female.

Through its connections to B15 $(1 + 0 + 5 \rightarrow 15)$ and B87 $(8 + 7 = 15)$, B105 addresses the shadow—that which is unacknowledged, repressed, or denied. Connected to the root and sacral chakras, B105 supports healing the shocks and discrimination that exist in our racial, tribal, and genetic lineages as well as the pain of repressed sexuality and unrequited love. At a cellular level there may be cellular consciousness of in-between states, between living and dying, between wakefulness and sleep. Through the healing and integration—the opportunity to become whole—encouraged by B105, we may understand the karmic seeds in our genetics and experience new insights and bliss. We may see with the eyes of another and understand their point of view.

The mica flakes and titanium, named for the Greek Titans, in B105 offer an iridescent reflectivity when light touches them. This veil of radiance seems to afford protection from external forces of habitual conflict and divisiveness similar to the protection offered by coral reefs to the vibrant sea life and the shoreline.

B105 helps us move beyond duality and our fear of separateness. B105 beckons us toward the alpha and omega (the A–Z of Azreal), toward the consciousness and universality of the Golden age and a transcendence into the fifth dimension beyond the space-time continuum.

B105 can be applied around the entire lower abdomen.

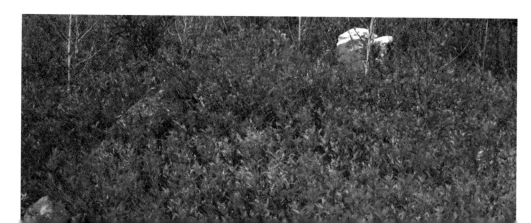

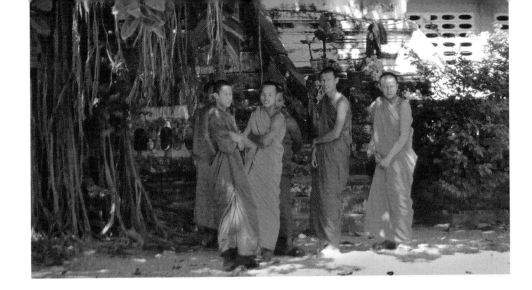

6

Connected Truths

Aura-Soma and Other Wisdom Teachings

It is reasonable to expect a system that describes truth to have a relationship and correspondence with other cosmologies that describes truth. This would be not an arbitrary connection made for the point of substantiating one or the other but a connection that is relevant to increased understanding. The systems may have an equivalence and, in that equivalence, may reveal something about each other. It is not necessary to search for an exact equality, although that may occur, but we can refer to the related cosmologies as gateways to understanding the same phenomena. As esoteric systems are related to one another, they facilitate discovery of a more complete understanding of the nature of reality. Each system can be seen in the light of its own inner truth and validity. Coincidences and synchronicities between systems are exciting and may indicate something more objective.

In some eras much of the esoteric knowledge was repressed. People were persecuted for embracing a particular philosophy or belief or for speaking the truth. Early Christians were thrown to the lions; the Albigensians were tortured by the Inquisition; individuals accused of being witches were burned at the stake. Throughout history, there have been times when it was important that information be hidden or encoded so that it could be protected and preserved until the time came for it to be revealed. In that way, those who understood or worked with occult information were protected from assault and persecution. Yet, always, those who have eyes to see and ears to hear can perceive the information. For example, the Dead Sea Scrolls were carefully hidden in caves around Qumran; the Masons have a secret handshake of recognition.

A straightforward way to hide information is through word-for-word equivalence; the use of the Navajo language, for example, was so effective during World War II for the Allies' top-secret communications that it defied the most expert of the Axis's code breakers. It is easy enough to encode information. Many children learn a kind of encoded speech called pig Latin. It is *othbay unfay anday easyay*. Computers work on coded information: all meaning and instructions are determined by sequences of on or off, and the sequences of bits are aggregated into bytes. From this little coded duality spaceships are guided to travel to Mars.

Above: Monks in Bangkok, Thailand.

As we enter into the Aquarian aeon, it seems to be time for ancient wisdom to be made available to everyone. Knowledge that had previously been reserved for certain groups, esoteric circles or the elite, is now available to us all. The more knowledge we share, the more knowledge we may receive. Morse code and radio communication, with a simple . . . - - - . . .—an SOS encoded as dot-dot-dot dash-dash-dash dot-dot-dot—can help people stranded at sea to reach the help that brings them home. Or, for a more colorful analogy, the semaphore language of waving brightly colored flags in front of the receiver, which is used for boats and airplanes, can direct a craft to safety. When presented to us externally, teachings can help establish a resonance within—a sense of familiarity or recognition that stimulates us to uncover our own gifts and qualities. As you embark on the process of choosing and working with your own color code, you may light your way back to yourself, unfolding your incarnational intention. This process of coming home presents the opportunity to share the truth of who you are in the world and to fully embrace your potential.

Ken Wilber is an American philosopher considered to have created a world philosophy that embraces essential truths of East and West. He suggests that there are three aspects, the "Big Three" basic disciplines, whereby we understand the world. One is through our senses—science, technology, and objective nature; one is through the mind or the intellect—morals, worldviews, and mutual understanding; the third is through the spirit—consciousness, self-expression, and truthfulness.[1] There are many examples for these categories. Each has its own disciplines, languages, and proofs. None of them is the whole truth in and of itself, as each describes only a part of reality. Each approach is a part of a whole and brings its own information.

Aura-Soma offers this type of integrative approach that is representative of a new paradigm and links these "Big Three." It is a gift from spirit that appeals to the senses and is based on formal concepts and intellectual constructs. While the ingredients of the Equilibrium bottles can be tested, the meaning of the bottles can be noted both experientially and theoretically.

Wilber goes on to say that in order to have access to the information and understanding of a discipline, we must engage in whatever is the initial protocol. For example, we could not understand *Hamlet* until we learned to read and could read well enough to read Shakespeare and have some understanding of drama. Only then could we comprehend and discuss the meaning of the play.[2] To understand spiritual truths, meditation might be an appropriate initial protocol; for example, describing nonduality (integrative rather than divisive thinking) to a physiologist, behav-

iorist, or physicist might be easier if you had first learned, through deep meditation, to experience emptiness and to take that experience back into yourself.[3] Aura-Soma, initially received through intuition and inspiration, helps us develop a consciousness about our purpose and a greater capacity to manifest it, with the support of the plant and mineral kingdoms and of spirit.

Wilber describes four quadrants, or ways, of experience: our interior experience, our exterior experience, the cultural context, and the social context.[4] Love, for example, might be felt or formulated quite differently in the Western world than it would in another era or region because cultural and societal context influences the experience. If you are in a state of romantic arousal, your body's response can be measured physiologically in regard to what is happening to your brain waves and to your body, but that certainly does not explain the whole experience. If we only measure brain waves when talking about love, we leave out the interior experience and the transformative power of love. An integrative understanding including all quadrants is important, particularly if there are problems or blockages (for example in expressing or receiving love). Any one system of analysis may not take into account the four ways of experiencing. The spiritual level is perhaps not respected or explored enough in the terms that our modern culture understands. Wilber says, "I don't think that partial approach will ever work. It seems instead that we need an integral approach that will include all four quadrants, all four faces of Spirit. Perhaps the secret to higher transformation involves the more balanced, complete, and integral approach."[5]

In the language of color, all four of these quadrants of experience—individual interior and exterior response and cultural and social context—are present. Color affords a means to converse about reality in a way that includes each quadrant and fosters integration of perception.

Vicky's vision was that by 2003 Aura-Soma would be available to anyone, anywhere in the world, who had need of it. Through Aura-Soma, people would have the opportunity to recognize who they are, what they are for, and what they are here to do in this lifetime. They might more easily fulfill their mission and purpose, while experiencing joy and love for life. Perhaps we are a little way off from fulfilling that aspiration, but Vicky's vision of helping people come into a fuller sense of who they are through the magic windows of color is an approachable goal.

In this aeon, it appears that the ancient and eternal truths are coming increasingly into consciousness. Aura-Soma seems to be a radical gift given from a Divine Source to help us understand and perceive these truths. Vicky would call it "old wine in new bottles," and in more than one sense it is. It is the language of color made available to anyone, regardless of race, creed, religion, or political background. In that language, in the sequence of the colors, in their association with numbers, with the tarot, and with the chakras, there are layers upon layers of truth to be revealed. These are available for anyone who is curious and wishes to cultivate the ability to perceive, and for all who love color, aroma, and inner adventure. The information is encoded in the colors, in the colors within the colors, in the sequence of colors in the four-bottle selection, in the numbers of the bottles, and in many other ways. It is all there to be uncovered and understood, revealed and restored.

The Aura-Soma system has been shown to correspond with other ancient systems that have in turn been tested and found to have integrity and reliability. Vicky and Mike were shown that Aura-Soma, through numerical and color equivalences, connects to the Kabbalah, the tarot, and the I Ching. Each of these systems offers a way to understand and perceive the nature of our reality. The I Ching, also known as the Chinese Book of Changes, is a contemplative study that guides us toward harmony with the forces of the cosmos. The Kabbalah, a Jewish mystical study, is a living experience of humanity's relation to the divine. The tarot, brought into the public eye in Europe in the Middle Ages, provides a pictorial description of the human journey of evolution. Each system sheds light on the others, giving more understanding and depth to each as they intermingle.

Matrices and the Tarot

When first presented with the range of Aura-Soma Equilibrium bottles, it is the colors of the upper and lower fractions that we find appealing and that call strongly to us. As you become more familiar with the meanings of the bottles and the colors, delving deeper into the system, it becomes apparent that the sequence in which these color combinations was given is also extremely important. The sequence, the number of each bottle, has information and relevance of its own. Studying the matrices—the pattern of the numbers of the bottles in your selection—individually and in summation, can allow you to see particular universal patterns emerging in your own life.

In this section we will focus on those bottles that relate to the major arcana, B0–B22 and B79–B99. The major arcana of the tarot chronicle the archetypal lessons of the soul, that which we all must encounter in one way or another as we journey and develop through our lives. We all may feel naïve and innocent at times—a fool as we rush into circumstances that have caught our attention; we all may feel skillful and competent at other times, as we master the

skills and tasks in front of us. At times we are powerfully in love with life itself and with each other, and at times we feel cast out into the harsh winters of isolation. And so it goes. But as we meet these experiences and find the resources within ourselves to grow through them, we achieve a level of capability and understanding that allows us to share our wisdom with others. The particular lessons of the major arcana are discussed below and in the descriptions of the individual bottles in chapter 5.

Behind each Equilibrium bottle is a story of the archetypal issues that the soul will encounter in the embodiment and experience of that Equilibrium bottle. While this is conceptual initially, it becomes understandable as we work with our particular color combination and trace the soul issues that we are meeting. There is a matrix, or a sequence, of numbers that each of the Equilibrium bottles belongs to, that resolves itself into one of the themes of the major arcana. There are nine matrices in all, which range from B9 to B17, from the Hermit to the Star, from the path of meditation to find the heart within the heart to the Aquarian aeon star beckoning and sharing its light with all. The nine matrices include the New Aeon Child Set (B11–B15) and two bottles on either side of this set. B87–B95 are the return journey bottles corresponding to the nine matrices.

There are three archangels particularly present and overlooking the matrices: Archangel Michael (B94), Archangel Gabriel (B95), and Archangel Raphael (B96). (See the table of the number patterns for each of the 104 bottles and note how often these Archangel bottles recur.) According to Steiner, Archangel Michael has taken primary responsibility, followed by Archangel Gabriel, for human evolution in consciousness at this time.

The fact that there are nine matrices presents an interesting correspondence with the Enneagram, which is composed of nine aspects in an open star formation. Just as each of the many Aura-Soma bottles resolve themselves into only nine matrices, similarly the great number of humans may be understood through the nine aspects of the Enneagram. The Enneagram and matrices also share a focus on essential life themes and character types. The Enneagram is an ancient system and a vast study in and of itself, a veritable key to the universe. One way it can be used is to gain understanding of ourselves and of different groups of people by determining with which of nine personality and soul types we most identify. Studying major trends and themes in our development can help us both to gain a perspective on our particular present-day life and to recognize our inclusion in a larger family of people and soul groups.

The numerical sequence behind each of the Equilibrium bottles is based on the laws of numbers. For

The Nine Matrices and Their Tarot Correspondences

Tarot Card	The Hermit	Wheel of Fortune	Strength	The Hanged Man	Death	Temperance	The Devil	The Tower	The Star
Matrix	9	10	11	12	13	14	15	16	17
Bottles Included	3	0	5	6	7	2	15	1	17
	9	4	11	12	13	8	18	16	20
	27	10	23	24	25	14	21	19	89
	30	22	29	33	34	26	69	79	98
	36	28	32	39	43	35	78	88	
	45	31	38	42	49	44	87	97	
	54	37	41	48	52	53	96		
	63	40	47	51	58	59	99		
	72	46	50	57	61	62	105		
	81	55	56	60	67	68			
	90	64	65	66	70	71			
		73	74	75	76	77			
		82	83	84	85	80			
		91	92	93	94	86			
		100	101	102	103	95			
						104			

The Outward and Return Journeys of the Nine Matrices

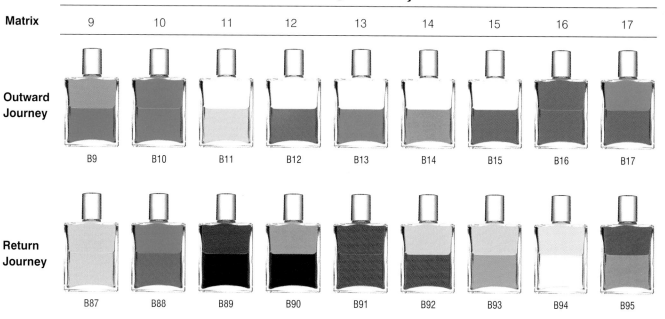

Matrix	9	10	11	12	13	14	15	16	17
Outward Journey	B9	B10	B11	B12	B13	B14	B15	B16	B17
Return Journey	B87	B88	B89	B90	B91	B92	B93	B94	B95

example, 23 is understood to have a relationship with 5 since 2 + 3 = 5. There is something about 23 that has to do with 5. Similarly 14 is related to 5, as 1 + 4 = 5. There is thence a relationship that 23 and 14 have through their shared connection to 5. The numerical sequence is also based on the outward and return journey of the major tarot, as indicated by their placement on the Tree of Life and as noted on each of the Equilibrium bottle pages related to the major arcana. The return journey is, with the exception of B0, the original number of the bottle with 78 added to it, as there are seventy-eight tarot cards. This represents how, once the soul has cycled through all the stages of development indicated by the tarot cards, we revisit these experiences from a different point of view. On this return visit we are hopefully wiser and able to give, or express, what we have learned or assimilated in our initial encounters with these lessons.

The bottle that you select determines into which of the nine matrices and where in the sequence you enter. Depending on where you enter the matrix sequence, as indicated by your bottle selection, the focus and emphasis will be slightly different; but the essential lessons and opportunities of the soul, at an archetypal understanding, will be similar. We will briefly discuss each of the matrices here.

The matrix sequence for B0 is as follows: B0 is the outward journey and the return journey is B22. This is the only one of the major tarot whose return journey is not indicated by the addition of 78—the number of a complete tarot set. The return journey of the Fool (B0) occurs at the end of the major arcana sequence of 0–21. Twenty-two can be represented as 2 + 2 = 4. B4 is the next bottle in the matrix sequence. The return journey of B4 is B82 (through the addition of the 78 cards of the Tarot). B82 can be represented as 8 + 2 = 10. B10 the outward journey is followed by B88 the return journey. B88 relates to 8 + 8 = 16. The B16 is the next bottle in the sequence with its return journey, B94. Again, B94 is connected to 9 + 4 = 13. B13 comes next in the matrix with its return journey, B91. Ninety-one leads us to 9+1=10. At this point there is a recurrence of a number that appeared earlier in the sequence and the matrix stops. In Aura-Soma we refer to B0 as being part of the ten matrix. This matrix brings the zero and the one together.

The matrix of B0 starts with the ordinary person, any and all of us, as the zero, the Fool in the tarot, who gains skill and understanding in the ways to use his energy. We ultimately will experience a rebirth in spirit: B22, the Fool's Mastership. At this point we are able to distinguish between knowledge and wisdom, what we have learned and what we have experienced and understood from that knowledge: B4. The wisdom that has developed in B4 grows into a more profound experience of insight that

we may then be able to express in a heartfelt way: B82. An instant understanding of the laws of karma, the laws of cause and effect, then occurs: B10. As we experience the consequences of cause and effect, we realize that it is not the seeds of the actions of the past that are most relevant, but the way that we do what we do, our dharma rather than our karma: B88. This leads us to an experience of metanoia, a complete change of our being, greater than just a change of our mind or of our feelings: B16. With this experience, and with the presence of the energies of Archangel Michael, B94, we develop an insight into the higher will. We develop an awareness of the Earth as a being and of the new consciousness that is unfolding upon the Earth. We go through a death: the dying of our identification with what we had adhered to in the past, B13. This helps us to bring a new quality into our life—in which death is, in a sense, invited into our life, B91—as we participate in the lessons of love and life, appreciating change and new growth. This leads us to a fresh experience of the wheel of life, the wheel of dependent origination, B10. At whatever point we enter this matrix described above, these will be some of the archetypal issues and experiences that we may encounter.

The matrix for B1 is as follows: The Magician, B1, begins his journey of learning to skillfully use the tools that he has. In the return journey, B79, the Magician learns about taking responsibility as a co-creator with all that is. This understanding leads to B16 (7 + 9 = 16), the Tower in the tarot, and metanoia, a complete change of being. At this point the soul would be experiencing the same patterns of learning as described in the B0 matrix. The return journey of B16 is B94, Archangel Michael inspiring insight into how our personal will can be expressed in harmony with Thy will. This leads to B13 (9 + 4 = 13), a death to that with which we have previously identified and an understanding of the hope that is ever present of new life and new possibilities of love, B91. We can come to an understanding of the lessons of karma, of the ups and downs of life, B10 (9 + 1 = 10), the wheel of fortune, and of the opportunities for dharmic expression, B88, that exist in life. This brings us again to B16, another great change of life experience, of our being. Here the matrix is complete, as B16 is the first repeat number in this matrix.

The matrix for B2 is a 14 matrix, because 14 is the number that repeats itself, bringing the matrix to a close. This matrix is the story of the Star in the tarot, B17, appearing for the first time in a sequence. Symbolically, the star may be connected to the High Priestess, B2. The High Priestess can be recognized as the high priestess of the silver star. The silver star represents the feminine principle, the Madonna, the Mother Mary, and the triple goddess of the

Matrix Tables

0/22 → 4/82 → 10/88 → 16/94 → 13/91 → **10**					53 → 8/86 → 14/92 → 11/89 → 17/95 → **14**
1/79 → 16/94 → 13/91 → 10/88 → **16**					54 → 9/87 → 15/93 → 12/90 → **9**
2/80 → 8/86 → 14/92 → 11/89 → 17/95 → **14**					55 → 10/88 → 16/94 → 13/91 → **10**
3/81 → 9/87 → 15/93 → 12/90 → **9**					56 → 11/89 → 17/95 → 14/92 → **11**
4/82 → 10/88 → 16/94 → 13/91 → **10**					57 → 12/90 → 9/87 → 15/93 → **12**
5/83 → 11/89 → 17/95 → 14/92 → **11**					58 → 13/91 → 10/88 → 16/94 → **13**
6/84 → 12/90 → 9/87 → 15/93 → **12**					59 → 14/92 → 11/89 → 17/95 → **14**
7/85 → 13/91 → 10/88 → 16/94 → **13**					60 → 6/84 → 12/90 → 9/87 → 15/93 → **12**
8/86 → 14/92 → 11/89 → 17/95 → **14**					61 → 7/85 → 13/91 → 10/88 → 16/94 → **13**
9/87 → 15/93 → 12/90 → **9**					62 → 8/86 → 14/92 → 11/89 → 17/95 → **14**
10/88 → 16/94 → 13/91 → **10**					63 → 9/87 → 15/93 → 12/90 → **9**
11/89 → 17/95 → 14/92 → **11**					64 → 10/88 → 16/94 → 13/91 → **10**
12/90 → 9/87 → 15/93 → **12**					65 → 11/89 → 17/95 → 14/92 → **11**
13/91 → 10/88 → 16/94 → **13**					66 → 12/90 → 9/87 → 15/93 → **12**
14/92 → 11/89 → 17/95 → **14**					67 → 13/91 → 10/88 → 16/94 → **13**
15/93 → 12/90 → 9/87 → **15**					68 → 14/92 → 11/89 → 17/95 → **14**
16/94 → 13/91 → 10/88 → **16**					69 → 15/93 → 12/90 → 9/87 → **15**
17/95 → 14/92 → 11/89 → **17**					70 → 7/85 → 13/91 → 10/88 → 16/94 → **13**
18/96 → 15/93 → 12/90 → 9/87 → **15**					71 → 8/86 → 14/92 → 11/89 → 17/95 → **14**
19/97 → 16/94 → 13/91 → 10/88 → **16**					72 → 9/87 → 15/93 → 12/90 → **9**
20/98 → 17/95 → 14/92 → 11/89 → **17**					73 → 10/88 → 16/94 → 13/91 → **10**
21/99 → 18/96 → 15/93 → 12/90 → 9/87 → **15**					74 → 11/89 → 17/95 → 14/92 → **11**
22 → 4/82 → 10/88 → 16/94 → 13/91 → **10**					75 → 12/90 → 9/87 → 15/93 → **12**
23 → 5/83 → 11/89 → 17/95 → 14/92 → **11**					76 → 13/91 → 10/88 → 16/94 → **13**
24 → 6/84 → 12/90 → 9/87 → 15/93 → **12**					77 → 14/92 → 11/89 → 17/95 → **14**
25 → 7/85 → 13/91 → 10/88 → 16/94 → **13**					78 → 15/93 → 12/90 → 9/87 → **15**
26 → 8/86 → 14/92 → 11/89 → 17/95 → **14**					79 → 16/94 → 13/91 → 10/88 → **16**
27 → 9/87 → 15/93 → 12/90 → **9**					80 → 8/86 → 14/92 → 41/89 → 17/95 → **14**
28 → 10/88 → 16/94 → 13/91 → **10**					81 → 9/87 → 15/93 → 12/90 → **9**
29 → 11/89 → 17/95 → 14/92 → **11**					82 → 10/88 → 16/94 → 13/91 → **10**
30 → 3/81 → 9/87 → 15/93 → 12/90 → **9**					83 → 11/89 → 17/95 → 14/92 → **11**
31 → 4/82 → 10/88 → 16/94 → 13/91 → **10**					84 → 12/90 → 9/87 → 15/93 → **12**
32 → 5/83 → 11/89 → 17/95 → 14/92 → **11**					85 → 13/91 → 10/88 → 16/94 → **13**
33 → 6/84 → 12/90 → 9/87 → 15/93 → **12**					86 → 14/92 → 11/89 → 17/95 → **14**
34 → 7/85 → 13/91 → 10/88 → 16/94 → **13**					87 → 15/93 → 12/90 → 9/87 → **15**
35 → 8/86 → 14/92 → 11/89 → 17/95 → **14**					88 → 16/94 → 13/91 → 10/88 → **16**
36 → 9/87 → 15/93 → 12/90 → **9**					89 → 17/95 → 14/92 → 11/89 → **17**
37 → 10/88 → 16/94 → 13/91 → **10**					90 → 9/87 → 15/93 → 42/90 → **9**
38 → 11/89 → 17/95 → 14/92 → **11**					91 → 10/88 → 16/94 → 13/91 → **10**
39 → 12/90 → 9/87 → 15/93 → **12**					92 → 11/89 → 17/95 → 14/92 → **11**
40 → 4/82 → 10/88 → 16/94 → 13/91 → **10**					93 → 12/90 → 9/87 → 15/93 → **12**
41 → 5/83 → 11/89 → 17/95 → 14/92 → **11**					94 → 13/91 → 10/88 → 16/94 → **13**
42 → 6/84 → 12/90 → 9/87 → 15/93 → **12**					95 → 14/92 → 11/89 → 17/95 → **14**
43 → 7/85 → 13/91 → 10/88 → 16/94 → **13**					96 → 15/93 → 12/90 → 9/87 → **15**
44 → 8/86 → 14/92 → 11/89 → 17/95 → **14**					97 → 16/94 → 13/91 → 10/88 → **16**
45 → 9/87 → 15/93 → 12/90 → **9**					98 → 17/95 → 14/92 → 11/89 → **17**
46 → 10/88 → 16/94 → 13/91 → **10**					99 → 18/96 → 15/93 → 12/90 → 9/87 → **15**
47 → 11/89 → 17/95 → 14/92 → **11**					100 → 10/88 → 16/94 → 13/91 → **10**
48 → 12/90 → 9/87 → 15/93 → **12**					101 → 11/89 → 17/95 → 14/92 → **11**
49 → 13/91 → 10/88 → 16/94 → **13**					102 → 12/90 → 9/87 → 15/93 → **12**
50 → 5/83 → 11/89 → 17/95 → 14/92 → **11**					103 → 13/91 → 10/88 → 16/94 → **13**
51 → 6/84 → 12/90 → 9/87 → 15/93 → **12**					104 → 14/92 → 11/89 → 17/95 → **14**
52 → 7/85 → 13/91 → 10/88 → 16/94 → **13**					105 → 15/93 → 12/90 → 9/87 → **15**

Outward and return journey number patterns for each of the 106 bottles.

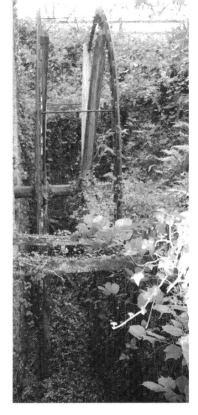

Water wheel from an old mill in Totnes, England.

virgin, mother, and crone. This feminine expression is part of our understanding of what B2 represents, and that which is awakened and experienced in the soul in B80, the return journey of B2. B8 follows B80 (8 + 0 = 8). Anubis, B8, is the guardian of the threshold between this world and the next, the guardian of the halls of initiation. Anubis weighs our heart. He balances the weight of our heart against a feather; when we are doing what we love, our heart may be lighter than a single feather. If our heart is heavy, if we are not doing what we love, many feathers are needed to balance our heart. Traditionally, Anubis travels to the underworld to procure feathers from Ma'at, collecting as many as are needed to balance the scales. Our light-body is symbolized by our wings. If our feathers are not needed to offset the weight of our heart, our wings may remain intact, and we may more easily develop our light-body. The return journey of B8 is B86. B86 indicates light being shone onto our process of individuation. We may begin to feel synchronicity unfolding, the experience of being in the right, the appropriate, place, at the right time, doing the right thing, all as a consequence of doing what we love to do. We are able to put the right energy into what we are doing, the energy that is in harmony with our own dharma and with the greater good. B86 leads us to B14 (8 + 6 = 14). If we consciously bring our attention to the golden area within ourself, where the true aura lies, we may begin to live from our star, from our innate wisdom. We are less inclined to let just our thinking or our feelings, our mind or our emotions, guide us. The return journey of B14 is B92, Gretel. As we trust our feminine intuition we

may overcome dogmatisms of the past and feel hope in a new quality of consciousness emerging. In this way we arrive at the gateway of B11 (9 + 2 = 11). B11 indicates taking greater responsibility for our thoughts and our feelings, acknowledging that each of our thoughts and each of our feelings creates an energy, a being. The return journey of B11 is B89. This bottle represents an opportunity that we, as humanity, have at this time. There is a window between that which has been and that which can be new, an opportunity to rescue the possibilities of humanity awakening. We may remember our potential and destiny as human beings, and value and fulfill the opportunities given by birth as a human. These Aquarian values are shone in B17 (8 + 9 = 17), the Star in the tarot and the Troubadour bottle. The troubadour experience to be released is of the persecution from the past for the expression of one's heart's truth. Then there is the opportunity to listen to the messenger of the star, to Archangel Gabriel, B95, who tells us of where to find the star, in the gold. B95 leads us back to B14 (9 + 5 = 14), where we may give conscious attention to the light shining into gold.

The matrix for B3 is a 9 matrix, hence a journey of meditation. Meditation is a path to the heart. B3 is called the Heart Rescue bottle. B9 is called the Heart within the Heart. As suggested by the Atlantean, the Lemurian, and the turquoise connections of both of these bottles, it has been a long time since the heart of the collective has been open. An opportunity for this may exist now, at the dawn of the Aquarian aeon. This is symbolized by B81, the return journey of B3, the awakening of the red as shown in pink. Pink can only be expressed through green or through turquoise, through the heart. This leads us to B9 (8 + 1 = 9), the Turquoise/Green bottle, the transcendental heart, the crystal cave within which many treasures exist. Pale Coral, B87, the return journey of B9, represents going beyond our fascination or preoccupation with ourself and bringing our orientation more into the community, the group, the interdependent context in which we live. In order to be able to penetrate, understand, and integrate the new consciousness, we each must face what lies in our shadow, in B15 (8 + 7 = 15), the Devil. Whatever we have denied, both individually and collectively, whatever we have said "no" to, needs to be addressed. Thus we may face, see, and accept our shadow. In the return journey of B15, B93, Pale Coral/Turquoise, we may step into the waters of the collective, while engaging fully in our individuation process. We may experience our creativity in the light of the new consciousness. This experience brings us to an initiatory step, B12 (9 + 3 = 12). Here, in the Hanged Man, we are in a new position; light has turned our world upside down. We may take a step beyond that which is ordinary. Our world is not as it was before; rescue is in order. If we place our attention in a conscious way on our golden area, we may refine the base material of our being into gold. B90, the return journey of B12, is the rescuing of our own wisdom. B90 returns us to B9 (9 + 0 = 9). We enter the heart within our heart as we refine the gold within ourselves.

The matrix for B4 resolves into a 10 matrix. The sequence is as follows: B4, the Emperor, is followed by the return journey, B82, Calypso. This leads to B10 (8 + 2 = 10), the Wheel of Fortune, with a B88 return journey, the Jade Emperor. He takes us to B16, the Tower (8 + 8 = 16), and the return journey of 16, which is B94, Archangel Michael. This is followed by an encounter with Death, B13 (9 + 4 = 13), and a new perspective on death and change, with the return journey, B91 (9 + 1), leading to another understanding of B10, the Wheel of Dependent Origination.

B4 and B0 are both part of the 10 matrix. Although there are certain themes that exist within each matrix as a whole, where you start or enter the matrix is extremely significant. The point at which you enter a matrix indicates the different ways of having learned life lessons. The multiplicity of experiences and life paths all ultimately lead to one of nine archetypal matrices of a soul's journey. The nine universal matrices point to a unified field—a realm where all is one, united harmoniously. If you enter the 10 matrix at B0 (Royal Blue/Deep Magenta) the emphasis on blue and red may be significant to your own life journey. Part of the opportunity of the Fool (B0), suggested by the blue and red colors, is to learn faith and detachment. B4 suggests power or control issues and the need to cultivate wisdom. By looking at where you enter a matrix, it is possible to see both the specific place at which you begin the journey and the overall archetypal themes of the matrix—in this case, an emphasis on the lessons of developing faith and the capacity to let go with trust and detachment.

Another pattern we can look for in any matrix is the colors that are involved. Using B4 as an example, we see that there is yellow present in all of the bottles except for B16, which represents a complete change of being. This could suggest that something about knowledge and wisdom, fear, power, control, and joy—all yellow issues—could be particularly significant. The first bottle in the sequence is Yellow/Gold, the Emperor, suggesting that we use our light and our knowledge, our wisdom and our power, skillfully and benevolently. The encounter with B16 might suggest that at this point in the sequence, we experience a complete change of point of view, of understanding, and of experience, with regard to our "yellow" issues. It is possible to consider each of the matrices in this way, seeing which particular parts of the journey are emphasized by the original bottle selection and the information of the language of color.

The matrix for B5 is as follows: B5, the Hierophant, has a B83 return journey. B5 reminds us of the importance of using our energy wisely and intelligently. B5 is attributed to the base chakra, wherein the potential for our awakening exists, at our root, the place from which the kundalini energy arises. B83, with its echoes of how wisdom was used in the past, encourages us to integrate the wisdom that we carry with our own individual experience and our own heart's feelings. Then, conscious of embodying and balancing those dynamics, we can express our wisdom with feeling. The turquoise/gold of B83 shows the process of individuation unfolding in the conscious mind as a consequence of bringing our awareness to the golden area of our being. B83 leads to B11 (8 + 3 = 11), a gateway. Eleven is the story of the star, the awakening of the earth star, and perhaps also the star that heralded the Christ consciousness awakening in humanity. A focus of B11 is responsibility, learning to take responsibility for what we think, what we feel, and the attitudes we hold. B11 is Essene bottle 1. In the Essene community, it was understood that each of our thoughts and our feelings creates an energy pattern, a being. The Essenes practiced the importance of working in harmony with the angelic world by invoking angelic presence and inspiration into every action and every thought. By this practice, our every action, our thoughts, and our attitudes may be inspired and informed with the best angelic intention and support. Within the Essene community, Mary, Jesus's mother, and his aunt, Elizabeth, received their training in the Essene way of life. Perhaps learning about some of these practices provided the fertile ground that helped bring the Christ into being. The return journey of B11 is B89, the Energy Rescue bottle. Here the magenta and the red are linked, the soul star and the root star. There begins to be an integration, grounding, and manifestation of all the potential that is held in the soul star. B17 is the next bottle in the sequence (8+9=17), followed by the return journey, B95, then B14 with its B92 return journey, leading ultimately to B11. The lessons and opportunities in the matrix for B5 are similar to the ones in the matrix of B2. The B2 matrix is a 14 matrix and the B5 matrix is an 11 matrix, as these are the first numbers that recur in the sequences. B5 places emphasis on the importance of grounding one's light with the strength and understanding of unconditional love.

For B6, the matrix resolves to a 12. B6, the Lovers, Red/Red, has the potential for initiation, for the awakening to commence from the red. The return journey of B6 is B84. The male/female energies within ourself become harmonious, with the pink of self-acceptance helping us to acknowledge and love all of who we are. A sense of mutual respect, both within and toward others, can occur as our intuitive and analytic abilities and our experiences of bliss and wisdom find a place in our life experience. There is a potential of union, of unified consciousness, a Tantric experience, in B84 as we become compassionate to all we see in ourselves. B84 leads to B12 in the sequence (8 + 4 = 12), showing that this is a matrix of the initiate, and specifically, because it originates in B6, the Lovers, a Tantric initiate. The return journey of B12 is B90, the Wisdom Rescue. An understanding of the initiate brought to the gold of B90 is that wisdom is refined from within, rather than acquired. The deep magenta offers an opportunity to refine wisdom through an understanding of what deep magenta means in the depth of one's self. B90 leads to B9. The appearance of nine in this matrix echoes the themes of the heart. B9 (heart within the heart) and B3 (Heart Rescue) both belong to the 9 matrix. The matrix that B6 (the Lovers) corresponds to (the 12 matrix) shares the heart issues, but from a Tantric point of view. The focus of B9 in this matrix is on integration of the male and female in relationship. This is another example of how the same bottle can have a different meaning or significance depending on what matrix it belongs to and at what point you enter. The return journey of B9 is B87. The pale coral of B87 represents the process of going within through the path of meditation, enabling you to then go out, compassionately, into the community. This leads to B15, the necessity of facing that which is in the shadow to emerge into the return journey, B93. There, the integration of the male and female energies within ourselves leads to an experience of individuation that also allows us to have access to the collective. This brings a birth of the new consciousness in the coral, which is of a singularity of view, an experience of the unified field and space. This brings the matrix to completion with the reappearance of B12, the illumination of the initiate who embodies a deep quality of peace.

The matrix for B7 is a 13 matrix. The 7 indicates a test. B7 is called the Garden of Gethsemene and represents the final test of faith. When our faith is tested, our light shines from within on our path of individuation, as in B85, the return journey of B7. B13 (8 + 5 = 13) indicates a death of our past identifications, allowing a new identity to be born now, one pertinent to present circumstances. By letting go of our current identities and of the thoughts we have about ourselves and about our roles, we may enter the flow of life more fully. We are able to be in the right place at the right time, "going with the flow." An awakening to the possibilities of new life and new growth occurs in B13's return journey, B91. Hope for the future is born of the holy spirit through trusting the empathetic, receptive leadership of our heart. This leads to B10 and the laws of cause and effect: as we plant, so shall we reap. B88, the return journey, stresses the importance of how we plant rather than what we plant, the quality and attitude that we bring to each

of our actions and thoughts. B16 (8 + 8 = 16) indicates a change of being that orients us to the higher will rather than our personal will, B94. Archangel Michael brings his sword of insight to illuminate what it is that is asked of us as service, that we may fulfill our purpose. It may become easier to let go of past identities (9 + 4 = 13) when we are able to make that connection to spirit and begin to express what is in our hearts and what is our higher purpose.

B8 is a 14 matrix, as is B2. Similarly B9–B14 also correspond to matrices already discussed. B15, however, yields a different sequence, a 15 matrix.

The 15 matrix emphasizes the importance of facing what is in the shadow and discovering what this process implies in terms of emergence. Part of each of our responsibilities has to do with dealing with our shadow and with the collective shadow. In the shadows we may find aspects of ourselves that are potentials and strengths. By connecting to these unacknowledged gifts we have the opportunity to develop toward the fulfillment of our dharma. Part of our individual expression is also in the context of community (the return journey of B15 is B93, Pale Coral/Turquoise). The challenge of B93 is to find a way to balance being a whole individual with living harmoniously in a relationship or community setting. This leads to B12 (9 + 3 = 12), indicating the suffering, sorrow, and aloneness of the initiate when facing the shadow, and the fear of looking at the depths in the shadow. There is an opportunity to learn from suffering and this brings the illumination that is possible along the path of initiation. The intensity of the light of the initiate (clear/blue) is inherently disorienting. Yet it could also bring forth distant memories of the perfect light of spirit from which we originated. The more peace we feel within, the more light comes: light shining is a consequence of increased calm and inner peace, which in turns brings a dawning of light in the mental and emotional planes of our being. As an awareness and consciousness of light develops, it settles in a point of gravity within our being, in the golden area. If we find the inner peace and calm of B12, we may gain access to the truth and wisdom inherent in the gold of the return journey, B90. Gold opens the door to joy that radiates at the center of our being. A sense of our potential and of our wisdom emerges. B9 (9+0=9) offers an opportunity to find the space to sense our individual nature—to prepare for our journey of awakening and of bringing our spirit into manifestation. We can question if there is a reason to embark on this journey; is it for temporary fulfillment or for temporary happiness? There is not a *way* to happiness, rather happiness is a way of being. B9 helps us take the space for inner reflection rather than for projection. B87 is the return journey of B9. When we look at what is going on beyond our own self-reflections, beyond the projections and transferences, this can lead to a new dawning and a new awakening, B87. B15 (8 + 7 = 15) provides the opportunity to perceive more of our conscious and subconscious patterns and to bring our spirit into manifestation.

The final matrix to discuss is 17, the Star. B17 is associated with Aquarius and the troubadours. Within 17 is movement from past persecution, when one has expressed the truth of one's heart, to the current epoch of opportunity for humanitarian independence and for individual development within the context of an awareness of the collective. The return journey of B17, the Star, is B95, Archangel Gabriel. Beginning the matrix with this combination emphasizes the potential for individual development in the Aquarian aeon and for being a messenger of that which has been learned. We are able to express something of what we have learned and refined from our own experience and from the wisdom that lies within. B95 (Magenta/Gold) links the soul star in the magenta with the incarnational star in the gold. The soul star represents our potential, and the incarnational star represents our current state. By linking them we may be able to manifest more of our potential. In B14 (Clear/Gold) awareness, or light, shines on the gold, illuminating (bringing understanding to) the incarnational star in the golden area of our being. The return journey of B14 is B92, in which the cosmic egg of our auric field begins to develop out of the hologram of the incarnational star expanding into the subtle energy fields that surround us. Through the stimulation of that hologram we begin to have access to all the beings we have been and to all the beings we are yet to be. In essence these aspects or potentials of our self become resources to help us respond most appropriately and with the greatest information moment to moment. In B92, the olive makes the space and helps to reduce the fear of trusting in our intuition. Rather than letting ourselves be manipulated or controlled by over-analysis, intuition may be the basis for our expression. We may experience a diminishing of dogma, of acquiescence to imposed philosophies, both perhaps lingering scars of the Piscean aeon, and an increase of relaxation as we trust our own resources and rely on our inner wisdom (B14). The pale coral in B92 is the new consciousness emerging, the reconciliation of our yearning for utopia with the experience of living in the material world. The integration of these two opposing tendencies is supported by qualities of feminine intuitive leadership. With the emergence of this reconciliation, we can stand for what we believe without an insistence on a utopian viewpoint and without holding on to false values, needs, and desires. Our potential qualities in the soul star in the magenta can infuse our life as we express the star that we are. B11 follows B92. The num-

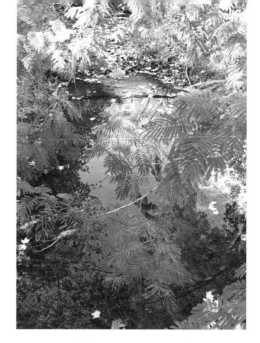

Dead Creek in Liberty Corner, New Jersey.

ber 11 is like the two pillars of a doorway. B11 can serve as a gateway to another dimension—allowing us to move through the pillars to a new level of understanding. Another part of the story of B11 is that we can be more susceptible to the harshness of dogma when we adopt someone else's point of view. When we stand on our own two feet, bringing light through us to our own earth star, there is a greater opportunity to express the strength of our light with caring and gentleness. B89, the return journey of B11, represents the time shift from the Piscean aeon to the Aquarian aeon. The strong red in this combination suggests the energy and power of awakening that exists in the deep magenta. The idea of potential is inherent in the deep magenta. It is the color of divine love, which can never really actualize. In addition, deep magenta contains all of the colors and so it has the potential of all the colors. As a Rescue bottle, we could say that the deep magenta has the potential to rescue the red (energy) out of the deep magenta. In B89 there is an enhanced opportunity for us to awaken from false dreams and from the mass hypnosis of society to bring conscious attention to the star within each of us. Whereas a devotional path was part of the Piscean aeon, the Aquarian aeon is a time for individuation, a time to stand up for what we know. The courage to do this, to move through this transformation, to articulate what is in our heart, is in the red in the violet of the lower fraction of B17. Red can be traced through each of the bottles in this matrix.

In this section, by studying the concept of the matrices, hopefully you have come to a new appreciation of the languages of color and number and how they can work together, and recognized both the complexity and simplicity inherent in the Equilibrium sequence. The archetypal themes of the matrices may help you perceive both the similarities and uniqueness of each of our paths and shed light on your own journeys.

A Number by Any Other Name

As we have seen, by studying the matrices, that which the Equilibrium bottles offer is also communicated through the number of each bottle. The bottles were given in a specific order, or unfolding, so that the number associated with each one has significance. Thus B1, Blue/Deep Magenta, has a reciprocal relevance to the number one tarot card, the Magician. Essentially, reciprocity and relationship exist inherently, in that one equals one equals one. Although this is basic number theory, it is also, curiously, the basis for the sacred kabbalistic teaching of gematria, the study of Hebrew as a numerological system. Vicky consciously knew nothing about gematria when she was guided to interweave these systems, but it was apparently something in which her father had been specifically trained.

As an example, let us take the number one further. In the tarot, the Magician is considered to have available all the tools of the four suits, which in turn relate to the four elements. The Magician is prepared to use the tools skillfully, creatively, and in harmony with divine order.

For several centuries there has been, in esoteric circles, recognition of the interface of the tarot with the Tree of Life.[6] Both B1 and the Magician card correspond to a path of movement on the Tree. On this path, raw creative energies are available from the source, Kether, initially to be contained and held as potential in the sephira Binah and later to be disseminated into the life force.

B1 in the Aura-Soma Equilibrium sequence has as its base fraction the color deep magenta representing the source of all that is possible. The deep magenta is available to be expressed through the blue in the upper fraction of the bottle; the blue means that it is expressed in the context of peace, clarity, and truth. B1 is the Physical Rescue bottle. It denotes that we are in touch with the soul star and the throat chakra, and that we can express caring and warmth in all that we do.

In the I Ching, the first hexagram is referred to as "the Creative" by Richard Wilhelm, "the Creative Principle" by John Blofield, and "the Initiating" by Master Huang. This hexagram is Heaven: Heaven below and Heaven above. It teaches us that when intent is good, in keeping with divine order, then when the Creative is successful the result is good.[7]

These four systems say something similar about the number one, or their first element. B1, the Magician, the corresponding path of the Tree of Life, and the first hexagram all describe qualities of creating and directing forces that, if activated in a benevolent and correct way, are helpful and transformative.

The number belonging to each Equilibrium bottle opens the door to other ways of understanding the relationships between the bottles and, for those interested in numerology and sacred geometry, provides insight to another level of communication contained within the Aura-Soma system. Number as well as color is a universal language. Numbers are at times directly related to language and in that way offer another way to communicate or to encode information. For example, the letter *a* could be equal to 1, *b* to 2, *c* to 3, and so on in the English alphabet. This could provide an amusing way to understand why you are at sixes and sevens, as the expression goes, if you do not know your ABC's: If you do not know your ABC's, you do not know your 1's, 2's, and 3's. $1 + 2 + 3 = 6$. The letter *s* is the nineteenth letter in the alphabet. Thus, "ABC's" $= 1 + 2 + 3 + 19 = 25; 2 + 5 = 7$. So if you do not know your ABC's, you are at sixes and sevens. Things are not in order and need to be straightened out.

Let us consider as an example B13, Clear/Green, Change in the New Aeon, whose main theme is illumination of the emotional side of life, enlightenment of the heart. Change is often marked by the death of something old and the beginning of something new. One complete year from its birth to its completion comprises thirteen lunar cycles. The thirteen-moon count is important in the Mayan calendar, which marks small and great cycles and epochs of time. The thirteenth tarot card is Death. In folklore, 13 is often considered unlucky, and some hotels and tall buildings skip over the number 13 when numbering their floors or rooms.

When the values of each letter in the Hebrew word for *one* are added together, the sum equals 13. The sum of the letters in the Hebrew word for *love* also is 13. Kabbalah teaches that two words having the same numerical value have an implied intimate relationship or in some way are synonymous. So in Hebrew, the words for *love* and *one* are related. And indeed, when we feel love for someone or something, we become bonded or more at one with that person or thing. The ultimate bond that brings everything to oneness or to unification is most likely the quality of love.

The task now is to relate these understandings about the number 13 so as to come to a greater understanding of B13. Through the process of death and change there is an inherent unity or oneness: our essence can continue. It may be that the quality and feeling of love help make that continuity and oneness more apparent. Enlightenment of the heart and illumination of and clarity about our feelings allow us to develop a new perspective on a situation. The notes on B13 suggest that we "let go of the past, set new goals, and plan for the right time to implement them." Selection of this bottle suggests that we may face an ending in one form or another. Perhaps the clue that 13 = Love = One can give us sustenance to face the constant of life: all things change. As we move through change we can be one with what has been, what is, and what will be.

How could this enhanced understanding apply when a person chooses B13? One person may be drawn to that bottle, and upon contemplation remember that at the age of thirteen he lost his beloved pet. Another person might choose Clear/Green and recall that, at the age of thirteen, she and her family moved back to their beautiful family farm, with acres upon acres of green pastures to explore on horseback. For apparently different reasons, both individuals may have a strong association with the bottle. Both experienced loss or change—a new direction or perspective for their lives. What they learned from these experiences might have different implications, but the themes of change and love are there.

The examples given are not unique, but are easy to understand and show how our intuition can be stimulated to perceive more about the meanings encoded in numbers and color. Sometimes one association with a color will initially seem most pertinent. Often over time those associations that might have seemed most far-fetched may come to have a more profound importance than was initially apparent. We invite readers to be open to all the possibilities inherent in a color combination, and to move through a process of exploration that is likely to bring profound growth, especially as a trigger to stimulate the deeper levels of intuition within ourselves.

It is as if each bottle were a radiating sun, a point of light that shines in many ways, giving visual impressions, inviting emotional responses, stimulating attitudes and reactions, implying connections, and revealing information. We can think in terms of astrological associations, reincarnational experiences, the archetypal story of the tarot, the meaning of the colors, and/or the connection to subtle anatomy. All the rays from a color combination are part of the picture. All can be referenced back to and become useful for the individual who responds to the bottle and says, "Yes, this one is me, this is the one I wish to identify with and which calls to me." As we use the ingredients in the bottle on our skin, we facilitate the resonance of insight within us. The Aura-Soma system is vast, both as it stands alone and as it interfaces with other systems. At the same time, it is accessible.

It may be difficult to believe that the 106 Aura-Soma Equilibrium bottles can contain so much information and be able to describe an individual in a way that is unique and pertinent. Yet if we consider the basic building block of life, the DNA double helix, we might have insight into how this is possible. The DNA strands within each living cell carry the genetic code for all life on Earth. This code is communicated through just four nucleic acids, which are assembled in pairs in varied sequences of three along the double helix. The magnificent multiplicity of humans, the billions and billions of us—as well as the millions of other species with populations large and small—is the product of these few nucleic acids grouping themselves in different ways, as into "chromo-somes." So, too, can the selection of dual-color combinations reveal, via our unique color code, the wonder and complexity of our soul's journey through time.

Aura-Soma and the Process of Individuation

As scientists are in the process of deciphering the genetic code of humans, animals, and plants, perhaps it is apropos that the color code of individual souls also becomes more apparent. Through Aura-Soma, our inherent soul path can be perceived and strengthened. "To thine own self be true," not only so that "thou canst not then be false to any man,"[8] but also so that we might co-creatively bring through the best potentials of the Aquarian aeon.

It is amazing that something so simple—the arrangement of a few nucleic acids—could produce the diversity of humans that exist on the earth. From a macroscopic perspective, recent studies of the Bible, facilitated by high-speed computers, indicate a similar complex conciseness. The Torah, a sacred Hebrew text, is written with the twenty-two Hebrew letters in a continuous sequence. There are no vowels. As described in books about this Hebrew scripture (e.g., *The Bible Code* by Michael Drosnin and *Cracking the Bible Code* by Jeffrey Satinover), it appears that through the process of permutations, sequential skips, and combinations of the letters of the Torah, it is possible to describe all that has been, is, and will be in human experience. As Vicky would say about Aura-Soma, "It is so simple, it is simply amazing."

There is a parallel between these multiplicities of outcomes and Aura-Soma. In our discussion of subtle anatomy (page 23), we spoke of the Jungian process of individuation. The turquoise area, the Ananda Khanda, is activated after each of the chakras is functioning and when we are connected to our earth star and soul star. At that moment, the turquoise starts to make its way toward the middle of the body to the emerald of the heart. Through this process of individuation, we are more able to fulfill our destiny on the earth, both individually and collectively.

This understanding from an Aura-Soma point of view has an interesting correspondence with Ken Wilber's research. Wilber recommends a developmental approach to describing different human values and worldviews, and an understanding that "one stage of development can only be defused by evolving to a higher level; and that only by recognizing and facilitating this evolution can social justice be finally served."[9] Furthermore, he describes these realities, worldviews, or deep structures in terms of color. Wilber suggests that people evolve through a progression of values, which are:

. . . various waves of existence (or stages of development) . . . [which] are not just passing phases in the self's unfolding; they are permanently available capacities and coping strategies that can, once they have emerged, be activated under the appropriate life conditions. . . .[10]

With regard to the stages, Wilber says, "The first six levels are 'subsistence levels' marked by 'first-tier thinking.' Then there occurs a revolutionary shift in consciousness: the emergence of 'being levels' and 'second-tier' thinking."[11] Wilber describes each of these levels in terms of a color. Bearing in mind our seven chakras and the Aura-Soma understanding of the emerald of the heart as the point where we can move off the cross of the time and space continuum, it is interesting to consider, with regard to the green meme or value, what Wilber says:

With the completion of the green meme, human consciousness is poised for a quantum jump into "second-tier" thinking. Clare Graves referred to this as a "momentous leap" where a "chasm of unbelievable depth of meaning is crossed." In essence, with second-tier consciousness, one can think both vertically and horizontally, using both hierarchies and heterarchies. One can, for the first time, vividly grasp the entire spectrum of interior development, and thus see that each level, each meme, is crucially important for the health of the overall spiral. Since each wave is "transcend and include," each wave is a fundamental ingredient of all subsequent waves, and thus is to be cherished and embraced.[12]

In Aura-Soma, turquoise, composed of blue and green, is known as the Abode of Bliss, and it is activated by simultaneous movement from the soul star and the earth star. Wilber describes the final wave of second-tier consciousness as turquoise, and as "relatively rare . . . the 'leading edge' of collective human evolution." Turquoise is:

Holistic: [a] [u]niversal holistic system . . . [that] unites feeling with knowledge (centaur); multiple levels interwoven into one conscious system. Universal order but in a living, conscious fashion, not based on external rules (blue) or group bonds (green). A "grand unification" is possible, in theory and in actuality. Sometimes involves the emergence of a new spirituality as a meshwork of all existence.[13]

There is a striking correspondence between Wilber's theories about consciousness, those of Carl Jung, and what Aura-Soma demonstrates. Aura-Soma supports the process of individuation so that we can fulfill our destiny on the earth in a collective context.

An Example: B5 and Aura-Soma

Vicky made B5, Yellow/Red, on the night Aura-Soma was born. It was the bottle that called to her the most, and it provides a good example of how a bottle speaks to both a person's unique path and the experience of a larger community.

Known as the Sunrise/Sunset bottle, B5 can be seen as the sun cresting or descending on the horizon of the red earth. B5's keynote is about the opportunity to use knowledge wisely in relation to the energies that we carry, with energy and passion (red) supporting the expression of knowledge (yellow). In the language of color, Yellow/Red might indicate a leader with a difficult but joyful path in relation to his or her mission, a person with strength (red) whose mission is grounded (red) with joy (yellow). All of this could describe Vicky.

Yellow and red shaken together create orange, the color of B26, Orange/Orange, known as the Etheric Rescue or Humpty Dumpty bottle. This suggests that the choice of B5 could indicate abuse, shocks, or difficult situations early in life. The orange connotes dependency and codependency issues, conditioned and addictive patterns, and liberation through the path of meditation to bring insight and bliss. Vicky's unique story, including the traumas and setbacks she experienced that tempered her soul, helped hone her strength and enabled her to ground her wisdom in something practical that could be shared with many. Thus the multiple meanings of this color combination could all be significant to her.

On a less individual scale, the keynotes to B5 mention that it may help establish contact with Tibetan and Chinese incarnations. Yellow/Red has a special relationship with the teachings and history of Tibetan Buddhism. The Dalai Lama and other Tibetan Buddhist monks wear robes of yellow and red, and the shrine room at the Karme Choling meditation center[14]—a major U.S. retreat in Barnet, Vermont, not far from the home of one of the authors—is painted with these colors. Often the students react quite strongly when they first see this room; it shocks and awakens visitors, breaking up habitual preoccupations. As Chogyam Trungpa Rinpoche, founder of Karme Choling, might say, it brings you "back to square one." After a while, students may come to crave the atmosphere in the shrine room.

Orange/Orange, which B5 shakes to, is intended to help with shock. It is the "get it together again" bottle and the healer of the timeline. Certainly the Tibetan Buddhists have suffered great shocks. In the case of the shrine room at Karme Choling, the positive consequence of shock is to startle the meditator into a state of wakefulness.

Moreover, we can imagine the monks in their saffron-colored robes as they go through their daily life. Through their practice of meditation, they may find a key to understanding that will help engender compassion and loving kindness and may help the evolution of humanity on the planet. Yellow, red, and orange are the colors of the first three chakras: the root, the navel, and the solar plexus. As we resolve the difficulties and energies of the first three chakras, the fourth chakra, the heart, may open.

Numerically, Yellow/Red connects to the fifth trump in the tarot, the Hierophant. Traditionally the Hierophant is considered to have been the chief priest in ancient Greece who presided at the celebration of Demeter and Persephone in the Eleusinian mysteries. Under the guidance of the Hierophant, the people were given the opportunity to grow in wisdom, a fitting connection to the bottle that helps us use our energies wisely. Within orange are yellow and red. Thus the experience of Yellow/Red can lead to insight (symbolized also by orange), and the practice of meditation (orange) can lead to knowledge of how to use our energies (red) wisely (yellow). Vicky herself practiced meditation, and she devoted herself to being of service in the world. She was given Aura-Soma, and under her initial guidance it became a system whereby she could serve others by assisting them on their path of awakening, a path that can lead to personal insight, a direct connection to the divine within, and the ability to wisely express their life force

B5, the sixth bottle in the Equilibrium sequence, also corresponds with *vov*, the sixth letter in the Hebrew alphabet. Vov occurs on the path of the kabbalistic Tree of Life just below Chokmah, the uppermost sphere on the masculine pillar where energies exist before they come into more concrete manifestation. Vov is the link between Chokmah and that which will come into being. One definition of this letter is "a hook, a nail, something that links together concepts or things that are seemingly separate." Chogyam Trungpa Rinpoche speaks about the pragmatic role of devotion in the process of reaching enlightenment, suggesting that it is the hook through which the teachers and the bodhisattvas can work with the human beings.[15] Vov also signifies uniqueness and the importance of fulfilling our own path.[16] When we think of Vicky's life, the significance of her bottles' relationship to this letter is apparent: she was a "hook," or one who fetched and received from the spiritual world the inspiration for Aura-Soma. In giving birth to Aura-Soma, Vicky was able to integrate seemingly divergent concepts, healing techniques, theories, and systems and make them readily available. In a practical way, the bottles are able to bring to the earth energies of a spiritual and inspired nature and to contain them in dual-color combinations that make them easily accessible.

At Karme Choling, the personal shock and awakening that occur through the practice of meditation can help students travel their unique path, to "hook" more firmly into their spiritual intention and to embody it in a practical way. In terms of devotion, shock, and wakefulness, Vicky Wall in England and the Tibetan meditation center in Vermont have a shared color story, one intriguingly held by B5 and B26. It is interesting to note that around the world B26 has consistently been the bottle purchased more than any other color combination. In fact, the name Aura-Soma equates to the number 26, using the basic numerical correspondence of the English alphabet. By kabbalistic tradition, this would imply that Aura-Soma and the number 26 have a special relationship or equivalence. By implication, Aura-Soma has been now offered from spirit to help us not only in releasing the traumas held in our own auric field and in the etheric but also in the healing of our individual and collective timeline. We may move into greater synchronicity and harmony. That B26 brings us to B8 ($2 + 6 = 8$) suggests that Aura-Soma is here now to help us each to develop our light-body, our wings.

Aura-Soma and the New Aeon

As we have seen, Aura-Soma is an evolving system. New bottles have been "born" or created from time to time as Vicky Wall and now Mike Booth received inspiration to bring them forth. The timing of these inspirations could suggest that the new bottles, the new color combinations, and even the new tints and hues arrive as the needs of humanity change. The arrival of unique color combinations seems to nurture personal individuation and to support, and perchance to lead, an evolution of humanity and a concurrent shift in consciousness in the collective.

The births of two bottles, B101 and B102, exemplify the synchronistic unfolding of the Aura-Soma system. B101, Archangel Jophiel, Pale Blue/Pale Olive, arrived December 14, 2000. Jophiel is known as the archangel who led Adam and Eve out of the Garden of Eden after they had eaten of the Tree of Knowledge. Perhaps Jophiel's appearance in the Aura-Soma sequence at the start of the new millennium is a hint that the time has come to return to a more harmonious, heart-centered life, to come into the wisdom within our being, to the incarnational star that resides in the golden area within our self. Our own grail cup may be filled to overflowing, and we may give to the world the essence of our talents, thereby helping us all to return to a unified field, to a oneness with one another.

Archangel Samael, Deep Olive/Deep Magenta, B102, arrived after Jophiel, and Samael's hues contrast markedly with the tints of B101. Perhaps, in the way that love may draw out everything unlike itself for the purpose of healing, the possibility of returning to the unified field brings to our awareness all the obstacles and shadow issues that we must deal with to reach harmony.

The circumstances surrounding the birth of B102 graphically demonstrate the synchronistic unfolding of the Aura-Soma system: During the Christmas season of 2000, Mike Booth mentioned that he felt another bottle was close to being born and that the narne he had been given for it was Archangel Samael. The spelling of the name was very specific, not to be confused with "Samuel" or other beings of similar names. Through the course of the winter, we researched what tradition says about the nature and role of Samael. Gustav Davidson, in *A Dictionary of Angels,* describes him as "a combination of 'sam,' meaning poison, and 'el,' meaning angel . . . regarded both as good and evil . . . the angel of death." Arthur Edward Waite, in *The Holy Kabbalah,* said that Samael is characterized as the "severity of God."[17]

According to Rudolf Steiner, Archangel Samael is associated with Mars, the planet or god traditionally associated with war and force. Steiner also associated Archangel Samael with the sixteenth tarot card, the Tower, as well as with the sixteen-petaled lotus, the throat chakra, the power of speech for expressing the Word, and the sword as a symbol of the Word.[18] As mentioned earlier, each of the major arcana of the tarot is traditionally associated with a particular path of the kabbalistic Tree of Life. The Tower is the path that joins together the pillars of mercy and severity by linking the seventh and eighth spheres, called Netzach and Hod, at the bottom of each pillar.

Through the course of the winter and spring of 2001, Mike felt the bottle approaching and then receding, as if the urgency for its birth would intensify and abate, almost like labor pains, or as if the energies of the bottle were in a period of gestation. Mike had several impressions of the bottle's possible color combinations, but he awaited further guidance. In August, he mentioned that he felt the bottle's birth to be close and that it might arrive around September 10 or 11, when he was next in England. On September 11, 2001, right after he heard the news that the twin towers of the World Trade Center had been hit, Mike felt compelled to go into the laboratory to make the new bottle.

The colors that presented themselves to him in a serendipitous visual combination on the laboratory table were different from what he had expected. Here for the first time was deep olive: a shade has been added to the Aura-Soma collection.

We are all familiar with the details surrounding September 11. In retrospect, the significance of Samael—the poison of God; the association with Mars, the god of war; even the connection to the Tower—is apparent. Those familiar with the Tower card, as depicted in the Rider-Waite deck, are aware of the similarity between the lightning-struck tower on the tarot card and the images, burned into many of our minds, of people falling from the twin towers as the towers themselves burst apart.

Even the astrological timing of the event had a significance of seemingly cosmic coincidence: the moon had been "void of course" in Gemini, the sign of the Twins. Moreover, both the Ethiopian and Coptic new year fall on the eleventh of September in the Gregorian calendar. Ancient Egypt's New Year's Day, when recalculated to modern calendars, is also the eleventh of September. This day was marked by the dawn rising of Sirius, the star sacred to Isis, the goddess who sustains life and healed Osiris, the wounded king and—in death—the lord of the underworld.[19]

In Egyptian mythology, Osiris, the king who needs healing and resurrection, is associated with the number 15. The fifteenth tarot card is Death. In the Aura-Soma sequence, Bottle 15 is Clear/Violet, and its main themes

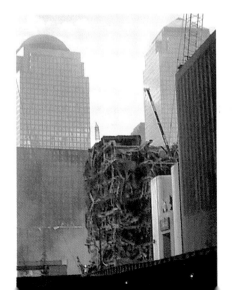

Mangled, twisted steel of the twin towers in front of the buildings of the world financial center that were left standing after 9/11/2001.

include healing in the New Aeon and elevation of the self through purification. Again we are given another association with the events of September 11—here, the need for an inspired (clear), transformative (violet) approach to them. The more we delve into the synchronicity between the birth of Archangel Samael and the events on September 11, 2001, the more powerful are the suggestions of a divine presence in Aura-Soma.

A principle of homeopathy is that the energetics of a bit of toxic material may stimulate a healing crisis. Perhaps the energy package of B102, the Archangel Samael, the poison of God, can have the homeopathic effect of stimulating a healing crisis through the response to the events of September 11 and help bring about a positive change in consciousness for humanity.

The colors of B102 suggest that this shift is possible. As noted in chapter 5, all the bottles with deep magenta in their base fraction are called "Rescue" bottles. Magenta is associated with divine love and grace; deep magenta is associated with the source of all that is, with energized compassion and deep caring, as well as with that which is in the shadow, in our unconscious. Olive symbolizes feminine leadership and empathy, leadership from the heart that releases bitterness and offers hope. It can assist cleansing and the clearing of negative emotions. From a subtle anatomy point of view, olive is the bridge to the heart from the golden part of our being. It is the step toward the opening of the emerald of our heart, as pink rises through the gold and the olive to facilitate that opening. As described earlier, a direct relationship exists between our human development and the development of the earth. As the emerald of our individual heart opens, so, too, is the grid system of the earth reinforced and the earth helped in her evolutionary step toward expressing herself as a planet of love.

Like most of the Equilibrium bottles, B102 is also related to both the tarot and a path on the kabbalistic Tree of Life. Each kabbalistic path corresponds to two specific tarot cards: an outward journey and a return journey. On the return journey, while still experiencing the learning of the outward journey, the traveler has developed increased insight about the specific archetypal lesson of the path and begins to offer to the world that which he or she has learned up to this point. Steiner denotes the importance of this stage of a person's growth thus:

> He does not learn in order to accumulate learning as his own treasure of knowledge, but in order to place this learning in the service of the world. . . . All the knowledge you pursue merely for the enrichment of your own learning and to accumulate treasure of your own leads you away from your path; but all knowledge you pursue in order to grow more mature on the path of human ennoblement and world-progress brings you a step forward.[20]

The return journey associated with the Tower is Archangel Michael, B94. With the arrival of Archangel Samael, this path may have gained a third level, B102. According to Steiner, in 1879 the Archangel Michael took over from Archangel Gabriel the responsibility of overseeing the evolution of consciousness on this planet. Archangel Michael is directly associated with the energetic grid lines on the planet, with sacred sites, and with awakening the consciousness of the planet itself. With the appearance of B102, it could be understood that Archangel Michael has called in the help of Archangel Samael.

With regard to the calling in of help, in the United States the emergency phone number is 911. While many associations may be made with these numbers, certainly 911 has taken on another significance since September 11. During the crisis, it was not only local police forces, firefighters, and Archangel Samael who were called in, but also over three hundred canine—K-9—rescue teams. It is fitting that *K* is the eleventh letter of the English alphabet. In a sense, the "11-9" unit was an emergency team coming on 9/11 to meet the 911 call for help. Perhaps a divine presence was at hand; "dog" spelled backward is, after all, "god" in English. Perhaps, as on the tarot card, when the Tower bursts and the eye of truer insight emerges, the deep olive and deep magenta of B102 indicate the possibility of a great hope for life, led from the heart, rescuing caring from the depth of darkness, the generative, operative principles following the destructive event.

Each Equilibrium bottle has such information and significance encoded in its color combination, all of which is part of the support the bottle offers to the person who chooses it and to the world at large. A thrill of Aura-Soma is that when we pick a color combination, we need have no conscious knowledge of that information. The significance is there, waiting to unfold for us as our connection to the bottle grows. Meanwhile, it is working on our behalf. There seems to be a beautiful perfection and internal consistency to what is offered to us through Aura-Soma.

Arctic sunset in Norway.

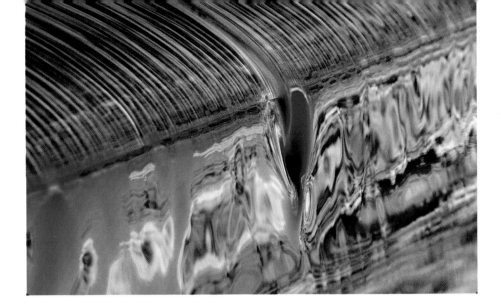

Resources

U.S. Practitioners and Distributors

For further information about Aura-Soma or referrals to practitioners in your area, contact:

Carol McKnight
Box 79
1306 Route 125
Ripton, VT 05766
802-388-6227
e-mail: cjmck101@sover.net

To purchase Aura-Soma products, contact:

Aura-Soma Products Limited
United Kingdom
011-44-150-753-3581
e-mail: info@aura-soma.co.uk
www.aura-soma.net

International Practitioners and Distributors

The Art and Science International Academy of Colour Technologies
Dev Aura
Little London
Tetford
Lincolnshire, LN9 6QL
United Kingdom
+44 (0) 1507 533218
e-mail: info@asiact.org
www.asiact.org

The Art and Science International Academy of Colour Technologies (AS I ACT) is a registered U.K. charitable trust established for the primary objective of education and understanding of color therapy. This objective is achieved through training courses, published educational materials, seminars and conferences, and research.

Aura-Soma Products Limited
South Road
Tetford
Lincolnshire, LN9 6QB
United Kingdom
011-44-150-753-3581
e-mail: info@aura-soma.co.uk
www.aura-soma.net

Publications

Aura-Soma: Self-Discovery through Color by Vicky Wall (published by Healing Arts Press in 2005) tells the story of Vicky's life and the innovation of the Aura-Soma Equilibrium bottles.

There are also many books about Aura-Soma available in other languages. Contact Aura-Soma Products Limited for further information.

Above: Blue-gold falling water at Connor's Pond dam in Petershan, Massachusetts.

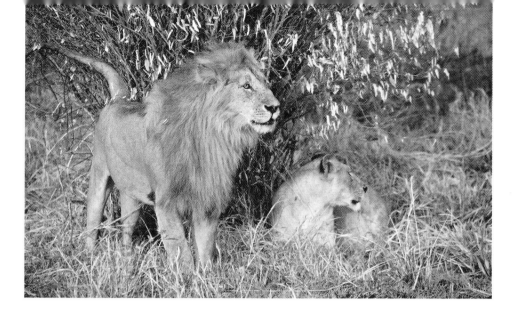

Notes

Introduction

1. Caroline M. Shreeve, *The Alternative Dictionary of Symptoms and Cures* (London: Rider, 1986), 489–97.
2. Rudolf Steiner, *Knowledge of the Higher Worlds* (London: Rudolf Steiner Press, 1969), 39–40.

Chapter 1

1. Every soul or consciousness that comes into human form has come as a part of the process of being attracted to a particular color frequency or ray and all of the qualities inherent in that particular color.
2. Seth Lerer, *The History of the English Language, Part I* (audiotape; Chantilly, VA: The Teaching Company, 1998). Professor Lerer is associated with Stanford University. The complete lecture series can be ordered on audiotape, audio CD, videotape, or DVD from The Teaching Company by phone at 1-800-832-2412 or on its Web site: www.teach12.com.

Chapter 2

1. Vicky Wall, *Aura-Soma: Self-Discovery through Color* (Rochester, VT: Healing Arts, 2005), 1.
2. Ibid., 57.
3. Ibid., 59, 67.
4. Vicky always said that Aura-Soma came from "Father," which was the way she referred to both her father and God.
5. Steiner, *Knowledge,* 22–23.

6. The Equilibrium bottles are known by color, name, and number. Thus, the bottle that sustained Vicky is known as Green/Green, Go Hug a Tree, and Bottle 10 (abbreviated B10).
7. A. P. Shepherd, *Rudolf Steiner: Scientist of the Invisible* (Rochester, VT: Inner Traditions, 1954).
8. Steiner, *Knowledge,* 39.
9. Shreeve, *Alternative Dictionary,* 489–97.

Chapter 3

1. Steiner, *Color* (Sussex: Rudolf Steiner Press 1992), 70.
2. Ibid., 177.
3. Ibid.
4. Johann Wolfgang von Goethe, *Theory of Colors* (Cambridge, MA: MIT Press, 1976), xxxvii.
5. Ibid., lvi.
6. Joseph Addison, *The Spectator* (England: 1711–1712).
7. Goethe, *Theory of Colors,* 307–8 .
8. Ibid., 321.

Chapter 4

1. Johann Wolfgang von Goethe, *Theory of Colors,* 310.
2. Steiner, *Color,* 118.
3. Ibid., 129–30.
4. For more information, visit the Web site www.paul-schatz.ch or www.oloid.ch.
5. As related by Paul Dicker, production, research, and development Aura-Soma Products Ltd., in a personal communication, July 22, 2005.

Above: Lion pair enjoying the light at the end of the day in East Africa.

6. Steiner, *Color*, 129–30.

7. Ibid., 65.

8. Information from *Aura-Soma: ArchAngeloi* by Mike Booth with deepest thanks to Carol McKnight and Iris Rebilas (Heiligenhaus, Germany: Seifert & Gries, 2004).

Chapter 5

3-a. A historical record of Atlantis is given in the *Timaeus* and *Critias* dialogues of Plato. These dialogues have been widely translated and published and are readily available.

3-b. Henriette Mertz, *Atlantis: Dwelling Place of the Gods* (Chicago: self-published, 1976).

7-a. "In the Garden of Gethsemane, Jesus began to feel terror and anguish. And he said to them, 'My soul is sorrowful to the point of death. Wait here, and stay awake.' And going on a little further he threw himself on the ground and prayed that, if it were possible, this hour might pass him by. 'Abba, Father!' he said, 'For you everything is possible. Take this cup away from me. But let it be as you, not I, would have it.'" (Mark 14:34–37) The Bible (New Jerusalem Version) (New York: Doubleday, 1985).

7-b. Lobsang Wangyal, "45 Years Ago, Witness to Dalai Lama's Flight Did Not Know History Being Made," *Tibetan News Update*, 2004; accessed March 12, 2005, at www.friends-of-tibet.org.nz/news/april_2004_update_20.htm.

7-c. Georges Serrus, *The Land of the Cathars* (Portet-sur-Garonne, France: Editions Loubatieres, 1990).

8-a. There are several interesting references for Egyptian myths and religions, one of which is *The Egyptian Book of the Dead*. Many English-language editions are available.

10-a. "Morris dances and Mumming plays . . . from the Middle Ages onward, became a principal expression of the human longing for the greening of life. . . . Hildegard of Bingen called this the *Veriditas,* the greening of the soul, showing that even within the mysteries of Christianity, the spirit of wildness was present." John Matthews, *Robin Hood: Green Lord of the Wildwood* (Glastonbury, UK: Gothic Image, 1993) 73.

11-a. For more information about the Essenes, consult any of the following:
Olivier Manitara, *The Essenes* (Montreal: Telesma Evida, 2005).
Brother Nazariah, D.D., "Introduction to the Ancient Essenes and the Modern Essene Church of Christ"; accessed March 7, 2005, from www.essene.org/Ancient_Essenes.htm.
Edmond Bordeaux Szekely, *The Teachings of the Essenes from Enoch to the Dead Sea Scrolls* (London: C. W. Daniel, 1978).

11-b. "They sent out healers and teachers from the brotherhoods, amongst whom were Elija, John the Baptist, John the Beloved and the great Essene Master, Jesus." (Edmond Bordeaux Szekely, *The Teachings of the Essenes from Enoch to the Dead Sea Scrolls* [London: C. W. Daniel, 1978], 13).

11-c. Edmond Bordeaux Szekely, *The Gospel of the Essenes* (London: C. W. Daniel, 1982).

15-a. Matthews, *Robin Hood,* 64.

16-a. Richard Cavendish, *The Tarot* (New York: Harper & Row, 1975), 54.

17-a. Guillaume de Machaut, *Foy Porter,* accessed April 10, 2005, from Study Guide for Medieval Love Songs www.wsu.edu:8080/~brians/love-in-the-arts/medieval.html.

17-b. Note that the Albigensians are related to the Cathars.

17-c. "Officially known as The Order of the Poor Knights of the Temple of Solomon, they were formed in 1118 by the French nobleman Hugues de Payens as knightly escorts to pilgrims to the Holy Land. . . . In 1307 came their inevitable fall from grace. The supremely powerful French king, Philip the Fair, began to orchestrate the downfall of the Templars with the connivance of the Pope. . . . [T]he Templars were rounded up on Friday 13ᵗʰ October 1307, arrested, tortured and burnt." Lynn Picknett and Clive Prince, *The Templar Revelation* (Reading, UK: Corgi Books, 1998), 125–28.

17-d. Varying dates are given for the beginning and end of the Piscean era. These dates were given by astrologer John Ramsey (johnpeniel45@hotmail.com), in an e-mail message to Carol McKnight, March 13, 2005.

18-a. These dates were given by astrologer John Ramsey, in an e-mail message to Carol McKnight, March, 13, 2005. Other authorities give varying dates for the beginning and end of the Piscean era and the Egyptian epoch within it. Ramsey also notes that the time of the more enlightened priest/kings was from 10,000 BC to 3500 BC.

20-a. The Buddhist concept of "right speech" mirrors Vicky's theory. An explanation of right speech is given on the Web site TheBigView.com as follows:

"Right speech is the first principle of ethical conduct in the eightfold path. Ethical conduct is viewed as a guideline to *moral discipline*, which supports the other principles of the path. This aspect is not self-sufficient, however essential, because mental purification can only be achieved through the cultivation of ethical conduct. The importance of speech in the context of Buddhist ethics is obvious: words can break or save lives, make enemies or friends, start war or create peace. Buddha explained right speech as follows: 1. to abstain from false speech, especially not to tell deliberate lies and not to speak deceitfully, 2. to abstain from slanderous speech and not to use words maliciously against others, 3. to abstain from harsh words that offend or hurt others, and 4. to abstain from idle chatter that lacks purpose or depth. Positively phrased, this means to tell the truth, to speak friendly, warm, and gently and to talk only when necessary" (www.thebigview.com/buddhism/eightfoldpath.html; accessed March 15, 2005).

22-a. "Jesus answered and said unto him, 'Verily, verily, I say unto thee, Except a man be born again, he cannot see the kingdom of God.' Nicodemus saith unto him, 'How can a man be born when he is old? Can he enter the second time into his mother's womb, and be born?' Jesus answered, 'Verily, verily, I say unto thee, Except a man be born of water and of the Spirit, he cannot enter into the kingdom of God.'" (John 3:3–5)

25-a. Barbara Montgomery Dossey, *Florence Nightingale: Mystic, Visionary, Healer* (Springhouse, Penn.: Springhouse, 2000), 237, 420–24.

25-b. Ibid., 33.

25-c. This dis-ease is known as chronic fatigue syndrome in the United States.

26-a. Ted Andrews, *Animal-Speak* (St. Paul, Minn.: Llewellyn Publications, 1996), 281–82.

27-a. For a broad historical biography of Robin Hood, see the description on Wikipedia.org. For a more in-depth account, see *Robin Hood: Green Lord of the Wildwood* by John Matthews.

32-a. "[B]y saying that with the resurrection of the cleaved Lucifer as the Human through the Mystery of Golgotha, and with the restoration of the primordial trinity of the holy Ghost, of Lucifer, Sophia, and Michael as the Human, the cognition, embodiment, and expression of cosmic intelligence could proceed without distortions or obstructions, and be established in the flesh of Earth. Another name for this restored cosmic trinity of the Human is the Virgin Sophia. That's because Sophia's purificatory catharsis takes place within the individual consciousness of each human as a result of the cleansing of the Old Moon astral body. When the human astral body no longer contains impure impressions of the physical world but has spiritual organs awake and competent for supersensible perception, then 'the pure, chaste, wise Virgin Sophia,' within the individual man or woman encounters the Cosmic Ego, the I-consciousness of the Christ Logos" (Richard Leviton, *The Imagination of Pentecost: Rudolf Steiner and Contemporary Spirituality* [New York: Anthroposophic Press, 1994], 401).

36-a. "And now abideth faith, hope, charity, these three; but the greatest of these is charity" (1 Corinthians 13:13).

44-a. "The Violet Flame, often called the Flame of Freedom because of its purifying and liberating qualities, is a function of the Seventh Ray, and is presided over and dispensed by the Elohim Arcturus, the Archangel Zadkiel, and the Chohan of the Seventh Ray, St. Germain. The use of The Violet Flame, when rhythmically invoked and directed with creative visualization into all aspects of individual and world conditions becomes a most useful method for Planetary Transformation and Transfiguration." The Violet Flame (recording). The Group, Route 9, Box 2370, Brooksville, FL 32512.

50-a. Each bottle in the Master Set is named after a Master Being. Though these Masters "have all passed through the human experience and are simply men who have achieved a relative measure of perfection, there are aspects of physical contact which They have completely transcended and utterly negated. There is nothing in the three worlds with which They have any affinity, except the affinity of life and the impulse of love for all beings. Recovery of certain facilities of activity has been deemed necessary. For instance, the five senses, where a Master is concerned, exist and are used at need, but the contact established and maintained with disciples and senior aspirants in the world (through whom They primarily work) is largely telepathic; hearing and sight, as you understand their uses, are not involved. The science of impression, with its greatly increased effectiveness over individual contact through the senses, has entirely superseded the more strictly human method. Except in the case of Masters working on the physical plane and in a physical body, the outer physical senses are in abeyance; for the majority of Masters Who still use these senses, the use is strictly limited; Their work is still almost entirely subjective and the mode of telepathic interplay and of impression is practically all the means which They employ to reach Their working agents" (Alice A. Bailey, *The Externalization of the Hierarchy* [New York: Lucis Publishing, 1989]).

50-b. The following definitions come from Mark Prophet, trans., *Intermediate Studies in Alchemy* (Los Angeles: Summit University Press, 1978).

Rays. "Beams of light or other radiant energy. The light emanations of the Godhead which, when invoked in the name of God or in the name of the Christ, burst forth as a flame in the world of the individual. Rays may be projected through the God consciousness of ascended or unascended beings as a concentration of energy taking on numerous God-qualities, such as love, truth, wisdom, healing, etc." (148)

Color Rays. "The light emanations of the Godhead; e.g. the seven rays of the white light which emerge through the prism of the Christ consciousness are 1) blue, 2) yellow, 3) pink, 4) white, 5) green, 6) purple and gold, and 7) violet. There are also five 'secret rays' which emerge from the white-fire core of being" (131).

50-c. For further exploration see Robert Wang, *The Qabalistic Tarot* (York Beach, Maine: Samuel Weiser, 1990), 50.

50-d. Good reference works about El Morya include the following:

Alice A. Bailey and Djwhal Khul, *Initiation, Human and Solar* (New York: Lucis, 1997).

"El Morya: Chohan of the First Ray," on the Web site of the Summit Lighthouse at www.tsl.org/masters/ElMorya.asp; accessed April 16, 2005.

"The Great and Holy Master Morya," on the Web site of the Sanctus Germanus Foundation at www.sanctusgermanus.net/great%20white%20brotherhood/Morya.htm; accessed March 10, 2005.

50-e. According to Michael Poynder, "the White Brotherhood is an esoteric brotherhood of light with which many of the Masters and many individuals are associated. . . . [The Brotherhood] is linked by soul consciousness from one being to another along the vibration of the light towards the purpose of the positive progression of the whole Earth in its cosmic journey. The interactions of the powers of God and good workings through each individual or group soul allow many strange and wonderful events to happen in everyday life to help hold the powers of darkness, ignorance, fear and untruth at bay" (Michael Poynder, *Pi in the Sky,* London: Random Century Group, 1992), 70.

The Web site of the Sanctus Germanus Foundation (www.sanctusgermanus.net) is another good resource for information about the White Brotherhood, explaining, "The Great Brotherhood of Light is a body of very highly evolved beings who have attained to much higher levels than the ordinary human being and penetrated more deeply behind the veil of nature. They have realized, through initiation into the Mysteries of the Ageless Wisdom, higher states of existence. Such beings are called Masters, and those of the highest grade are believed to have attained the most sublime wisdom and knowledge that is possible for humanity in its present stage of evolution. As the spiritual Executives of God's plan, they oversee human and planetary affairs. . . . [T]hey act as Messengers of the Wisdom of God, Custodians of the truth as it is in Christ, and Those Whose task is to save the world, to impart the next revelation, and to demonstrate divinity" (Sanctus Germanus Foundation, "Welcome and Introduction," www.sanctusgermanus.net/great%20white%20brotherhood/great_white_brotherhood.html; accessed March 12, 2005).

50-f. For a more complete description, see Rabbi Adin Even Yisrael (Steinsaltz), "Miriam, the Big Sister," at www.jewish-holiday.com/miriam.html; accessed April 11, 2005.

51-a. Good reference works about Kuthumi in his various incarnations include the following:

Alice A. Bailey and Djwhal Khul, *Discipleship in the New Age*, volume 1 (New York: Lucis, 1985).

"The Great and Holy Master Kuthumi (Koot Hoomi)," on the Web site of the Sanctus Germanus Foundation at www.sanctusgermanus.net/great%20white%20brotherhood/Kuthumi.htm; accessed March 12, 2005.

52-a. See also H. P. Blavatsky, *The Voice of the Silence*, 1889; various published editions are available. This work is based on excerpts from the *Book of the Golden Precepts*, an Eastern scripture.

53-a. Collins, Mabel. *Light on the Path*. Covina, Calif.: The Theosophical University Press, 1949.

53-b. For more information about Master Hilarion, see Alice Bailey and Djwhal Khul, *The Rays and the Initiations* (New York: Lucis, 1971), part 2, section 2.

For further discussion of the Way, see Annie Besant, *The Masters* (Chicago: Theosophical Publishing, 1977); more recent editions are available as well. This volume discusses many aspects of the Way and sheds light on the steps that are necessary for us to reach an understanding of our soul and our purpose. *Light on the Path* is discussed beginning on page 79 of Besant's work.

For more about Theosophy, visit the Web site of the Theosophical

Society in America at www.theosophical.org. The society's basic definition of the practice is this:

"Theosophy . . . is a tradition found in human cultures all over the world and at all times in history. . . . The three basic ideas of Theosophy are (1) the fundamental unity of all existence, so that all pairs of opposites—matter and spirit, the human and the divine, I and thou—are transitory and relative distinctions of an underlying absolute Oneness, (2) the regularity of universal law, cyclically producing universes out of the absolute ground of being, and (3) the progress of consciousness developing through the cycles of life to an ever-increasing realization of Unity" (Theosophical Society of America, www.theosophical.org/theosophy/faqs/index.html#Q1; accessed March 15, 2005).

54-a. "One other Master may here be briefly mentioned, the Master Serapis, frequently called the Egyptian. He is the Master upon the fourth ray, and *[T]he great art movements of the world, the evolution of music, and that of painting and drama, receive from him an energizing impulse*" (emphasis added; Alice Bailey and Djwhal Khul, *Initiation, Human and Solar* [New York: Lucis, 1997]; reproduced from http://netnews.org/bk/initiation/init1023.html, accessed March 15, 2005).

55-a. Richard Leviton, *The Imagination of Pentecost: Rudolf Steiner and Contemporary Spirituality* (New York: Anthroposophic Press, 1994).

55-b. See Richard Leviton, *The Imagination of the Pentecost: Rudolf Steiner and Contemporary Spirituality* (New York: Anthroposophic Press, 1994), 222–24.

56-a. For more information about Saint Germain and his various incarnations, see:

Mark Prophet, trans., *Intermediate Studies in Alchemy* (Los Angeles: Summit University Press, 1978), 102.

"Saint Germain's Embodiments," on the Web site of the Summit Lighthouse–Poland, at http://tslpl.org/StGermain_embodiments.html; accessed August 2, 2005.

57-a. Roy Willis, ed., *World Mythology* (New York: Henry Holt, 1996).

58-a. "Perhaps second only to the Big Dipper in Ursa Major, the constellation of Orion is one of the most recognizable patterns of stars in the northern sky. Orion, the hunter, . . . is accompanied by his faithful dogs, Canis Major and Canis Minor. According to Greek mythology, Orion was in love with Merope, one of the Seven Sisters who form the Pleiades, but Merope would have nothing to do with him." (www.astro.wisc.edu/~dolan/constellations/constellations/Orion.html; accessed April 17, 2005).

The Wikipedia Web site (www.wikipedia.org) explains the Orion myth as follows: "In one version, Orion claims himself to be the greatest hunter in the world. This is heard by Hera, the wife of Zeus, and she decided to send a scorpion after Orion. Orion is stung to death by the scorpion. Zeus felt sorry for Orion and put him onto the sky. The scorpion is also taken up to the sky, becoming the constellation Scorpius. It is an interesting fact that when one of the two constellations rises from the horizon, the other would have already set. So the two rivals can never see each other again (http://en.wikipedia.org/wiki/Orion_%28constellation%29; accessed April 18, 2005).

58-b. Lemesurier, Peter, *The Great Pyramid Decoded* (New York: Barnes & Noble, 1996), 160.

For a detailed analysis and commentary on this alignment idea, see Chris Tedder, "Stars and the Giza Pyramids," 2002, www.kolumbus.fi/lea.tedder/OKAD/sky2475.htm; accessed April 18, 2005.

58-c. Jane Grayson, *The Fragrant Year* (London: Aquarian/Thorsons, 1993).

59-a. William Shakespeare, *The Merchant of Venice,* act 4, scene 1.

60-a. Raghavan Iyer, "The Pledge of Kwan-Yin," *Hermes* (November

1979); accessed April 22, 2005, on the Theosophy Library Online Web site at http://theosophy.org/tlodocs/PledgeKY.htm.

60-b. Lao Tzu, *The Way of Life, the Wisdom of Ancient China* (New York: New American Library, 1955).

60-c. The Eyes of Kwan Yin, www.mykwanyin.com/kwgoddess.html, accessed March 11, 2005.

61-a. Sanat Kumara is an Ascended Master and "one of the seven holy Kumaras who came to earth aeons ago to keep *the threefold flame* of life on behalf of mankind after their expulsion from Eden. Sanat Kumara established his *retreat* at Shamballa, an island in the Gobi Sea, now the Gobi Desert. The first to respond to his flame was Gautama *Buddha,* then *Lord Maitreya.* Sanat Kumara held the position of Lord of the World until his disciple Gautama Buddha reached sufficient attainment to hold that office. On January 1, 1956, Gautama Buddha was crowned Lord of the World and Sanat Kumara returned to Venus and to his *twin flame,* the lady Master Venus" (Mark Prophet, trans., *Intermediate Studies in Alchemy* [Los Angeles: Summit University Press, 1978], 150).

62-a. "The Maha Chohan is the personification of the Third Person of the Trinity—of Father, Son, Holy Spirit and the Divine Mother. The Maha Chohan is the representative and the incarnation of the Holy Spirit. This does not mean that he is the Holy Spirit, but that he of all Ascended Masters most ably represents the Holy Spirit as we enter the age of Aquarius." Prophet, Elizabeth Clare. "Lesson One: Who and What Is the Holy Spirit?" Environment of the Soul Conference. Reproduced online at www.tsl.org/Masters/maha_chohan/ and accessed April 17, 2005.

63-a. For more information about Djwal Khul, consult "The Great and Holy Master Djwal Khul," on the Web site of the Sanctus Germanus Foundation at www.sanctusgermanus.net/great%20white%20brotherhood/Djwal%20Khul.htm; accessed March 10, 2005.

For more information about Hilarion, consult the Web site www.crystalinks.com/hilarion.html.

66-a. William Shakespeare, *As You Like It,* act 2, scene 7.

68-a. The following definitions come from Gustav Davidson, *A Dictionary of Angels* (New York: Free Press, 1971):

Angel. An angel is a divine spirit, a courier or a messenger (20).

Archangel. "The term archangel applies generically to all angels above the grade of (the order of) angels; it also serves to designate a specific rank of angels in the celestial hierarchy. . . . [T]he greatest angels are referred to as archangels, as in the Old Testament . . ." (51).

Gabriel. "Means 'God is my strength.' . . . He is the angel of annunciation, resurrection, mercy, vengeance, death, revelation" (117).

70-a. For further exploration of the astral plane, see Alice Bailey's *Ponder on This* (1971); several editions have been published.

72-a. "The essential circus clown is a big man with a sad smile and a strong sense that his jokes are more bitter than they seem.

"Leoncavallo's *Pagliacci,* composed in 1892, takes this tradition to its logical conclusion. It concerns a troupe of traveling actors, and in its famous central aria, *Vesti la Jiuba,* the tenor sings that though he has to put on his make-up for the show, his heart is broken. His wife is planning to run away with her lover and yet he has to go on stage and play the funny man." Bradley Winterton "Opera for Everyone," *Taipei Times,* Friday, September 24, 2004.

78-a. For further exploration of the relationships between Aura-Soma and astrology, see *Esoteric Astrology*, by Alice Bailey and Djwal Khul (1951); several editions are available.

82-a. "Unlike most religious and Christian groups that tend to stress conformity towards the powers-that-be, Rastafari stresses nonconformity and peaceful rebelliousness towards what it terms Babylon, which is the modern society where we live. Rastafari grew up amongst very poor people, to whom society had nothing to offer except more suffering. Rastafarians see themselves as conforming to a vision of how Africans should live, reclaiming what they see as a culture stolen from them when they were brought on slave ships to Jamaica, birthplace of the movement. Their religion is difficult to categorise, because Rastafari is not a centralised organisation; and it is left to the individual Rastafarians to work out the truth for themselves, resulting in a wide variety of beliefs entering beneath the general umbrella of Rastafari" (Answer.com Web site, www. answers.com/topic/rastafarianism; accessed June 29, 2005).

84-a. "Loneliness was tough

The toughest role you ever played

Hollywood created a superstar

And pain was the price you paid

Even when you died

Oh the press still hounded you

All the papers had to say

Was that Marilyn was found in the nude."

(from the album *Goodbye Yellow Brick Road*; lyrics by Bernie Taupin, as reproduced at www.eltonography.com/songs/candle_in_the_wind.html; accessed March 11, 2005).

87-a. "In the twentieth century, we stand at a major turning point in which the etheric body, weak and relatively powerless within the physical head organization, will emerge again, free itself from the gravity of the physical—that "three pound universe," as some neuroscientists jokingly refer to the human brain—and reclaim its cosmic, thought-filled independence. In essence, this loosening of the tight bond between etheric and physical body is the major change Steiner indicated the etheric body would start to undergo in our time. The loosening of the etheric body from the physical is the rightful task of the consciousness soul epoch. It is also what will bring forward that natural etheric clairvoyance destined to unfold in humanity starting in the mid-twentieth century. This natural, etheric clairvoyance providing wakeful cognition will be the legitimate fruit of the consciousness soul. Once again we find Christ is the orchardist. In our time the etheric body will be revitalized, Steiner indicated, and this re-energization of the thinking, picture-weaving life body, in which thoughts are, once again, real, living forces, is connected with the new revelation of Christ. 'When the etheric body is revitalized, man finds Christ'" (Richard Leviton, *The Imagination of Pentecost: Rudolf Steiner and Contemporary Spirituality* [New York: Anthroposophic Press], 64).

89-a. For further exploration of the codices, see Jose Arguelles, *The Mayan Factor* (Santa Fe, N.M.: Bear and Company, 1987).

91-a. One recent version of this transformation is the movie *Meet Joe Black* (1998), in which Death comes to life and falls in love with a woman, who in turn shows Death what love is. Through this, Death changes his relationship with life. This movie beautifully portrays the olive energy.

92-a. See Ellen Cannon Reed, *The Witches Qabala* (York Beach, Maine: Samuel Weiser, 1997), 51.

94-a. For further exploration, see John Barnwell, *The Arcana of the Grail Angel* (Bloomfield Hills, Mich.: Verticordia Press, 1999), especially page 509.

95-a. "During the rulership of the Archangel Gabriel, the forces of heredity were the dominant aspect of human culture, with the different groups of people having a much greater tendency to act out of a response to their ancestral ties" (John Barnwell, *The Arcana of the Grail Angel* [Bloomfield Hills, Mich.: Verticordia Press, 1999], 501).

96-a. Davidson, Gustav. *A Dictionary of Angels*. New York: Free Press, 1971.

97-a. See *The Little Prince* by Antoine de Saint-Exupéry. Several editions are available.

101-a. Also of interest to the reader may be Michelangelo's painting *The Fall of Man and the Expulsion from the Garden of Eden*.

102-a. See John Barnwell, *The Arcana of the Grail Angel*, 475.

102-b. Ibid.

Chapter 6

1. Ken Wilber, *The Collected Works of Ken Wilber,* volume 7 (including *A Brief History of Everything* and *The Eye of Spirit*; Boston: Shambhala, 2000), 164.

2. Ibid., 140.

3. Ibid., 675.

4. Ibid., 119.

5. Ibid., 127.

6. Richard Cavendish, *The Tarot* (New York: Harper and Row, 1975), 54.

7. Chaih-hsu Ou-i, *Buddhist I Ching,* translated by Thomas Cleary (Boston: Shambhala, 1987), 1.

8. William Shakespeare, *Hamlet,* act 1, scene 3, lines 82–84.

9. Wilber, *Collected Works,* 7.

10. Ibid., 8.

11. Ibid., 9.

12. Ibid., 11.

13. Ibid., 13.

14. www.karmecholing.org.

15. Chogyam Trungpa, *The Heart of the Buddha* (Boston: Shambhala, 1991), 60.

16. Edward Hoffman, *The Hebrew Alphabet* (San Francisco: Chronicle Books, 1998).

17. Both quotations are from Gustav Davidson, *A Dictionary of Angels Including the Fallen Angels,* 255.

18. John Barnwell, *The Arcana of the Grail Angel,* 321.

19. David Wood, *Genisis* (Tunbridge Wells, U.K.: The Baton Press, 1985), 37.

20. Steiner, *Knowledge,* 30–31.

Selected Bibliography

Bailey, Alice A. *The Reappearance of the Christ*. New York: Lucis Publishing, 1948.

———. *A Treatise on White Magic*. New York: Lucis Publishing, 1974.

Baquedano, Elizabeth. *Aztec, Inca and Maya*. New York: Alfred A. Knopf, 1993.

Barnwell, John. *The Arcana of the Grail Angel*. Bloomfield Hills, MI: Verticordia Press, 1999.

Bartlett, John. *Familiar Quotations*. Boston: Little, Brown and Company, 1955.

Berenson-Perkins, Janet. *Kabbalah Decoded*. Hauppauge, NY: Barron's Educational Service, 2000.

The Bible (New Jerusalem Version). New York: Doubleday, 1985.

Blofeld, John. *Bodhisattva of Compassion*. Boston: Shambhala, 1978.

Bremness, Lesley. *Herbs*. New York: DK Publishing, 1994.

Brown, Sarah, and David O'Connor. *Medieval Craftsmen Glass-Painters*. London: British Museum Press, 1993.

Cavendish, Richard. *The Tarot*. New York: Harper and Row, 1975.

Church, W. H. *Edgar Cayce's Story of the Soul*. Virginia Beach: A.R.E. Press, 1989.

Cotterell, Arthur. *The Encyclopedia of Classic Mythology*. London: Lorenz Books, 2003.

Davidson, Gustav. *A Dictionary of Angels Including the Fallen Angels*. New York: The Free Press, 1971.

Dawkins, Peter. *Francis Bacon: Herald of the New Age*. Warwickshire, UK: Francis Bacon Research Trust, 1997.

de Purucker, G. *Occult Glossary: A Compendium of Oriental and Theosophical Terms*. Pasadena, Calif.: Theosophical University Press, 1956.

Drosnin, Michael. *The Bible Code*. New York: Simon and Schuster, 1997.

Fishcher-Rizzi, Susanne. *Medicine of the Earth*. Portland, OR: Rudra Press, 1996.

Goethe, Johann Wolfgang von. *Theory of Colors*. 1810. Cambridge, MA: The MIT Press, 1976.

Guiley, Rosemary Ellen. *Encyclopedia of Angels*. 1st edition. New York: Checkmark Books, 1996.

Hamilton, Edith. *Mythology*. Boston: Little, Brown and Company, 1942.

Hart, George. *Ancient Egypt*. New York: Alfred A. Knopf, 1990.

Hoffman, Edward. *The Hebrew Alphabet*. San Francisco: Chronicle Books, 1998.

Lerer, Seth. *The History of the English Language*. Chantilly, VA: The Teaching Company, 1998. (Audiocassette series.)

Matthews, John. *Robin Hood: Green Lord of the Wildwood*. Glastonbury, UK: Gothic Image, 1993.

Pearson, Anne. *Ancient Greece*. New York: Alfred A. Knopf, 1992.

Philip, Neil. *Myths and Legends*. New York: DK Publishing, 1999.

Above: Sun setting over the Nile.

Poynder, Michael. *Pi in the Sky*. London: Random Century Group, 1992.

Price, Simon, and Emily Kearns. *The Oxford Dictionary of Classical Myth and Religion*. UK: Oxford University Press, 2003.

Rinpoche, Sogyal. *The Tibetan Book of Living and Dying*. San Francisco: HarperCollins, 1994.

Rosenberg, Donna. *World Mythology, an Anthology of the Great Myths and Epics*. 2nd edition. Lincolnwood, IL: NTC Publishing Group.

Rudhyar, Dane. *Astrological Timing: The Transition to the New Age*. New York: Harper & Row, 1972.

Saint Germain dictated to the messenger Mark L. Prophet. *Intermediate Studies in Alchemy*. Los Angeles: Summit University Press, 1978.

Satinover, Jeffrey. *Cracking the Bible Code*. San Francisco: HarperCollins, 1998.

Serrus, Georges. *The Land of the Cathars*. Portet-sur-Garonne, France: Editions Loubatières, 1990.

Shakespeare, William. *A Midsummer Night's Dream*. Reprinted in *The Complete Works of William Shakespeare* edited by Clark and Wright. New York: Doubleday, n.d.

Shepherd, A. P. *Rudolf Steiner: Scientist of the Invisible*. Rochester, VT: Inner Traditions, 1990.

Shreeve, Caroline M. *The Alternative Dictionary of Symptoms and Cures*. London: Rider, 1986.

Steedman, Scott. *Ancient Egypt*. New York: DK Publishing, 1995.

Steiner, Rudolf. *Color*. 1914–1924. Sussex, U.K.: Rudolf Steiner Press, 1992.

———. *The Course of My Life*. 1923–1925. New York: Anthroposophic Press, 1928.

———. *Knowledge of the Higher Worlds*. 1904–1905. London: Rudolf Steiner Press, 1969.

Trager, James, ed. *The People's Chronology*. New York: Holt, Rinehart and Winston, 1979.

Trungpa, Chogyam. *The Heart of the Buddha*. Boston: Shambhala, 1991.

Wall, Vicky. *Aura-Soma: Self-Discovery through Color*. Rochester, VT: Healing Arts Press, 2005.

Watts, Alan W. *The Way of Zen*. New York: Random House, 1999.

Wilber, Ken. *The Collected Works of Ken Wilber*, volume 7 (including *A Brief History of Everything* and *The Eye of Spirit*). Boston: Shambhala, 2000.

Willis, Roy, ed. *World Mythology*. New York: Henry Holt, 1996.

Wood, David. *Genisis*. Tunbridge Wells, U.K.: The Baton Press, 1985.

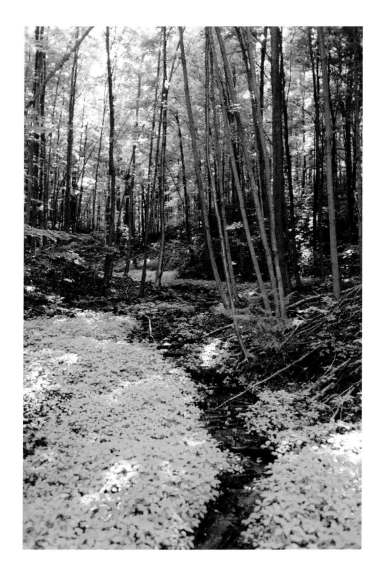

The way beckons, Orangeville, Canada.

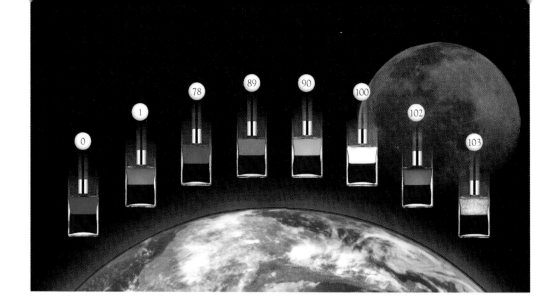

Illustration Credits

David Allaway: 107 (top)

Tiki Archambeau: 2, 38, 91, 95 (top), 137

Ryan Barolet-Fogarty: 79

Claudia Booth: 29 (top left), 29 (right), 30, 31, 150 (left), 181 (bottom), 213 (bottom), 230 (bottom right)

Mike Booth: 24 (with Jakael and Issette Tristram and Carol McKnight), 28, 37 (bottom right), 89, 148, 155, 157, 206, 209 (top right), 224 (top left), 247 (upper left), 248, 268 (top left)

Professor John Buckeridge, Head of the School of Civil, Environmental and Chemical Engineering at Royal Melbourne Institute of Technology University in Melbourne, Australia: 98, 113 (bottom left), 166 (left), 170

Ariel Kaile Burgess, "The Getco Says Fue": 18, 81 (bottom), 127 (bottom left), 129 (bottom left), 131 (bottom), 149 (top), 176, 180, 181 (top), 183 (bottom), 204, 207 (top), 223 (top right), 236, 266 (bottom left)

Michael Burgess: 7 (bottom left), 16, 34 (bottom), 58 (left), 66 (left), 74, 82 (left), 123 (bottom), 144, 160, 161 (top), 182, 225 (top right), 231 (bottom), 242, 345 (top)

Robert Lee Cohen, courtesy of Dianne Cohen McInerney: 132, 253 (top right)

Kameron Decker Harris and Dawn Decker: 65 (top), 186

John Dillon-Guy: iii, 17, 119 (right), 164, 209 (left bottom), 267

Mary Farrell: 232

Keith Fielder: 73

Russell C. Hansen of Lincoln, Vermont (www.birdsinflight.net; birdsinflight@mac.com). Russ's photographs, unique in the world of wildlife photography, have appeared in many periodicals and books. His exhibit "Birds in Flight" has been traveling to museums throughout the U.S. since 1992. Courtesy of Martha S. Hansen. Russ's photograph appears on page 215.

William Kolker: 173

Andrea Lloyd: 59, 158, 183 (top), 258, 265 (top)

Carol Jean McKnight: 2, 11, 13 (bottom right, courtesy of Deborah LaFramboise and Kirsten Talmage), 14 (right), 19, 21, 22, 24 (with Jakael and Issette Tristram and Mike Booth), 27, 63, 65 (bottom), 66 (right), 68 (left), 70 (left, courtesy of Richard Brigham), 76, 77, 80, 83, 85 (left), 85 (right), 87, 88 (left), 88 (right), 93 (top), 93 (bottom), 95 (bottom), 96 (left), 97 (top), 99, 100, 101 (top), 103, 109 (top), 112 (left), 115 (right), 116, 125 (bottom), 128, 133 (bottom), 142, 143, 145 (bottom), 149 (bottom), 151, 152 (right), 159 (bottom left), 161 (bottom right), 162, 165 (top), 167, 168, 171 (bottom), 175 (top), 187, 188, 199 (bottom left), 201, 210, 211 (top right), 216 (with Annabelle Westling Williams), 220 (left), 222, 224 (bottom), 225 (bottom left), 228, 229, 231 (top), 233 (bottom left), 234 (bottom left), 235 (bottom), 237 (top), 237 (bottom), 240, 243, 247 (bottom left), 256, 259, 262, 276, 279, 285, 292, 294 (with Nick Vittum and Jakael and Issette Tristram)

Judi McLaughlin (www.35mmMagic.com) is a professional photographer whose true passion is photographing exotic locales. For the photographs appearing in this book she used the beautiful darkness of night to capture Alaska's magical Aurora Borealis; photographed majestic Bengal tigers at close range while riding an elephant in Khana National Park, India; revealed the power of nature in the photograph taken from a helicopter over an erupting Hawaiian volcano;

Above: The part of the Rescue Set with deep magenta in the lower fraction.

and caught the playfulness of seals while following the trail of Darwin in the Galapagos Islands. Her photographs have been published in *Nature Photographer Magazine* and *Digital Photographer Magazine* among others. Her photographs appear on pages vi, 34 (top), 47 (top), 47 (bottom), 60, 67, 70 (bottom right), 75 (left), 86, 90, 96 (right), 108, 110 (left), 110 (bottom), 113 (top right), 114, 118, 124, 125 (top), 129 (top right), 130, 131 (top), 139 (bottom), 140, 141, 147 (top), 153, 156 (right), 163, 165 (bottom), 166 (right), 169 (bottom left), 171 (top), 195 (top), 197, 200, 205 (top), 205 (bottom), 227, 233 (top), 239 (top), 241 (top), 245 (bottom), 249, 264, 265 (bottom right), 270, and 284.

Alma Midgehope's original art appears on page 122

Helen Newman: 203 (bottom)

Larry Neumann: 145, 219, 254

Lindsay Raymondjack: 190 (right)

Kris Root: 134, 147 (bottom)

Michele de Santis, a full-time dentist with an interest in the uncommon view: 3, 6, 23, 127 (top right), 154 (right), 199 (top right), 218, 234 (bottom right)

Tay Sloan: 75 (right), 196 (right)

Sansea Sparling: 61 (bottom), 138, 196 (left)

Thalia Morrow Sparling: 58 bottom left, 193, 214, 221

Colin Talmage: 112 (right), 230 (bottom left)

Erin Talmage, naturalist: 62, 71, 78, 115 (bottom left), 123 (top), 172 (left), 192, 194, 212, 238, 239 (bottom right), 257

Kirsten Talmage: 111 (original art work), 217 (top)

Judy Taylor (www.agpix.com/judytaylor, www.photosourcefolio.com/1254, www.judytaylor.photosourcegroup.com) enjoys photographing nature as well as people at home and at work, often in historic sites that are part of their everyday lives. She spends as much time as she can in the field in an ongoing quest for the perfect photograph. Her photographs appear on pages 7 (bottom right), 14 (left), 37 (top), 49, 82 (right), 92, 94, 105, 109 (bottom), 133 (top), 136, 169 (top right), 177, 185, 190 (left), 191, 195 (bottom), 211 (bottom), 217 (bottom), 235 (top), 250, 251 (top), 252, 255, 263, 266 (bottom right), 268 (bottom), 269, 286, 287.

Mark Taylor: 12 (bottom left), 13 (top left), 12 (top right), 15, 26, 97 (bottom), 106, 121, 161 (bottom left), 253 (top left)

Pardon Elisha Tillinghast VII, Professor Emeritus in History at Middlebury College in Middlebury, Vermont: 61 (top), 72 (left), 72 (right), 84, 119 (bottom left), 135, 184, 244, 246, 251 (bottom).

Doug Todd (www.dougtodd.com) is a professional photographer now living in New York City: 203 (top)

Issette and Jakael Tristram, graphic designer (jkl@triple-ring.com): 2 (with Carol McKnight), 24 (with Carol McKnight and Mike Booth), 198, 294 (with Carol McKnight and Nick Vittum)

Nick Vittum: 101 (bottom, courtesy of Nasa), 102

Charles von Bruns: 174–175 (bottom)

Elaine Lasker von Bruns: 208

Scott Wayne, Principal of SW Associates, LLC—Sustainable Development through Tourism (www.sw-associates.net). Mr. Wayne has managed a broad range of tourism development programs and projects focusing on economic development through tourism coalition-building and international government relations. He is the author of seven travel books for Sierra Club Books and Lonely Planet. His photographs appear on pages 120 and 207 (bottom).

Debra Jo Whitcomb: 68 (right), 178, 293

Annabelle Westling Williams: 64, 69, 95 (bottom), 117 (bottom), 126, 139 (top), 154 (left), 216 (with Carol McKnight), 220 (right), 223 (bottom), 260, 261

Tanya Williams: 107 (bottom), 156 (left)

Rick Winslow: 152 (left), 159 (top right), 202, 213 (top), 226

Lynn Yarrington and Michael Mode: 81 (top), 104, 117 (top), 172 (right), 189, 241 (bottom)

The Equilibrium Bottles

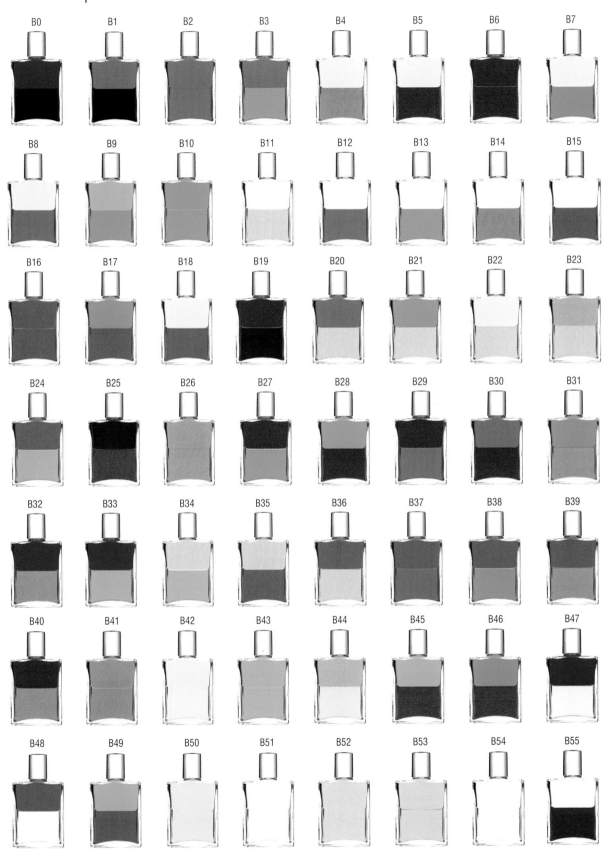

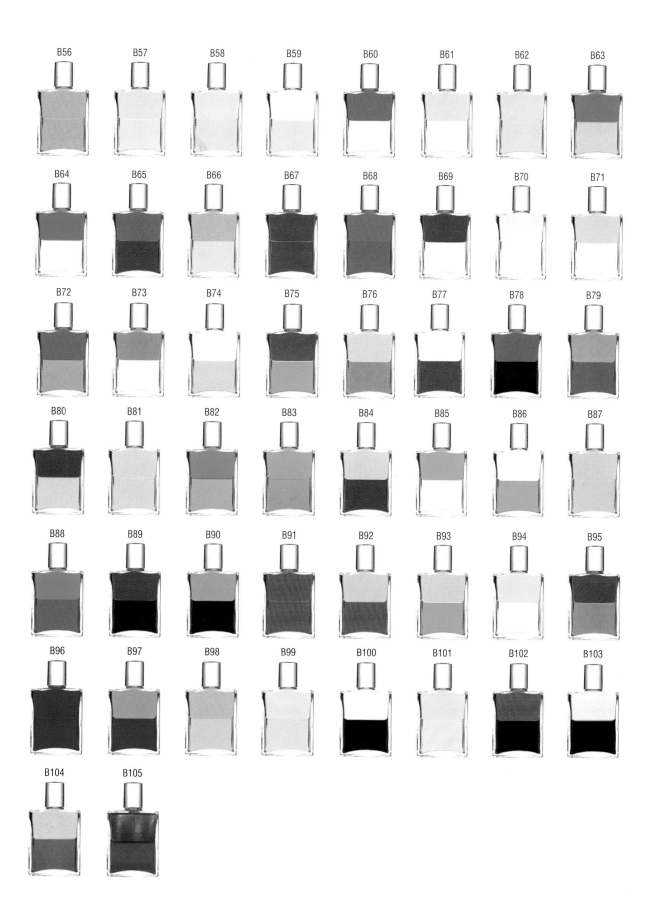

Books of Related Interest

Aura-Soma
Self-Discovery through Color
by Vicky Wall

The Healing Power of Color
Using Color to Improve Your Mental, Physical, and Spiritual Well-Being
by Betty Wood

Himalayan Salt Crystal Lamps
For Healing, Harmony, and Purification
by Clémence Lefèvre

The Metaphysical Book of Gems and Crystals
by Florence Mégemont

Advanced Aromatherapy
The Science of Essential Oil Therapy
by Kurt Schnaubelt, Ph.D.

The Healing Intelligence of Essential Oils
The Science of Advanced Aromatherapy
by Kurt Schnaubelt, Ph.D.

Aromatherapy for Healing the Spirit
Restoring Emotional and Mental Balance with Essential Oils
by Gabriel Mojay

Hydrosols
The Next Aromatherapy
by Suzanne Catty

Discover Your Soul Template
14 Steps for Awakening Integrated Intelligence
by Marcus T. Anthony, Ph.D.

Inner Traditions • Bear & Company
P.O. Box 388
Rochester, VT 05767
1-800-246-8648
www.InnerTraditions.com

Or contact your local bookseller